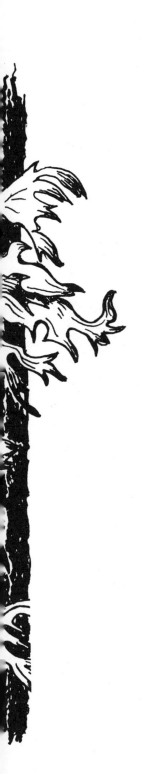

THE
PERFUME
HANDBOOK

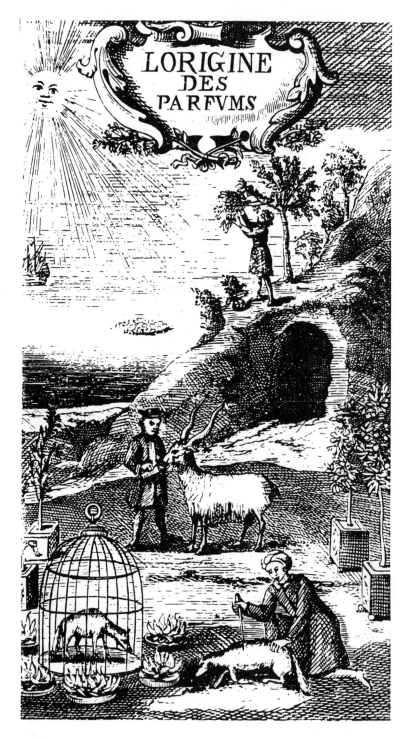

The sources of perfume materials, as depicted in an early book on perfume – *Parfumeur Francoys* (Paris, 1680). They include civet cats and a goat, from the beard of which labdanum is being combed. Floating on the sea is ambergris.

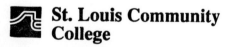

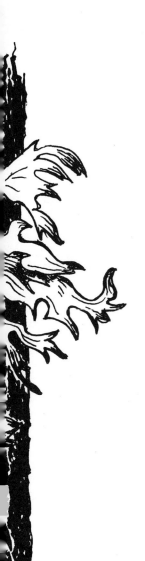

THE
PERFUME
HANDBOOK

NIGEL GROOM

CHAPMAN & HALL

London · Glasgow · New York · Tokyo · Melbourne · Madras

Published by Chapman & Hall, 2-6 Boundary Row, London SE1 8HN, UK

Chapman & Hall, 2-6 Boundary Row, London SE1 8HN, UK

Blackie Academic & Professional, Wester Cleddens Road, Bishopbriggs, Glasgow G64 2NZ, UK

Chapman & Hall Inc., One Penn Plaza, 41st Floor, New York NY 10119, USA

Chapman & Hall Japan, Thomson Publishing Japan, Hirakawacho Nemoto Building, 6F, 1-7-11 Hirakawa-cho, Chiyoda-ku, Tokyo 102, Japan

Chapman & Hall Australia, Thomas Nelson Australia, 102 Dodds Street, South Melbourne, Victoria 3205, Australia

Chapman & Hall India, R. Seshadri, 32 Second Main Road, CIT East, Madras 600 035, India

First edition 1992
Reprinted 1994

© 1992 Nigel Groom

Typeset in 10/12pt Palatino by Best-set Typesetters Ltd., Hong Kong
Printed in Great Britain by St Edmundsbury Press, Bury St Edmunds, Suffolk

ISBN   0 412 46320 2

A catalogue record for this book is available from the British Library

∞   Printed on acid-free text paper, manufactured in accordance with ANSI/NISO Z39.48-1992 and ANSI/NISO Z39.48-1984 (Permanence of Paper).

Contents

Preface

In 1948 I was posted, as a Political Officer, to a remote part of south-west Arabia on the edge of the great desert called the Empty Quarter. In valleys made fertile by seasonal flood-waters lay the remains of an ancient civilization. I found inscriptions and the ruin sites of towns, palaces and temples. Almost buried under the sand dunes were the tumbled walls of a great city. From here, two thousand years before, huge camel caravans had trudged their way along 1600 miles of burning sand and rocks to Petra and Gaza, burdened with a most precious cargo – frankincense, myrrh and other perfume materials for the courts, temples and perfume shops of Rome.

My book *Frankincense and Myrrh* delved into the details of this romantic trade and led to a broader interest in the perfumes of ancient times. Then, researching on behalf of a perfume house into the Arab contribution to perfumery, I came across the collection of perfume recipes assembled by the Arab philosopher–scientist Yaqub al-Kindi, which have never been translated into English (some, which I have translated myself, are now included in an appendix to this book). I realized that in that work I had found key evidence to demonstrate how the medieval Arab perfume makers had been the bridge in perfume history between ancient and modern times. Perfumery could now be seen as an art with a continuous history of development since the dawn of civilization. This book has been compiled for a multitude of purposes, but among them is the object of affirming this continuity in the long story of perfumery. There is, therefore, no incongruity if an entry about a great 'classic' perfume of the 20th century appears next to one describing an unguent of ancient Greece; besides, both may well be found to contain some of the same exotic ingredients as were loaded on to camels in the spice market of that city in south-west Arabia all those centuries ago.

But it is for the person with a general interest in the perfumes of modern times that this book is principally intended, especially for the women (now about 40% of all women in this country) and, increasingly, the men, who like to use fragrances as a normal part of the process of getting dressed. Hitherto, they have been faced with a bewildering range of fragrances but have had little information to guide their selection of them. This book aims to help them choose their fragrances more confidently and to enable them to talk about the whole subject of perfumery more intelligently. Others for whom it is hoped this book will be of value include those people who may wish to try making fragrances themselves. For them brief guidance notes, under the heading 'Perfume Making at Home', supported by an appendix of recipes and formulas, will provide an introduction into a fascinating occupation. Among other general monographs which will be found grouped together under the broad heading 'Perfume' is one on 'Perfume Containers', designed to help the growing number of persons who now follow the hobby of collecting perfume bottles. Throughout this work I have tried to give due recognition to the artists and craftsmen who design and manufacture the elegant and striking flacons in which perfumes are now contained.

There has always been a mystique in perfumery, but in modern times it has been overplayed. Many couture designers, concerned with nebulous objectives like the 'image' of their fashion houses, have preferred to keep the art of perfumery obscure, sometimes even so that it will appear they have personally created the fragrances they market. Thus the skill of the highly trained perfumer, who alone is capable of assembling the multiple ingredients of a modern perfume into a satisfying compound (see the entry for 'Perfume Creation'), has tended to be hidden under a cloak of anonymity. It is hoped that this work will go some way towards reasserting the importance of the trained perfumers and reaffirming them as artists.

I have sought to make this work technically acceptable to the botanist. In preparing entries for the many hundreds of plants used in perfumery which are recorded here, I have therefore, for the sake of accurate, scientific identification, given botanical names; but this inevitably leads to the problem of the constant changes of nomenclature as botanists discover, for example, that a plant found in one part of the world is identical with a plant found elsewhere and already named differently. Where more than one botanical name has applied I have therefore quoted them all, using the conventional equation format, but I have not sought to put the currently definitive botanical name first in the equation, as that would have been too onerous and beyond my competence. I am grateful to Nigel Hepper, of the Royal Botanic Gardens, Kew, for his help and advice over some botanical aspects, including the spelling of some of the botanical names, but he has seen only a portion of the text and errors in it are my own.

Inevitably in the writing of a book of this sort, there will be omissions and inaccuracies. For these I apologize. I would also be very grateful to hear of them, through the publishers, in the hope that they can be rectified should a second edition of this book be possible.

Nigel Groom
Fulham, London

Illustrations

The atomizer featured on the front cover is French, *c.* 1930, and is in the National Museum of Perfume, Grasse. The photograph is by Claude Muzzin of Grasse.

Line drawings are by the author except where otherwise stated.

The design on the title page and section headings depicts Oak Moss (see page 162).

Perfume bottles shown in the tail-piece drawing at the end of some of the alphabetical sections (also reproduced below) are as follows (left to right): Patou ('1000'); Levy ('Escada'); Guerlain ('Shalimar'); Guerlain ('Mitsouko'); Dior ('Diorissimo'); DeVilbiss atomizer (*c.* 1928); Hermes ('Caleche'); Matchabelli (1927); Lelong ('Mon Image', *c.* 1928); Giorgio Beverly Hills ('Red'); Balenciaga ('Le Dix'); Bijan; Amouage.

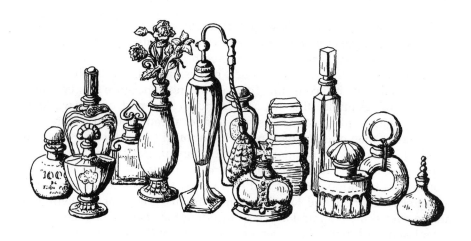

Acknowledgements

The author wishes to thank the following for assistance and advice, volunteered or given with great willingness in response to his queries: Juliette Bogaers of Bonhams; Liliane Cohen of Azzaro, Paris; Douglas Cope of Floris; Amanda Farnish of Floris; Paul M. Griffin of Amouage; Nigel Hepper (Royal Botanic Gardens, Kew); Diana Moore of Dior; Jay Morley of Harrods Perfume Hall; Sophie Peter of Lacroix; and A.J. Tettifer of the British Society of Perfumers.

He also wishes to thank the following, who have so helpfully met his requests for information about their companies and products, or assisted him to obtain it, or have provided photographs: Susan Albury of Giorgio, Beverly Hills; Shawn Allen of Parim (Lancôme); Karen Alli of Giorgio, Beverly Hills; Jeannie Balleu of Lanvin; John Boorman of Wassen-Europ (Gucci, Worth, Grès and Léonard); Christina Boyes of Dior; Susan Boylan of Revlon; J. Brennan of Cussons; Mary Ann Buckler of Quest; Nadine Chelly of de Varens, Paris; Gina Cherrett of Caroline Neville Associates (Givenchy); Caroline Clark of Bijan; Diane Condon of Creative Fragrances (Rochas); Francis Cubbon of Prestige & Collections (Armani, Cacharel, Lauren, Picasso and Laroche); Suzie Cunningham of St Laurent; Aurélie de Fournaux of Scannon, Paris (Gucci); Jane Dobson of Dobson Communications (Ricci); Ann Eaden-Allen of Charles of the Ritz; Lisa Eagle of Dobson Communications (Ricci); Mary Elliott of Caroline Neville Associates (Cartier); Victoria Ewen of Hermès; Jill Fraysse of L'Artisan Parfumeur; Sarah Griffiths of Estée Lauder; Diana Harris (Boots Press Office); R.W. Harris of Roure; Angela Hart of Yardley; Pauline Harvey of Max Factor; Chris Hawksley of Les Senteurs; Brian Hepburn of Dana; Melanie Herfet of Revlon; Samantha Higham of Hermès; Elizabeth Hindle of Selective Beauté International (Vanderbilt); Kate Histed of the P.R. Workshop (Puig, Rabanne, Herrera, Dali and Rocher); Nathalie Hollingworth of Yardley; Tatia Hudson of Caroline Neville Associates (Givenchy); Jacqueline Hurley of Shiseido; Graham Hurst of Givaudan, Geneva; Michelle Ionadi of Fine Fragrances and Cosmetics (Caron, Raffles, Hardy Amies); Barbara Jacquesson of Guerlain; Miriam Kelaty of Patou (Patou, Scherrer, Benetton, Jacomo, Lacoste, Cerutti, Capucci, Boucheron and Balmain); Roger Kennedy of Quest; M. Kent of Elida Gibbs; Carri Kilpatrick of Prestige & Collections (Armani, Cacharel, Lauren, Picasso and Laroche); Anne Klahn of Selective Beauté International (Lancôme,

L'Oréal); Nathalie Lamande of Brosse, Paris; Jan Lawrence of IFF; Patricia
Ling of Caroline Neville Associates (Cartier); Janet Marshall of Aramis;
Bernie McBridge of The Fragrance Group (UK) (Balenciaga, Bogart,
Lapidus); Jane McCorriston (Revlon); Nanda Mengjhi of La Femme
Cosmetics (Perfumers Workshop); Lauren Munton of Penhaligon's;
Francesca Muscroft of Dior; Rosanna Palmer of Ungaro; Jane Phillips
of Vivienne Tomei PR (Goutal); Bernadette Randle of Chanel; Barbara
Rathe of Yardley; Jane Raven of Crabtree & Evelyn; Seema Ray of Bergal
(Molyneux, Roger & Gallet, Van Cleef & Arpels and de la Renta); Alison
Reynolds of Revlon; Christopher Rhodes of Boss Advertising (Amouage);
members of Janine Roxborough Bunce Associates (Elizabeth Arden, Fendi,
Lagerfeld); Amanda Sage of Network Management (Balmain and Desprez);
Ch. M. Saloman of Givaudan, Geneva; Vicky Smith of Avon; Kerry
Sparkes of Chanel; Jo Spink of Jo Spink PR (Molinard, Sinan, Van Gils
and Morabito); Heather Stacey of Lenthéric-Morny; Sally Stevens of Sally
Stevens Associates (Lalique); Janice Swales of Houbigant; Carole Sykes
of Riverhouse (Lagerfeld); Chris Tamlyn of Firmenich; Vivienne Tomei
of Vivienne Tomei PR (Goutal); Laura Topping of Creative Fragrances
(Rochas); Karina Van Hunnik of IFF; Philippa Varney of Beauty Inter-
national (Coty); Lisa Webster of Czech & Speake; Karen Whitehead of
Mary Chess; David Wiffen of IFF; Andrea Witty of Max Factor; Jackie
Woodcock of Prestige & Collections (Paloma Picasso); and Michel Wortham
of Baccarat, Paris.

The author and publishers are grateful to the following for permission
to reproduce copyright perfume recipes in Appendix B:

Darton, Longman & Todd/The Herb Society. Recipes nos. 22, 23, 27, 28
and 29. From Ivan Day: *Perfumery with Herbs* (1979);
Dorling, Kindersley, London. Recipes nos. 3, 4 and 8. From Penny Black:
The Book of Pot Pourri (1989);

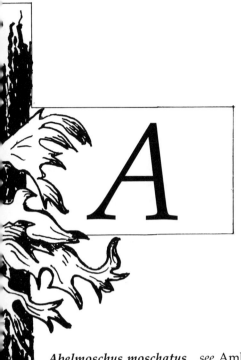

A

Abelmoschus moschatus   *see* Ambrette
Abies alba   *see* Silver Pine Needle Oil
      balsamea   *see* Canada Balsam
      canadensis   *see* Canada Balsam
      pectinata   *see* Silver Pine Needle Oil
      pichta   *see* Siberian Pine Oil
      siberica   *see* Siberian Pine Oil

Abir   Also Abeer. A scented talcum powder sprinkled on clothes and linen in India. Composition of the powder varies; one variety is reportedly made from sandalwood, aloes, rose petals, zedoary, civet and kapur-kachri; another from curcuma, cardamon, cloves and sandalwood.

Absinthe Oil   *see* Wormwood Oil

Absolute   The essential oil of scented flowers and other aromatic plant parts in its purest and most concentrated form; this is obtained after stearoptene has been removed from the concrete by extraction with alcohol. It is extremely expensive. Among the most important oils used in an absolute form are cassie, champac, clary sage, geranium, ylang-ylang, jasmine, labdanum, lavender, lily, mimosa, orange flower, rose, tuberose, violet and violet leaf.

Acacia   Different species of acacia produce cassie, mimosa and gum arabic. But the term 'acacia' is also used for a particular type of compound perfume, made to various formulas, with an intense flowery fragrance reminiscent of a blending of hawthorn with orange blossom.

Acacia cavenia   *see* Cassie

dealbata   *see* Mimosa

farnesiana   *see* Cassie

floribunda   *see* Mimosa

gummifera   *see* Gum Arabic

nilotica   *see* Gum Arabic

senegal   *see* Gum Arabic

sorts   *see* Gum Arabic

Accord   In perfumery this signifies a combination of a number of different scents which blend together to produce a new fragrance.

Acerra   A small box in which the Romans kept, and sometimes burned, incense used in the temples during a sacrificial ceremony. In ancient Greece it was called *libanotris*. See Roman Perfumes.

Achillea agoratum   *see* Maudlin

decolorans   *see* English Mace

moschata   *see* Iva

Acorus calamus   *see* Calamus

Adiantum amabile   *see* Scented Maidenhair

Aframomum melegnata   *see* Grains of Paradise

African Myrrh   *see* Bdellium

Agar Wood   *see* Aloewood

Agastache anethiodora   *see* Giant Hyssop

pallidiclora   *see* Giant Hyssop

Aglaia   The flowers of a tree *Aglaia odorata*, known to the Chinese as Yu-chu-lan, are highly regarded in China for their exquisite fragrance and are used there for making joss sticks and scented necklaces and for flavouring tea. They retain their perfume when dried and are widely used in sachets and pot pourri.

Agrimony   The dried flowers and leaves of Scented Agrimony (*Agrimonia odorata*), a perennial herb native to N. Europe, including Britain, are used for scenting pillows and in pot pourri.

Agrumen Oils   The collective term in perfumery for the essential oils of citrus fruits (bergamot, colobot, cravo, grapefruit, lemon, lime, mandarin, bitter orange, sweet orange and tangerine). See also Hesperides.

Agua Mellis   *see* Honey Water

Ague Tree   *see* Sassafras

Ailanthus malabarica   *see* Mattipaul

Ain Gum   A fragrant gum obtained from the bark of the Ain tree (also called Asna, Sain, Saj and Laurel) of India (*Terminalia tomentosa*). It is used in cosmetics and as an incense.

Ajowan   Also called Ajvan and True Bishops Weed. An erect herb

(*Carum copticum = Ammi copticum*) cultivated in Egypt, Iran and India. The seeds have a strong thyme-like scent and an oil obtained from them is used as an antiseptic and to aid digestion. The crushed seeds are dried for use in sachet powders and pot pourri.

An oil called Ajowan Oil, sometimes known as Oman Water, is also distilled from the seeds of *Ptychotis ajowan*, cultivated in India. The seeds are used locally as a spice and the oil is occasionally used in soaps.

Ajuga chamaepitys   *see* Ground Pine

Akar Laka   A vine (*Dalbergia junghuhnii = D. parviflora = D. zollingaria*), related to the rosewood tree, which grows in India and Malaysia. The heartwood of the stems and roots is scented and used for making joss sticks and as an incense in temples.

Alant   *see* Elecampane

Alabastrum   A vessel or pot used in Roman times to hold perfumed oils and unguents. They were usually made of alabaster or related stone (agate or onyx), but the term was also used to describe such vessels made of other materials (Theocritus speaks of 'golden alabastra'). Those for oils were usually tapering in shape, with a long narrow neck. See Roman Perfumes.

Aldehyde   An important group of chemicals, derived from alcohol and some natural plant materials. They form one of a number of chemical groups known as benzenoid compounds which were discovered at the end of the 19th century and are used in manufacturing synthetic materials for modern perfumes. Anisic aldehyde, for example, provides the scent of hawthorn, while decylic aldehyde is used in reproducing the odours of violet, orris, neroli, cassie flowers, rose and orange. Aldehydes can also give perfumes a distinctly individual fragrance of their own. In their pure state aldehydes possess such a powerful and persistent odour that a single drop spilt on a person's clothes will make them so odoriferous as to be objectionable. They have therefore to be used with extreme care and discretion and in minute quantities, when they are of great value to a perfumer, providing fragrances with a new richness and strength. The use of aldehydes in perfumes was developed by Ernest Beaux for Chanel, leading to the first aldehydic perfume – 'Chanel No. 5'.

Alecost   *see* Costmary

Alectoria jujuba   *see* Horsehair Lichen
           usnesides   *see* Fragrant Moss

Alehoof   *see* Ground Ivy

Aleroot   *see* Ground Ivy

Alespice   *see* Costmary

Algerian Oil   *see* Rue Oil

Alhagi camelorum   *see* Aspalathus

Alkanet   Also known as Dyer's Alkanet, Dyer's Bugloss, Orchanette and Anchusa. A small perennial herb (*Alkanna tinctoria*) native to south-east Europe and Turkey but now grown widely. It has a large root from which a red dye, called Alkanna or Alkanet, is extracted by maceration in oil, fat or alcohol. The dye was used to give perfumes an attractive red colour by the ancient Egyptians, Greeks and Romans. In the 17th century, French women made a cosmetic ointment from it to give their cheeks 'an oriental glow'. It is still used for colouring infused oils and pomatums.

A similar dye is also taken from *Macrotomia cephalotus*, a herb found from Greece to Asia Minor, Syria and the Caucasus, which is known as Syrian Alkanna and Turkish Alkanna.

Allheal   *see* Valerian

'Alliage'   A trend-setting 'green' perfume introduced by Estée Lauder in 1972. Green top notes cover a spicy, resinous heart which includes galbanum and nutmeg, with hints of rosewood, pine-needle and thyme, and a base note dominated by oak moss. The bottle was designed by Ira Levy.

Allspice, Oil of   *see* Pimento

Allspice, Carolina   *see* Calycanthus

Aloe   The juice of aloe (*Aloe vera*, *A. succotrina* and related species), a succulent plant found in East Africa, Arabia, Socotra and S. Africa, was used by the women of ancient Egypt to perfume their bodies. It is thought to be the *ahaloth* of the Bible (*St John* 19:39), in which it was a perfuming agent, and was much used in ancient times as an ingredient of incenses. But some scholars have suggested that the references to aloes in the Old Testament related to sandalwood. Aloe vera oil is still used in cosmetics, particularly as an emollient in skin-care preparations.

Aloewood   Also called Aloeswood, Lignum Aloes, Oriental Lignaloes, Xylaloes, Eaglewood, Columback Wood, Agar Wood and Lignum Rhodium. One of the most valuable of all perfume materials since it was introduced into Europe by the early Arabs during the 8th century AD.

Aloewood is the aromatic, resinous heartwood of a large evergreen tree (*Aquilaria agollocha*, also *A. malaccensis*), native to Assam, Malaysia and China. The wood becomes resinous and fragrant due to a disease which makes part of the heartwood black, oily, very hard and heavier than water. Aloewood Oil is distilled from the infected wood and has an odour reminiscent of ambergris and sandalwood. The early Arabs, who first obtained it from China, regarded it as one of the most desirable of all perfume materials and recognized ten different varieties. It was soon highly valued in Europe and became an important ingredient of pomanders. Most Aloewood Oil made today is distilled in India, where it is called Agar Attar or Chuwah, but the wood is becoming increasingly rare and the oil extremely expensive, so that it is now little used in western perfumery. The dried wood left after distillation was used in sachets and pot pourri. The Eaglewood tree of Cambodia and Annam (*Aquilaria crasna*) produces a fragrant resin in the same manner.

Aloewood should not be confused with Aloes. Suggestions that it was the Aloes of the Bible are discounted.

Aloysia citriodora   *see* Verbena

   triphylla   *see* Verbena

Alpine Rose   A rose-like essential oil obtained from the roots of the Rusty-leaved Alprose (*Rhododendron ferrugineum* = *Chamaerhododendron ferrugineum*), which grows in Alpine Europe. It is occasionally used in perfumery.

Alpinia galanga   *see* Galingale

   malaccensis   *see* Galingale

   officinarum   *see* Galingale

Amantilla   *see* Valerian

Amaracus dictamus   *see* Dittany

Amarante   A name given to a type of compound perfume. The word means cock's comb or prince's feathers. Perfumes so named usually contain synthetic muguet, with rose, sandalwood, musk and jasmine to round off the bouquet.

'Amarige'   A quality floral perfume, with woody undertones, launched by Givenchy in 1991. Created by Dominique Ropion of Roure, its main ingredients are neroli, rosewood, violet and mandarin leaf oil in the top notes, with gardenia, mimosa, cassie and ylang-ylang prominent in the heart, finishing with a base which includes sandalwood, musk, ambergris, vanilla and tonka.

Amaryllis   A name given in perfumery to perfumes of the lily type, usually with added traces of rose and neroli.

'Amazone'   A light floral fruity perfume with green notes first introduced by Hermès in 1975 and relaunched in 1989 with a revised formula created by Hilton McConnus. The dominating fragrances in the heart are rose and jasmine. In the top notes narcissus is supported by bergamot, lemon, orange and blackcurrant buds. The base notes are underlined by sandalwood and cedar. The flacon was designed by Jean Rene Guerrand Hermès and Joël Desgrippes.

Amber   An abbreviated form of ambergris. In perfumery this is nothing to do with the semi-precious fossilized resin of the same name which is used in jewellery. The word denotes a fragrance found not only in ambergris itself but also in several other natural materials, such as labdanum. It is also sometimes used to describe the fragrance of oak moss, and sometimes used to designate the family of perfumes more usually called 'oriental'. See Perfume: Classification of Fragrances,

Perfume Families and Perfume Notes. For 'Artificial ambers' see Ambres.

Amber, Sweet   *see* St John's Wort

Ambergris   Since antiquity, one of the most valuable of perfume ingredients and also one of the most legendary. Ambergris is found in oily, grey lumps floating in the sea, mainly in the Indian Ocean, or cast on to its shores. Speculation about the origin of this material persisted until the 19th century. The substance is excreted by the sperm whale (*Physeter macrocephalus*) after it has been feeding on cuttle fish. The lumps usually weigh a pound or two, but may be up to seventy pounds weight and occasionally much larger. Its odour is most unpleasant in the raw state and it has to be considerably diluted, by dissolving in alcohol, when it becomes highly fragrant, with a scent which has a similarity with labdanum. It is usually used in the form of a tincture. The fragrance is very persistent. The weathering of ambergris while it is in the sea is an important factor in its fragrancy; ambergris removed directly from the body of a whale, or freshly expelled from it, is nauseating and must be aged over several years before it can be used in perfumery.

Ambergris was not known to the Greeks and Romans and appears to have come into use during early Arab times. It was included in a list of items sent as tribute from the Yemen to the Persian Emperor in the 6th century AD, and al-Kindi, early 9th century AD, used it in a number of his perfume recipes. It also appeared in a Byzantine list of perfumes permitted to be sold in Constantinople in about 895 AD. It enjoyed a reputation as an aphrodisiac.

Solid ambergris is said to retain its perfume for three centuries or more. In Elizabethan times it was used to perfume gloves because its scent remained on them despite repeated washing. For centuries it has been very highly valued by perfumers as a fixative. However, because of the growing scarcity and consequent costliness of 'floating' ambergris and environmental objections to obtaining it by killing whales, it is now rarely used in perfumery other than in a synthesized form. Quality perfumes which contain ambergris include 'Amouage', 'Miss Dior', 'Parure' and 'Vol de Nuit'.

Ambon Sandalwood   The scented wood of the Ambon Sandalwood tree, also called Sasooroo and Rozemarijinhout (*Osmoxylon umbelliferum*), native to Indonesia, is burnt as an incense.

Ambrein   A substance extracted from purified labdanum which has an ambergris-like fragrance and is of considerable value in perfumery as a fixative.

Ambres   Also called Artificial ambers. A name given in perfumery to a group of powerful fixatives of similar type which generally contain an animal material, such as musk, civet or castoreum, together with labdanum or balsam of Tolu or Peru. See also Amber.

Ambrette Oil   An oil with a floral, musk-like fragrance, steam-distilled from the seeds of the Musk Mallow (*Hibiscus abelmoschus* = *Abelmoschus moschatus*), also called the Target-leaved Hibiscus, an evergreen tropical or subtropical shrub, cultivated for the oil in India, Egypt, Indonesia and the West Indies, and closely related to Okra. A particularly fragrant variety grows in Martinique. The seeds, sometimes called Musk Seeds, Musky Seeds, Abelmosk Seeds, Ambrette Seeds or Amber Seeds, hold their scent for a very long time and were once much used by perfumers for scenting gloves, mattresses and pillows. Today they are used in sachets and for adulterating musk. The oil, extracted by volatile solvents, is expensive and used in quality perfumes.

Ambroisia   An essential oil with a geranium-like fragrance, also called Baltimore Oil, American Wormseed Oil or Chenopodium Oil, which is distilled from the herb Mexican Wormwood (*Chenopodium ambroisiodes* = *C. anthelminticum*), also called American Wormseed, Mexican Tea and Jesuit's Tea. The plant, a perennial weed growing up to about 2 feet high, is found in S. America, Mexico and southern and eastern parts of the USA.

American Balsam   *see* Balsam of Tolu

American Liquidamber   *see* Storax

American Sea Lavender   *see* Marsh Rosemary

American Sweet Gum   *see* Storax

American Wild Ginger   *see* Canadian Snakeroot

Ammi copticum   *see* Ajowan

Ammoniacum   The Ammoniacum of the ancients, which was used as an incense, probably came from the African Ammoniacum plant (*Ferula communis* and *F. marmarica*) found in N. Africa. Dioscorides described Ammoniacum as the juice of a giant fennel found in Libya, especially near the temple of Ammon, in Cyrene.

Gum Ammoniacum of modern times is a resin collected from insect punctures in the stem of the Persian Ammoniacum plant (*Dorema ammoniacum* = *Diserneston gummiferum*), which grows up to 7 feet tall in Arabia, Iran, Turkestan, India and S. Siberia. The resin, a white latex which soon hardens, is known as Tear Ammoniacum when collected off the stem and Lump Ammoniacum when picked up from the ground (when it usually contains dust and grit). It has an odour resembling castoreum, for which it is sometimes used as a substitute, and is ground up for use as a fixative in pot pourri and sachets; it also has medicinal uses.

Amomium   *see* Cardamom

Amomum zingiber   *see* Ginger

Amonis jamarcensis   *see* Pimento Oil

Amouage   A company founded by the Hamood family of the Sultanate

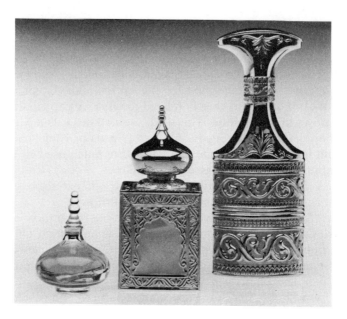

'Amouage'.

of Oman in 1983 to revive the ancient association of Arabia with high class perfumes. The company now sells 'Amouage' perfume worldwide at the top level of international quality perfumes. Created by Guy Robert, 'Amouage' is a floral–oriental fragrance unique for its range of over 120 natural ingredients (it contains unusually few synthetics); many of these are rare and costly, making it one of the most expensive perfumes on the market. The floral–fruity top note includes rose (three varieties), jasmine, geranium, orris, bergamot and tuberose, blended with peach, apricot and lime. The spicy heart contains, with many other constituents, patchouli, sandalwood, labdanum, myrrh, frankincense and ylang-ylang. Among the most dominant lower notes are vanilla, vetiver, ambergris, civet and musk. It is marketed in containers of gilded silver and semi-precious stones developed by Aspreys, and is also now sold in flacons made by Baccarat and Brosse. In 1991 it was selected as 'Star Product of the Year' at Cannes.

'Amour Amour' A classic floral perfume with fresh, fruity top notes brought out by Jean Patou in 1925. The heart is a flowery bouquet based on rose, jasmine and carnation, with top notes of neroli, blackcurrant buds, narcissus and bergamot, and lower notes dominated by vetiver. The perfume was relaunched in 1984 and is now sold in a flacon modelled after the original by Louis Süe.

Ampelopsis grana paradisi *see* Grains of Paradise

Ampulla *see* Aryballos

Amygdalus communis   *see* Bitter Almond
        persica   *see* Peach
Amyris balsamifera   *see* Sandalwood
        opobalsamum   *see* Balm of Gilead
        punctata   *see* Sassafras

'Anais-Anais'   A fresh floral perfume introduced in 1979 by Cacharel, for whom it was created by Firmenich perfumers. In 1989 it was the top-selling perfume in Britain. It is named after Anaitis, the ancient Persian goddess of love. The heart, based on rose, jasmine and iris, with hints of tuberose, ylang-ylang and other flower fragrances, is delicately floral. The top notes are leafy green, and the base notes contain vetivert, oak moss and patchouli. The original bottle, with a silver cap, was designed by Annegret Beier.

Ananus comosus   *see* Pineapple
        sativus   *see* Pineapple

Anchusa   *see* Alkanet

Andropogon aromaticus   *see* Ginger Grass Oil
        citratum   *see* Lemon Grass Oil
        flexuosus   *see* Lemon Grass de Cochin
        nardus   *see* Citronella
        odoratus   *see* Ginger Grass Oil
        schoenanthus   *see* Lemon Grass Oil

Anethole   A white crystalline solid found in the oils of aniseed, star anise, fennel and some other plants. It is occasionally used in perfumes and soaps.

Anethum foeniculum   *see* Fennel
        graveolens   *see* Dill

Angelica   Also called Garden Angelica, Archangelica and Root of the Holy Ghost. A tall biennial plant (*Angelica archangelica* = *A. officinalis* = *Archangelica officinalis*), believed native to Syria but now naturalized in temperate areas from Europe to the Himalayas. There are about 30 varieties. Angelica has a considerable place in N. European folklore, being regarded since the Icelandic sagas as a powerful charm against evil spirits and infectious diseases. It is said to have been introduced into England from Scandinavia in the Middle Ages as a valuable antidote to bubonic plague, one legend holding that this property was first revealed by an angel. In addition to its uses in medicines and flavourings, an essential oil is steam-distilled from the root (Oil of Angelica Root) and seeds which has a strong musky, benzoin or juniper-like odour and is used in perfumery, especially in chypre and fern-like perfumes, sometimes as a fixative. The dried roots and seeds are also used in pot pourri and sachets, and a resinoid extracted from the roots is used as a fixative.

Angelica levisticum   *see* Lovage

Angostura Beans   *see* Tonka Beans
Aniba rosaeodora   *see* Linaloe
　　　　terminalis   *see* Rosewood Oil
Animal Perfume Materials   A few materials derived from animals have been used in perfumes since antiquity and some are still highly valued by perfumers, most of them being exceptionally powerful and excellent fixatives. The main ones are:

>**Ambergris**　(from the sperm whale)
>**Castoreum**　(beaver)
>**Civet**　(civet cat)
>**Hyraceum**　(hyrax)
>**Musk**　(musk deer)
>**Propolis**　(bee)
>**Sweet Hoof**　(marine snail)

Animalic   A term used in perfumery to describe a fragrant material of animal origin, or the fragrance coming from that material, or a fragrance from a plant source or made synthetically which resembles such material.

Anise   Also known as Aniseed and Roman Fennel. A small annual (*Pimpinella anisum = Anisum vulgare = A. officinarum*) growing to about 18 inches high and native to Egypt, Asia Minor, Greece and Crete. The medical properties of anise were well known to the Greeks and Romans, who also used it as a spice. Its cultivation spread into central Europe and as far as England during the Middle Ages, when it was believed to avert the 'evil eye'. Oil of Anise is distilled from the seeds and occasionally used in perfumery. Both the oil and the seeds are sometimes added to pot pourri and sachets. Anise should not be confused with Star Anise, from which Aniseed Oil is obtained.

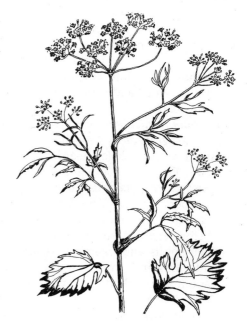

Anise (*Pimpinella anisum*).

Aniseed Star   *see* Star Anise
Annick Goutal   Born in France, a successful concert pianist and model, Annick Goutal is one of the few women who have become 'noses'. She

took up perfumery in 1977, creating her first fragrance, 'Folavril', in 1979 and opening a perfume shop in Paris in 1980. Her company, which bears her name, now has a world-wide business in association with the Tattinger Group. Her perfume creations, using high-quality natural materials, include 'Passion' (1980), 'Heure Exquise' (80), 'Parfum de Femme' (82) and 'Gardenia Passion' (89), together with a number of fragrances for men and the first fragrance for babies 'Eau de Bonpoint'. The perfumes are sold in a signature spherical flacon featuring a butterfly on the stopper.

'Antaeus' A fragrance for men created for Chanel in 1981 by Jacques Polge. It is named after an invincible hero of Greek mythology. Its principal ingredients are clary sage and myrtle, providing aromatic notes, patchouli and sandalwood to give woody notes, and labdanum to add an amber/leather touch.

Anthemis nobilis   *see* Camomile

Antofle   *see* Clove Oil

Anyme Oil   An oil obtained by distillation of the wood of an Australian tree – *Myoporum crassefolium*. It has a woody odour and is occasionally used in soaps.

Apium carvi   *see* Caraway

　　　　graveolens   *see* Celery Seed Oil

Aplotaxis lappa   *see* Costus

'Apogée' An innovative floral–chypre perfume introduced by the perfumers 'Les Senteurs' of London in 1989. Created for Les Senteurs by Francois Robert (the son of Guy Robert), it contains in the top note lily of the valley, jasmine and (unusually for a top note) frankincense, with a heart built on rose and sandalwood and a base in which patchouli, oak moss and amber are the main ingredients.

Apple   The early Arabs used apples (from *Malus pumila* = *M. communis* = *Pyrus malus*) in some of their perfumes; Syrian apples feature in several perfume recipes recorded by al-Kindi. In modern perfumery the aroma is obtained by distillation of the fruit juice or, more usually, by synthesis.

Apple Mint   *see* Mint

Appura   *see* Cedar

Apricot   Early Arab perfume recipes recorded by al-Kindi include the use of oil and flesh extracted from apricot kernals, from the Apricot tree (*Prunus armeniacus* = *Armeniaca vulgaris*) found in central and S.W. Asia and in Mediterranean regions. In modern perfumes the fragrance of apricot is created synthetically; it is often used to provide a fruity effect (e.g. 'Femme'), while Apricot Kernal Oil is used in toiletries.

Aptandra spruciana   *see* Sandal Oil

Aqua Angeli   A perfumed water first made for scenting the shirts of King Louis XIV of France (1638–1715). It was composed of aloewood, nutmeg, clove, storax and benzoin boiled in rosewater, with added jasmine, orange flower and musk.

Aquilaria bancana   *see* Ramin

      agollacha   *see* Aloewood

      malaccensis   *see* Aloewood

Arab Perfumes   The Arabs have been associated with perfume since the dawn of history. Frankincense and myrrh were collected by the Egyptians from the Land of Punt, which may have included south Arabia, from at least as early as 1500 BC (see Egyptian Perfumes), and Herodotus recorded in about 450 BC that Arabia was 'the only place

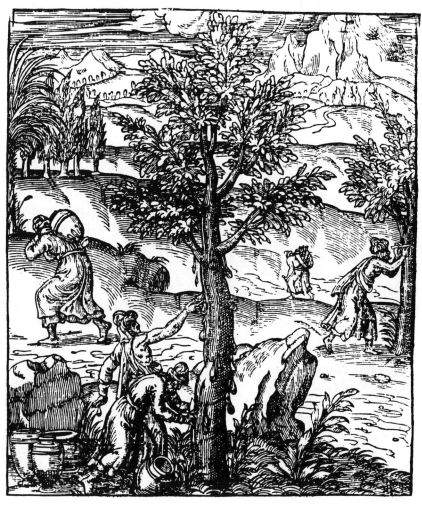

Arabs collecting incense
(*source* Andre Thevet, *Cosmographie Universelle*, 1575).

that produces frankincense, myrrh, cassia, cinnamon and the gum called ladanon', observing also that the Arabs sent several tons of frankincense every year to the Persian emperor Darius as a tribute. Theophrastus, too, noted these materials as coming from Arabia, and Pliny provided a detailed account of the very substantial Roman trade in aromatics from south Arabia, which were taken either overland to Petra or by sea, together with spices from India, through Egyptian Red Sea ports. Arabia also produced other perfume materials such as balsam of Makkah. Calamus and costus were used in early south Arabian incenses and may have been locally grown. Pliny commented that the Arabs liked to burn the wood of 'storax brought in from Syria'. But the cinnamon and cassia of the early accounts do not appear to have been the same materials as we know by those names today.

After the collapse of the Roman Empire the Arabian trade in frankincense and myrrh continued on a reduced scale. At the same time Arab perfume makers, especially those in Aden, began to make their name (it is recorded that Indian merchants even sent their ingredients to Aden to be made up into perfumes). With the advent of Islam in the 7th century AD, and subsequent wide-scale Arab conquests, came the Golden Age of Arab civilization, particularly under the Abbasid Caliphs of Baghdad (8th to 10th centuries AD), the period remembered in the *Arabian Nights Tales*. The Caliphs controlled Persia, where perfume-making was already an art, and their ships, trading directly with India, the East Indies and China, began to bring back new perfume materials. Sophisticated techniques of distillation were devised by the Arabs of this time, enabling attars, particularly of rose, to be manufactured on a large scale. The Persians sent 30 000 bottles of rosewater to Baghdad as a tribute every year. With the Caliphs encouraging the lavish use of perfume in their courts, Baghdad became the centre of a substantial perfume industry, and Arab perfume makers set up their shops in all parts of the Arab Empire. From Islamic Spain and Sicily, and in the luggage of returning crusaders, Arab perfumes crossed the borders into the Christian world. As Shakespeare testified, the 'perfumes of Arabia' were unexcelled in Europe until the 16th century.

Much of our knowledge of early Arab perfumes derives from a book of perfume recipes compiled by al-Kindi (c. 850 AD). From this it is evident that most of the principal ingredients of Egyptian, Greek and Roman perfumes were used by the Arabs, together with many materials previously unknown in Europe, notably the animal perfumes, ambergris, castoreum, musk and, a little later, civet, and Far Eastern plant products such as aloewood and camphor. Fruits, like apple, apricot, mahaleb cherry, citron, myrtle, peach and quince, were used. Floral ingredients included hollyhock, hyacinth, jasmine, jonquil, lily, narcissus, pandanus, rose, violet and wallflower. But the Arabs also had a strong liking for the fragrance of herbs and spices and employed a wide range of them. Among the more extraordinary fragrant materials used were sweet hoof, pissasphalt and hyraceum. Oils employed as a base included bitter almond, ben, cotton, olive and sesame. Most perfumes were coloured for good appearance, and for this the dyes included alkanet, emblic, dragon's blood and safflower. Several standard compound perfumes were produced widely, including Ghāliya, Khalūq (a recipe quoted under this heading shows the complexity of some of the Arab perfumes), Rāmik, Sukk and Naddah (a particularly luxurious incense). Some notion of the extravagant manner in which wealthy medieval Arabs used perfume is given in the 15th century Arab book of erotica *The Perfumed Garden*, where the advice to a man preparing for a (successful) seduction reads: 'Fill the tent with a variety of different perfumes: ambergris, musk and all sorts of scents, such as rose, orange flowers, jonquils, jasmine, hyacinth, carnation and other plants. This done, have placed there several gold censers filled with green aloes, ambergris, *naddah* and such like'.

Aramis   An Italian company based in Florence which was established in 1965 and is now a part of the Estée Lauder group. It specializes in men's toiletries. Fragrances include 'Aramis', a trend-setting chypre-type eau de cologne launched in 1965; its main ingredients are aldehydes with artemisia in the top note, jasmine and patchouli in the middle note, and oak moss and leather fragrance in the base. Other Aramis fragrances include 'Aramis 900' (73), 'Tuscany' (89) and 'New West' (90).

Arar Tree   *see* Sandarac

Araucaria Oil   A viscid, rose-scented oil distilled from the wood of a tree growing to about 30 feet high, *Neocallitropsis araucarioides*, found in New Caledonia. It is used as a fixative in cosmetics and soaps.

Arbor Vitae Oil   Also called Oil of White Cedar, Cedar Leaf Oil and Thuja Leaf Oil. An oil with a balsamic, pine-like fragrance which was once used medicinally and is still used occasionally in perfumes (especially as a fixative). It is distilled from the leaves of the Eastern Arbor Vitae tree (*Thuja occidentalis*) of the eastern USA, also called White Cedar, False White Cedar, Swamp Cedar and Tree of Life. The tree was introduced into Britain in about 1566. See also under Cedar.

Archangelica   *see* Angelica

Archangelica officinalis   *see* Angelica

Arden   *see* Elizabeth Arden

Arillus Myristicae   *see* Mace

Aristolochia clematatis   *see* Birthwort

Armani   *see* Giorgio Armani

Armenia vulgaris   *see* Apricot

Armenian Paper   A paper saturated with an aromatic solution so that it can be burned as an incense. (See Appendix B, recipe no. 34.)

Armoise   *see* Artemesia

Aromachology   A branch of aromatherapy concerned with the physio-
logical effects of scents. Current research, mainly in Japan, is concerned
with the selection of scents with calming or uplifting effects and the
physical measurement of those effects. Applications being developed
in Japan, principally by Shiseido, include an aromatic alarm clock,
designed to emit satisfying odours at the time of awakening, and the
emission of perfumes in work environments designed to refresh and to
relieve stress among office and operational staff.

Aromanthemes   A name used in perfumery to describe highly concentrated natural flower perfumes.

Aromatherapy   A method of therapeutic treatment developed during
the present century, but mostly based on herbal remedies evolved
over many centuries, in which the essential oils of aromatic plants are
applied to the body by massage, in aromatic baths, or in compresses, or
the aroma of them is inhaled. Experiments in 1991 at an NHS hospital
have used the scent of lavender oil to induce sleep. The word was
first used (in French as *Aromatherapie*) in 1928 by René Gattefossé, a
French chemist working in his family's perfume company. See also
Aromachology.

Aromatic Quinquina   *see* Cascarilla

'Arpège'   A classic, trend-setting
aldehydic perfume created by
André Fraysse and first issued
by Lanvin in 1927. Aldehydic
top notes, with hints of bergamot, neroli and peach, yield
to a floral heart, principally
jasmine, rose, camellia and lily
of the valley, with woody base
notes including ambrein, benzoin, musk, sandalwood and
vetiver. It is sold in a distinctive
black, ball-shaped flacon in Art
Deco style, designed by Armand
Rateau, and in a bottle by Brosse.

Arrace   *see* Orris

Artabotrys   The flowers of a
climbing plant *Artabotrys odoratissima*, native to India and
Indonesia, are used locally
in making perfume. Their
fragrance resembles ripe
apples.

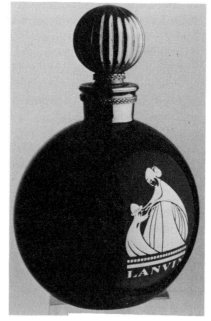

'Arpège'.

Artemisia Oil   Also called Armoise. An oil steam-distilled from the dried plants of two species of Artemisia (*Artemisia vulgaris* and *A. alba*), which are closely related to tarragon. They grow widely in temperate areas and are cultivated for this oil in Algeria, Morocco, France and Yugoslavia. The oil has a spicy fragrance and is used in many types of perfumes (e.g. 'Macassar', 'Aramis', 'Quorum' and 'La Nuit').

Artemisia abrotanum   *see* Southernwood

absinthium   *see* Wormwood

dracunculus   *see* Tarragon

pallens   *see* Davana Oil

pontica   *see* Wormwood

Arvensis Peppermint Oil   *see* Peppermint

Aryballos   A small flask used in ancient Greece, especially in the period 600–500 BC, to hold a perfumed unguent. It was round-bodied, with a very narrow mouth, so that the oil could be poured out drop by drop; usually it was made of terracotta and was carried hanging from the owner's wrist by a small strap. Athletes used it when washing after performing in the Olympic Games. Some types of aryballos remained in use into Roman times, when they were known as Ampullae and were usually carried together with a *'strigil'*, a form of comb for scraping the skin, used while perspiring in the public hot baths.

Asafoetida   Also called Devil's Gum, Devil's Dung, Stinking Gum, Food of the Gods and Silphium. A gum obtained from a tall evil-smelling (due to sulphurous compounds) plant of this name (*Ferula assafoetida* and *F. narthex*) originating in Iran and Afghanistan. The gum was used as a spice and medicine by the ancient Egyptians and Greeks and was known to the Romans as Persian Silphium. It is still used, as a fixative, in oriental-type perfumes after removal of the sulphurous content. An oil with an intense onion-like odour is steam-distilled from the gum and used in both medicines and perfumery.

Asarabacca   Also called Hazelwort, Wild Nard and European Wild Ginger. A species of Birthwort, *Asarum europaeum*, growing in Europe and Asia Minor. The fragrant roots, used medicinally and in the preparation of snuff, resemble spikenard and were an ingredient in some early Arab perfumes. See also Birthwort.

Asarum canadense   *see* Canadian Snakeroot

Ash Twig Lichen   A lichen (*Ramalina fraxinea = Lobaria fraxinea*) found in temperate zones of Europe and sometimes used in the manufacture of perfumes and cosmetics.

Ashanti Pepper Tree   *see* Cubeb

Asna   *see* Ain

Aspalathus   A perfumed plant mentioned by Theophrastus and Dioscorides and also in the Book of Ecclesiasticus. It has no connection with the genus Aspalathus of modern times, which is native to S.

Africa, nor with Rhodium, which is sometimes called 'Aspalathus'. It is thought most likely that the Aspalathus of ancient times came from varieties of Camel's Thorn (*Alhagi camelorum*) found in the Middle East and N. Africa, or from a shrubby herb *Cytisus lanigerus*. See Kypros.

Asperula odorata   *see* Woodruff

Assam, Oil of   *see* Patchouli

Astragalus gummifera   *see* Tragacanth

Atherosperma moschatum   *see* Sassafras

Atomizer   Also called Spray and Vaporizer (French: *Vaporasiteur*). A perfume bottle made with a pressure device, often operated by squeezing a rubber bulb, which discharges its fragrance as a fine spray. Originally developed as medicinal throat sprays, atomizers, notably those made by the American firm DeVilbiss, were used for perfumes from about 1910. Fine examples are now much sought after by collectors.

Attar   Also known as Otto. A fragrant essential oil derived from a flower by distillation. The word comes from Arabic *'Itr*, meaning a perfume (also *'Atr jul* in Persian, meaning 'fat of a flower'. It is applied in particular to the essential oil of the rose. The term is sometimes used loosely to signify any essential oil.

Auklandia costus   *see* Costus

Australian Santal Tree   *see* Sandalwood

Avens   A common wayside plant (*Geum urbanum*) growing up to 2 feet high and found in temperate Europe, N. America, Asia and Australia. The botanical name *Geum* originates from a Greek word meaning 'to yield an agreeable fragrance'. The plant has many country names, including Avens Root, Clove Root, Colewort, Goldy Star, Caryophyllata, Wood Avens, Wild Rye and Herb Bennett (a corruption from 'the blessed herb' because of the belief that it could ward off evil spirits and wild beasts). The rhizomes have a clove-like fragrance and are dried for use in sachet powders and pot pourri as well as for flavouring and medicinal purposes. In 17th century England they were strewed among clothes to provide fragrance and keep away moths. They were once thought to counter bubonic plague. The leaves, also dried for use in pot pourri, have a sweet, clover-like smell.

Avocado Oil   An oil obtained by expression from the dried fruits of the Avocado tree (*Persea gratissima*), which grows to about 20 feet high and is native to tropical America. The tree is now cultivated widely in tropical areas. The oil is one of the most penetrating oils known. It is used in cosmetics and soaps.

Avon   Founded in the USA in 1886 by David McConnell, a travelling book salesman who liked to give his customers a gift of inexpensive perfume. The company was first called The California Perfume Company, becoming Avon Products Inc. in 1939 (the name is after

Stratford-on-Avon). It is now one of the largest manufacturers of fragrances, cosmetics and toiletries in the world. It opened in Britain, as Avon Cosmetics Ltd, in 1959, selling to the mass market directly through its representatives, the 'Avon ladies'. Avon fragrances, of which two or three new ones are introduced every year, are sold as sprays at eau de toilette concentration and include some long-standing lines such as 'Moonwind' (1971) and 'Charisma' (1968). Many of them are created for Avon by one or other of the large wholesale fragrance manufacturers (see Perfume Manufacture). The company's main headquarters and factory complex is at Suffern, in California, and a factory in Northampton manufactures products sold in Britain and Europe. In 1987 Avon entered the quality perfume market by acquiring Giorgio Beverly Hills.

Aydendron rosaeodora *see* Linaloe

Azalea The flowers of several species of Azalea, shrubs of the genus *Rhododendron*, are fragrant, but perfume with the fragrance of Azalea is made synthetically.

Azalea Oil *see* Linaloe

'Azzaro pour Homme' A trend-setting fougere-type men's fragrance brought out by Loris Azzaro in 1978. A creation of the fragrance firm Naarden (now Quest), its principal ingredients are lavender, with other fresh, herbaceous elements, in the top note, patchouli with some woody elements in the middle note, and amber and musk in the base note. The bottle was designed by Pierre Dinand.

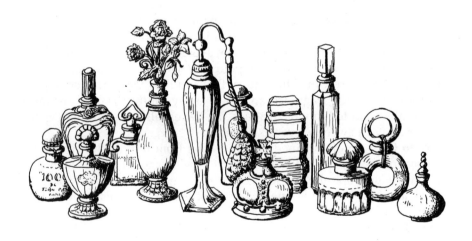

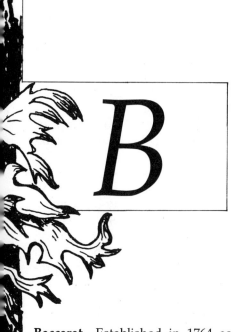

Baccarat Established in 1764 as a wood-burning glassworks, Baccarat has been making lead crystal at the village of Baccarat, in Lorraine, since 1817 and is now one of the world's foremost manufacturers of high quality crystal ware. Baccarat started to provide flacons for perfume early in the 19th century, and with the great expansion of the perfume industry at the end of that century it began to supply many of the major perfume houses, its early clients including Pinaud, Houbigant, Coty, Guerlain and, later, Roger & Gallet, Bourjois and Jean Patou. In subsequent years almost all the major perfume houses sold fragrances in Baccarat flacons. The company's current clients include Amouage, Bijan, Paco Rabanne, Dior and Jean Patou. See also Perfume Containers.

Baccharis dracunculifolia   *see* Vassoura Oil

Bachelor's Buttons   *see* Feverfew Chrysanthemum

Backhousia Oil   A lemon-like essential oil distilled from the leaves of the Citron Myrtle tree (*Backhousia citriodora*), also called Native Myrtle and Scrub Myrtle, which grows in Australia. It is used in perfumes and soaps.

Back Note   *see* Low Note

Badiane   *see* Star Anise

Bahama White Wood   *see* Canella

'Balahé'   A fresh–floral perfume introduced by Léonard in 1983.

It was created for Léonard by Givaudan perfumers. Fruity, aldehydic top notes, with mandarin and bergamot, head floral middle notes, principally of jasmine, rose, ylang-ylang, iris and tuberose. The lower notes include sandalwood, vanilla and vetivert. The flacon was designed, as a black 'moonstone', by Serge Mansau.

Balanos   An oil derived from the fruit of a thorny tree known as the Egyptian Plum tree (*Balanites aegyptiaca = Ximenia aegyptiaca*) once abundant in the Nile valley. It was a popular base oil in ancient Egyptian perfumes, fragrant flowers or herbs being steeped in it to impart their scents. Theophrastus described Balanos, coming either from Egypt or Syria, as the oil most used in perfumery, noting that it was a good fixative. See also Ximenia and Egyptian Perfumes.

'Bal à Versailles'   A classic top quality oriental-type perfume, one of the most expensive marketed, brought out by Jean Desprez, its creator, in 1962. It contains some 300 ingredients, mostly natural. Rose, jasmine and orange flower in the top note herald a middle note which includes patchouli, sandalwood and vetivert, with musk, civet and amber among the base notes. It is presented in a variety of hand-polished crystal flacons, designed by Pierre Dinand and carrying a label which reproduces a painting by Fragonard, contained in silk-brocaded boxes.

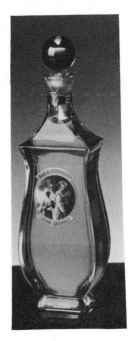

'Bal à Versailles'.

Balenciaga   Parfums Balenciaga was founded by the Spanish-born Paris couturier Cristobal Balenciaga (1895–1972) with the launching of his first perfume, 'Le Dix', in 1947. The success of this led to 'Quadrille' (55, relaunched 89), followed by 'Cialenga' (73), 'Michelle' (80), 'Prélude' (82) and 'Rumba' (88), together with men's fragrances which include 'Ho Hang' (71) and 'Eau de Balenciaga Lavande' (73). After acquisition by the German group Hoescht, the company was in 1986 taken over by J. Bogart.

Balm   Oil of Balm is taken from the leaves of Balm, a perennial lemon-scented herb of medium height (*Melissa officinalis*), also called Melissa, Lemon Balm, Lemon Nettle, Common Balm, Garden Balm, Sweet Balm and Bauline, which originated in S. Europe and S.W. Asia and now grows widely. Commercial Oil of Balm is usually distilled with Oil of Lemon. Once an ingredient of Carmelite Water, it is used in perfumes, toilet waters, ointments, liqueurs and furniture polishes, and the dried leaves are used in sachets and pot pourri. The plant was introduced into Britain by the Romans. It should not be confused with the Melissa plant of ancient times, used in medicine and for bees, which probably came from a Mediterranean herb *Prasium majus*. The word 'balm' is an abbreviation of 'balsam' and the two words are often used synonymously; it indicates a honeyed sweetness.

Balm of Gilead   A balm, or balsam, referred to in the Old Testament, notably in reference to 'a company of Ishmaelites from Gilead with their camels bearing spicery and balm and myrrh...into Egypt' (Genesis 37:25) (on this text see also under Labdanum). For centuries this balm has been confused with Balsam of Judaea, with which it is not connected. The plant from which it was derived is unknown; possibly it was the balsam known as Balsam of Makkah, but it may have been resin from the terebinth or lentisk.

The term Balm of Gilead is sometimes used for the buds of the Scented Poplar (*Populus balsamifera*), a N. American tree, and for a shrub *Cedronella tryphylla*, found in the Canary Islands, and also for some other plants with a balsamic fragrance.

Balm of Gilead Buds   *see* Tacamahac
Balm of Peru   *see* Balsam of Peru
Balmain   The Balmain fashion house, which now sells a wide variety of products, was opened in Paris in 1945 by Pierre Balmain (1914–83), who produced his first perfume, the innovative 'Vent Vert', in the same year. This was followed by 'Jolie Madame' (53), 'Miss Balmain' (68) and 'Ivoire' (79), together with men's fragrances 'Ébène' (67) and 'Eau de M. Balmain' (64). After various ownerships, the company was purchased in 1991 by the Canadian businessman Erich Fayer.

Balsam   A viscous, resinous exudation from certain trees and shrubs, with a consistency which is thick but not solid. The principal balsams used in modern perfumery are Balsam of Peru, Balsam of Tolu, Balsam of Copaiba, Storax and Balm of Gilead. They have in common a vanilla-like odour. The words Balsam and Balm are often used synonymously. The word Balsam is also used for certain flowering plants of the genus *Impatiens*.

Balsam of Copaiba   Also called Copaiba Resin, Copaiva, Balsam of Capivy, Campaif, Colocai and Gamelo. An essential oil distilled from the resin of the Copaiba tree (*Copaifera lansdorfii* = *C. officinalis*) and other related species, including *C. reticulata* and *C. guyenensis*, of Brazil and other parts of S. America. The oil is sweet and balsamic, with a peppery overtone. One tree may yield up to 12 gallons of oil, and the trees have even been known to burst under the pressure of the oil inside them. The oil is an excellent fixative, and is used in incenses, pomander beads and pot pourri as well as in perfumes. The resin of a tree *Daniellia thurifera*, found in tropical Africa, is also sometimes called Balsam of Copaiba (other names being Liiorin Gum, Illorin Copal, Hardwickia Balsam, and Ogea Gum of Sierra Leone) and is used as a perfume. A similar balsam used medicinally and sometimes in per-fumery comes from *Hardwickia pinnata*, native to India, and from *Oxystigma mannii* of tropical Africa, the balsam of which is called West African Copaiba. See also Bois d'Olhio.

Balsam Fir   *see* Canada Balsam

Balsam Herb   *see* Costmary

Balsam of Judaea   The botanical identity of the plant providing this balsam, by far the most valuable of all the perfume materials of the ancients, is not known. It is usually, but incorrectly, identified with Balsam of Makkah and Balm of Gilead. Pliny stated that 'every scent ranks below the balsam'. Several classical authors have related that from as early as the time of Alexander the Great it was only known as a cultivated plant growing in Judaea, in two irrigated plantations near Jericho which belonged to the king and which Cleopatra took over from Herod after her marriage to Anthony. Josephus held that the first seeds were brought to Solomon by the Queen of Sheba. The Romans, who subsequently expanded the cultivated area in Palestine, regarded it so highly that branches of it were carried in triumphal processions in Rome. The plant was described as a small, vine-like bush with leaves like rue, and the balsam resin, called opobalsamum, exuded slowly in tiny drops which were collected in a shell, one man taking a whole day to fill his shell. Between them the two original plantations only produced about 40 pints of opobalsamum a year. So rare and sought after was the perfume that in the time of Theophrastus it cost more than twice its weight in silver, and in Pliny's time it was worth 1000 denarii a pint, or about 170 times as much as the costliest frankincense. The whole plant was fragrant, with the berry (carpobalsamum) and wood (xylobalsamum) (the branches were kept pruned) also having their uses in medicines, perfumes and incenses. Pliny described an unguent with xylobalsamum among its ingredients. A 12th century Arab recorded that in his time one small garden of balsam bushes had survived in Egypt, but that they no longer grew in Palestine. There is uncertain record of the existence of the perfume in the 13th century, but no subsequent account of it. Various suggestions have been made as to the identity of Balsam of Judaea, but none satisfactory, and it would appear that this most romantic of perfume plants may well have become extinct.

Balsam of Makkah (Mecca) Also called Balsam, Makka Myrrh, Balm of Gilead and Opobalsamum. A balsam taken from the Arabian balsam tree (*Commiphora gileadensis* = C. *opobalsamum* = *Balsamodendron gileadensis* = B. *ehrenbergianum* = *Balsamea meccanensis*), which grows to about 12 feet tall and is found in Arabia, Somalia and Ethiopia. In Arabia the tree is known as *Bashām* or *Balasān* (cf. the word 'balsam'). For a very long time this plant has been much confused with Balsam of Judaea and Balm of Gilead, the botanical names reflecting early beliefs that these plants were all the same. Identity with Balm of Gilead is possible but not certain. The balsam produced by it had a vogue in medieval times, when it was mainly gathered from trees in the area of Makkah and when unsuccessful attempts were made to cultivate it in Egypt. 'Carpobalsamum', from the berry (see Balsam of Judaea), was used in the 17th century for scenting wine. It is little used today and not at all in western perfumery. See also under Myrrh.

Balsam of Peru Also called Balm of Peru. An oleo-resin with a cinnamon-like fragrance obtained, by treatment with alcohol, from the fruits and bark of a large tree (*Myroxylon balsamom* var. *pereirae* = M. *pareira*), mainly found in San Salvador and shipped from Peru. The balsam from the fruit pods, which is superior, is sometimes known as Myrocarpin. A similar balsam is also derived from the trunk of a species of Cabreu tree (see Cabreu Oil). An oil is distilled from the balsam and is the substance now mostly used in perfumery (e.g. 'Shalimar' and 'Fidji'), but usually in modified form to meet modern safety standards (see Perfume Creation). The fragrance is vanilla-like. Balsam of Peru is a good fixative and is used in many types of perfume, making a good base for oriental-type perfumes. It is also used in soaps, cosmetics and incenses.

Balsam Poplar *see* Tacamahac

Balsam of Tolu Also called Tolu Balsam, American Balsam and Opobalsam (see Balsam of Judaea). A balsamic resin tapped from the trunk of a tall tree (*Myroxylon balsamum* = M. *toluiferum*), found in Venezuela, Columbia and Peru. It has a vanilla or benzoin-like fragrance and the balsam hardens as it ages. An oil is steam-distilled

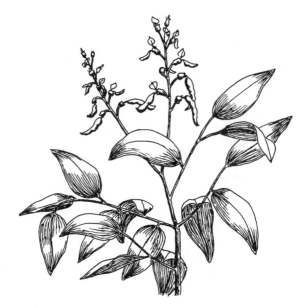

Balsam of Tolu (*Myroxylon balsamum*).

from the resinoid. It is a good fixative and used in incenses and perfumes (e.g. 'Youth Dew' and 'Chamade') and in preparing soaps and toilet waters. When dissolved in a minute portion of liquor potassa the fragrance changes to that of clove-pink.

Balsamic Note   A term used in perfumery to describe the sweet, soft and warm fragrance of balsams and resins. See Perfume Notes.

Balsamaea meccanensis   *see* Balsam of Makkah

Balsamita Foemina   *see* Maudlin

Balsamita major   *see* Costmary

Balsamodendron ehrenbergianum   *see* Balsam of Makkah
          gileadense   *see* Balsam of Makkah
          myrrha   *see* Myrrh

Baltimore Oil   *see* Ambroisia

Banana   The aroma of banana is obtained by distillation of the juice of the fruit of the Banana tree (*Musa sapientum*), native to S.E. Asia but now grown widely in tropical areas, and the Horse Banana tree (*M. paradisiaca*), also called Adam's Banana, and Plantain, native to tropical Asia. Though called trees, these plants are large herbs.

Banana Shrub Oil   A banana-scented oil extracted from the flowers of the Banana Shrub (*Michelia fuscata*), which originated in China but is now cultivated widely. It is used in scenting hair oils.

Barosma betulina   *see* Buchu Leaf Oil
          crenulata   *see* Buchu Leaf Oil

venusta   *see* Buchu Leaf Oil

Base Note   See Low Note

Basil   Also called Sweet Basil, Common Basil and Basilicon. A plant cultivated for its essential oil and also used in pot pourri and sachets as well as in cookery and flavouring. The name Basil derives from the Greek meaning 'king', indicating the high esteem in which it was held. Orthodox Greeks still regard it as a holy plant. The plant is an annual, growing to about 3 feet high (*Ocimum basilicum*) and is thought to have originated in India. It is now cultivated widely for its essential oil, obtained from the leaves. The fragrance is sharp and spicy, with some similarity to mignonette, and is used in quality perfumes (e.g. 'Nina' and 'Rumba'). Other varieties are also found, one with a scent of citron, another with that of tarragon. An Indian species (*O. sanctum*) has the fragrance of cloves and is a holy herb to the Hindus. The early Arab perfume makers used the oils of *O. basilicum*, which they called 'French musk', of a N. Arabian variety called 'Nabataean Basil', and of Bush Basil (*O. minimum*), their name for which (*Shāhsiferam*) derived from Persian meaning 'king of the fragrant plants'. It was once believed that a sprig of basil left under a pot would in time turn into a scorpion.

Basil Thyme   *see* Calamint

Bastard Cinnamon   *see* Cassia

Bastard Bullet Tree   *see* Houmiri

Batteuse   A machine used by the perfume industry in the south of France for extracting the perfume from concretes by means of alcohol.

Baur, Albert   A German chemist who patented the first synthetic musk perfume, Musk Baur, in 1888 and was responsible for other formulas for synthetic musk (Musk Ketone and Musk Ambrette). See Synthetic Fragrances.

Bay, Oil of   Also called Laurel Leaf Oil. A spicy fragrant oil, sometimes used in perfumery to provide a masculine note, which is steam-distilled from the leaves of the Bay tree (*Laurus nobilis*). An example of its use in a modern quality perfume is 'Knowing'. The tree, native to the Mediterranean area, is also called Laurel, Sweet Bay, Bay Laurel, True Laurel, Roman Laurel, Noble Laurel and Daphne. It grows up to 25 feet high in the UK, but up to 60 feet in warmer climates. The dried leaves are used in sachets and pot pourri and as a flavouring. The Bay was much venerated in classical and biblical times, being regarded as beneficial to health and happiness. The Greeks and Romans dedicated it to Apollo and to Aesculapius, the god of medicine, and used it in crowns and garlands as a symbol of victory. Throughout history it has been used as a strewing herb both for its scent and for its antiseptic properties. A fat, Bay Fat, is extracted from the berries to make soap, as also is an oil known as Oil of Bays. The early Arabs used oil obtained from both the leaves and the berries in their perfumes.

A similar spicy oil, known as Oil of Bay and Oil of Myrica, is obtained from the Bois d'Indes tree.

Bay Pine Tree   *see* Oyster Oil

Bdellium   An aromatic gum obtained from certain species of trees of the genus *Commiphora* (once classified as *Balsamodendron*), which also encompasses Myrrh and Balsam of Makkah. Several sorts of bdellium are used in perfumery, most importantly that called Opoponax (q.v.), from *Commiphora erythraea* var. *glabrescens*, found in Ethiopia. Other bdellium trees include *C. hildebrandtii*, from the Dunkal tree of Somalia; *C. africana*, the African Myrrh tree, found in Ethiopia, Sudan and Arabia; and *C. mukul* (= *C. wightii* = *C. roxburghii*), the Mukul Myrrh tree, found from Arabia to India, the bdellium from which is called Mukul and sometimes Indian Bdellium. Bdellium was known to the Romans and is referred to twice in the Old Testament, but there is still uncertainty about which of the trees were regarded in ancient times as producing bdellium and which as producing myrrh.

Bead tree   *see* Melia

Bearded Usnea   *see* Tree Moss

'Beautiful'   An Estee Lauder floral perfume launched in 1986. Green top notes from thyme and clary sage introduce a floral bouquet, mainly of rose, jasmine, carnation and orange flower, with a background accord in the lower note which includes vetivert, patchouli, frankincense, myrrh, tonka, vanilla, oak moss, orris and beeswax. The flacon was designed by Ira Levy.

Beaux, Ernest   Famous in perfume history as the man who created 'Chanel No. 5'. Beaux, a chemist, met 'Coco' Chanel when he was experimenting with ways of fixing aldehydes for use in perfumery. She encouraged his work and, in 1921, he presented her with two sets of sample fragrances using aldehydes, labelled Nos 1–5 and 20–25. From these she chose No. 5 for her new collection. Other successful perfumes created by Beaux for Chanel included 'Gardenia' (1925), 'Bois des Isles' (1926), 'Cuir de Russie' (1929) and 'Chanel No. 22' (1926), all relaunched in 1989. He also created 'Soir de Paris' for Bourjois.

Beaver Musk   *see* Castoreum

Beaver Oil   *see* Castoreum

Bee Balm   *see* Bergamot

Bee Glue   *see* Propolis

Beene, Geoffrey   *see* Sanofi

Beeswax   The wax used by bees in making honeycombs. It is used in cosmetics and ointments, principally to thicken essential oils, and appears occasionally as an ingredient in perfumes (e.g. 'Beautiful'). See also Propolis and Honey.

Behan Oil   *see* Ben Oil

Ben Oil   Also called Ben-nut Oil, Behan Oil, Horseradish Oil and

Moringa Oil. An essential oil expressed from the winged seeds of the Horseradish tree (*Moringa oleifera* = *M. pterygosperma*), a deciduous soft-wood tree indigenous to N. India, but now cultivated widely. The oil is clear and odourless, does not go rancid, and readily accepts other fragrances added to it, making Ben Oil an excellent base oil for perfumes and valuable in enfleurage and maceration. It has been used in perfumery, cosmetics and medicines since the days of ancient Egypt when it was taken from the Egyptian species of the tree, *M. peregrina* (= *M. aptera*) (see Balanos and Egyptian Perfumes). Pliny noted different varieties of the tree growing in Arabia, Egypt and Ethiopia, the Arabian providing the best-quality oil and the Egyptian the highest yielding. It appeared in many of the perfumes of the early Arabs.

Benckiser Following acquisitions since 1990, this is now the largest German company in the fragrance industry. Its perfume houses include Jil Sander, Joop, Lancaster, Margaret Astor, Monteil and Perera.

Bene Oil *see* Sesame Oil

Benjamin *see* Benzoin

Benzaldehyde A synthetic prepared from either benzyl or benzyl chlorides. The material is present in Bitter Almond Oil, with which it is almost identical, and in some other natural oils. Benzaldehyde is sold as an artificial almond oil. It is used in small amounts in violet and heliotrope types of perfume, and in soaps.

Benzene A substance derived from coal tar, used in the manufacture of synthetic rose scents and many other artificial fragrances.

Benzoin Also called Benjamin, Gum Benjamin, Sumatra Benzoin, Head Benzoin, Belly Benzoin and Benzoin Gum. A sweet-smelling oleo-resin obtained from a number of related species of trees found in S.E. Asia, more especially *Styrax benzoin* and *S. tonkinense* (= *S. macrothyrsus*). *S. benzoin* was first described in the 14th century by Ibn Battuta, who found it in Sumatra. The resin from it has a storax-like fragrance. The more highly valued resin from *S. tonkinense*, which grows mainly in Thailand, is sometimes called Siam Balsam and has a vanilla-like fragrance (it contains Vanillin). Benzoin oil is extracted from the gum with alcohol or benzene. The Arabs call benzoin *Luban Jawi*, meaning Frankincense of Java, from which the names Benjamin and Benzoin derive. Benzoin was for long an important ingredient in pomanders and was used in incenses and soaps as well as to give 'body' to many perfumes. Examples of its use in modern quality perfumes are 'Chamade', 'Crêpe de Chine' and 'Opium'. It is an excellent fixative and is added to sachets and pot pourri. It is also an ingredient in Friar's Balsam.

Benzoin aestivalis *see* Spicewood

Benzyl Acetate A colourless liquid with a fruity, jasmine-like odour which occurs naturally in the oils of ylang-ylang, hyacinth and gardenia but can also be manufactured synthetically. In perfumery it is regarded as one of the most useful synthetic materials available, being inexpensive to produce, and is a basis of almost all jasmine perfumes.

Benzyl Alcohol   An alcohol used in perfumery which occurs naturally in many essential oils, including jasmine, tuberose, wallflower and ylang-ylang. It is also synthesized chemically.

Bergamot   Also called Bee Balm, Red Bee Balm, Oswego Bee Balm, Oswego Tea and Scarlet Monarda. In origin a N. American swamp herb (*Monarda didyma*), this plant is now cultivated widely and grows up to 2 feet high in Britian. Flowers and leaves have a sharp flavour and fragrance similar to that of the Bergamot Orange. The essential oil is called Monarda Oil, to distinguish it from Bergamot Oil, and sometimes also Oil of Thyme. The oil is described as reminiscent of lavender and ambergris, and is used in perfumery and hair preparations, the dried leaves and flowers also being used in sachets and pot pourri. In N. America the leaves are also used as a tea.

Bergamot Mint   A herb (*Mentha citrata = M. aquatica = M. odorata*) now found in N. America, Asia, S. Europe and N. Africa, from the leaves of which is distilled an essential oil with a lemon and lavender-like fragrance resembling Bergamot Oil. Theophrastus noted its use in 300 BC as an ingredient in Greek perfumes. The oil is used in perfumery and the dried leaves in sachets and pot pourri. See also Mint.

Bergamot Oil   An orange-scented essential oil extracted by expression from the fruit peel of the Bergamot Orange tree (*Citrus bergamia = C. aurentium* var. *bergamia*). The tree, which originated in tropical Asia, is cultivated for the oil in S. Italy, Sicily and Spain and also, to an extent, in S. America and W. Africa. The name Bergamot is believed to derive from the Turkish *beg-armudi*, meaning 'the prince's pear', because the fruit is pear-shaped. The oil, one of the rarer and more valuable perfume materials, has a fresh, fruity fragrance; it contains linaoöl and is also produced synthetically (see Perfume Creation); it is much used in modern perfumery, appearing in about 34% of all women's perfumes (e.g. 'L'Heure Bleue', 'Balahé' and 'Crêpe de Chine') and 50% of all men's fragrances, and is also found in Eau de Colognes and hair preparations. It should not be confused with Monarda Oil extracted from the Bergamot plant. See also Bitter Orange Oil and Neroli.

Betula alba   *see* Birch Bud and Birch Tar Oil
    lenta   *see* Sweet Birch Oil

Bible Leaf   *see* Costmary

Bible Perfumes   The Bible gives us details of many of the perfume plants used in Palestine and its environs over a considerable period and is a valuable supplement to our knowledge from other sources about Egyptian, Greek and Roman perfumes. From early times it is apparent that the Hebrews esteemed the use of perfume. 'Ointment and perfume rejoice the heart' says the Book of Proverbs, a statement better translated in today's idiom as: 'Perfumes and incenses rejoice the heart'.

Some 25 different perfume materials are mentioned in the Bible, but the identification of some of them is by no means certain. Difficulties in translating from the ancient texts have sometimes led to plants being incorrectly named (e.g. the 'myrrh' of Genesis – see under Balm of Gilead – was probably labdanum); sometimes the same name may have been given to more than one perfume plant; in some cases, such as cinnamon, the name may have transferred over the passage of time, so that the cinnamon of the Old Testament may have derived from a different plant to that mentioned in the New Testament.

Frankincense and myrrh feature consistently in both Old and New Testaments. Israelite women wore a sachet underneath their clothes containing myrrh and other substances, which would release their fragrance from the warmth of the wearer's body. The special appeal of myrrh is reflected in many places in the Bible, and the Book of Esther reveals that girls selected for the Persian court were prepared over a twelve-month period, 'six months with oil of myrrh and six months with sweet odours'.

Other perfume plants mentioned in the Bible include aloes, balm, calamus, camphire, cassia, cinnamon, galbanum, labdanum, myrtle, saffron, spikenard, stacte and storax, all in contexts indicating a reference to them as perfume plants. Certain other plants used in perfumery, such as lily, bdellium, mint, anise, cumin and coriander, are mentioned without being related to perfume. The rose, which is referred to frequently, is now thought to have covered several different flowers. A number of oils used as perfume bases are also mentioned (e.g. olive oil).

Of compound perfumes, we know (from Exodus 30:23) that the holy anointing oil of the early Hebrews consisted of myrrh, 'cinnamon', calamus, 'cassia' and olive oil, while the holy perfume (incense), 'a confection after the art of the apothecary', was made from equal parts of stacte, onycha, galbanum and frankincense. Neither of these compounds was allowed to be used for secular purposes.

Bigarade Orange   *see* Bitter Orange Oil and Neroli

Bigroot Geranium   *see* Zdravets

Bijan   An American men's wear fashion company, started by Bijan Pakzad in Beverly Hills in 1976, which in 1981 launched its first fragrance, 'Bijan for Men', as a concentrated perfume sold in a crystal flacon made by Baccarat. 'Bijan Fragrance for Men', a Cologne to the same formula, followed in 1987, together with 'Bijan Perfume for Women'. The latter, a floral-oriental perfume created by Peter Bohm, has ylang-ylang, narcissus and orange-flower in the top notes, with a heart of jasmine, lily of the valley and Bulgarian rose, underlined by patchouli, oak moss and sandalwood in the base; it is sold in a ring-shaped flacon.

Bilsted   *see* Storax

Birch Bud Oil   An essential oil with a balsamic odour distilled from the leaf buds of the European Birch tree (Common Birch tree) (*Betula alba*), which grows widely in Europe and temperate Asia. The oil was also once known as Russian Leather Oil, being imported from Russia and used for scenting and preserving book leather. See also Birch Tar oil.

Birch Tar Oil   A thick bituminous liquid with a woody, tarry, smoky odour, obtained by distillation from the bark of the European Birch tree (Common Birch tree) (*Betula alba*), which grows widely in Europe and N. Asia. It is similar to Oil of Gaultheria (Wintergreen) and used mainly in masculine fragrances (e.g. 'Cuir de Russie'). See also Birch Bud oil.

Bird's Foot   *see* Fenugreek

Birthwort   A trailing shrub (*Aristolochia clematatis*), which grows wild in Europe, N. America and Japan. The early Arab perfumers used it in making a base for solid perfumes. There is some evidence that it was used in ancient Egypt, principally for medicinal purposes and in connection with child birth. See also Asarabacca.

Bissabol Myrrh tree   *see* Myrrh and Opoponax

Bitter Almond Oil   An essential oil derived from the fruit of the Bitter Almond tree (*Amygdalus communis* var. *amara*). The best is obtained from the S. of France, Sicily and N. Africa. It is sometimes used in perfumes today, but mainly in medicine. Bitter Almond Oil was one of the ingredients of the famous Metopium perfume oil of ancient Egypt and was used as a base oil for scented materials (see Balanos). Theophrastus noted that some of the perfume makers of ancient Greece regarded it as the best base for making unguents, although it was not very long-lasting. The early Arab perfume makers used it as a base for jasmine oil. See Benzaldehyde.

Bitter Orange Oil   An oil obtained by expression from the orange peel of the Bigarade Orange tree, also called Seville Orange or Sour Orange tree (*Citrus aurantium* var. *dulcis* and *C. aurantium* var. *amara*), the flowers and leaves of which produce respectively Neroli and Petitgrain. See also Bergamot Oil. The oil is mostly produced in Sicily and Italy, but also in California, W. India and N. Africa. It is used in Eau de Colognes, in some perfumes, especially of a chypre type, and also in soaps. It is also produced synthetically (see Perfume Creation).

Black Balsam   *see* Labdanum

Black Cumin   *see* Gith

Blackcurrant Bud Oil   Also called Cassis. A fragrant essential oil obtained from the flower buds of the Blackcurrant bush (*Ribes nigrum*), native from Europe to central Asia and now cultivated widely. It is usually extracted by volatile solvents as a concrete which gives a high yield of absolute. It is used in high-quality perfumes to provide a special effect (e.g. 'Amazone' and 'Jardins de Bagatelle').

Bloodwort   *see* Milfoil

'Blue Grass'   A famous classic perfume by Elizabeth Arden, first brought out by the founder of that firm, Florence Graham, in 1936 and named to recall the view from her home in Virginia. The perfume was created by Georges Fuchs of Fragonard, the Grasse perfume makers, and was relaunched in 1989. The top note is fresh and aldehydic, with a middle note of various flower fragrances built on jasmine, rose and lavender and given a spicy touch by clove, pepper and nutmeg. The base note is chiefly sandalwood, with suggestions of vetiver and Virginia cedar.

Bog Myrtle   Also called Candleberry Myrtle and Sweet Gale. A plant (*Myrica gale*) growing to about 3 feet high which is found in N. America and Europe. A wax, sometimes called Myrtle Wax, is drawn from the berries and used to make fragrant candles.

Bogart, Jacques   A perfume company founded by Jacques Konckier in 1975, in conjunction with the Paris couturier Jacques Bogart, to launch the men's fragrance 'Bogart'. This was followed by 'One Man Show' (80) and 'Furyo' (88). In 1984 the company acquired Parfums Ted Lapidus, launching 'Creation by Ted Lapidus' in that year and 'Lapidus pour Homme' in 1987. In 1986 it acquired the firm of Balenciaga.

Bois de Rose   *see* Linaloe

Bois de Siam   Also called Coffin-wood Oil. An essential oil distilled from the roots of the Coffin-wood tree, a species of cypress (*Cupressus hodgsinii = Fokiena hodgsinii*) and two other conifer trees (*Cunninghamia sinensis* and *Dacrydium elatum*) found in S. China and Vietnam, where they are known respectively as Pe-mow, Se-mow and Hoang-da. The oil is sweet and cedar-like. The wood, which is also aromatic, is used for making jewel boxes and coffins.

'Bois des Isles'   A mellow early perfume by Chanel, introduced in 1926, which was one of the first aldehyde perfumes. It was created by Ernest Beaux. The central bouquet of jasmine, rose, ylang-ylang and cassie has a top note which is principally bergamot, with suggestions of petitgrain and coriander, and a base note of musk, tonka, vanilla and sandalwood. It was relaunched in 1989.

Bois d'Inde   A tree (*Pimenta acris = Myrica acris*) native to the W. Indies but now cultivated in Sri Lanka, Kenya and W. Africa for a spicy oil distilled from the leaves. The oil is similar to Oil of Bay and is called Oil of Bay or Oil of Myrica. It is used in soaps and perfumes and, as Bay Rum, in hairdressing preparations.

Bois d'Olhio   An essential oil distilled from the wood of the Oleo Vermelho tree (*Myrospermum erythroxylon*), grown in Brazil and Japan.

The fragrance lies between rose, cedar and sandalwood and is used in soaps. The name Oleo Vermelho is also given to the resin of one of the trees producing Balsam of Copaiba and used to treat skin diseases.

Boldea Oil   An essential oil with a cinnamon-like fragrance distilled from the leaves and young wood of a tree (*Peumas boldus* = *Boldea fragrans*), native to Chile. The pea-sized fruits are dried and used locally to make scented necklaces.

Boronia   A small, woody plant (*Boronia megastigma*) native to Australia and Tasmania. A spicy, lemon-like essential oil is extracted from the flowers and leaves and produced as an absolute for use in high-class perfumery, particularly those of chypre and fougere type ('Diorissimo' is an example). Boronia absolute is one of the most expensive of modern perfume materials.

Boswellia bhau-dajiana   *see* Frankincense

                carteri   *see* Frankincense

                frereana   *see* Frankincense

                glabra   *see* Frankincense

                papyrifera   *see* Frankincense

                sacra   *see* Frankincense

                serrata   *see* Frankincense

                thurifera   *see* Frankincense

'Boucheron'   A high quality semi-oriental–floral perfume brought out in 1988 by the well-known firm of Paris jewellers founded by Frederic Boucheron in 1893. It was created by Firmenich perfumers. Top notes of mandarin, bitter orange, galbanum, tagetes, basil and apricot are followed by a floral heart composed of broom, ylang-ylang, tuberose, jasmine, orange flower and narcissus, with sandalwood, ambergris, vanilla, civet and tonka in the base notes. The flacon, in the form of a giant ring with a cabochon-like stopper of sapphire blue, is a Boucheron design produced in association with Joel Desgrippes.

Bouquet   A mixture of different floral notes in a perfume. Also a perfume composed of a combination of perfumes from different Perfume Families. Also a blend of different essences (see Essential Oil and Glycine).

Bourjois   Established in Paris in 1863 by Alexandre-Napoleon Bourjois to manufacture theatrical make-up and face powders. In 1929 the company launched its classic perfume, 'Soir de Paris', and subsequently produced many others, including 'Kobako', 'Mon Parfum' (in a flacon by Baccarat) and 'Clin d'Oeil' (84).

Bouvardia   A name given to a popular early 19th century fragrance resembling jasmine which was made from synthetic materials.

Boy's Love   *see* Southernwood

Box Berry   *see* Gaultheria

Bridewort   *see* Meadowsweet

Broom   The honey-scented flowers of Spanish Broom (*Spartium junceum*), also called Weavers' Broom, which grows in the southern parts of France and Spain, are used to make a perfume ingredient extracted by volatile solvents as a concrete or absolute. The plant, known in France as *Genêt*, is cultivated in Provence for this purpose, having been harvested for use in perfumes by maceration as early as the 16th century. The fragrance of *Genêt* is described as sweet, floral and hay-like. It is used in quality perfumes (e.g. 'Boucheron' and 'Madame Rochas').

Brosse   One of the principal manufacturers of luxury glass and lead crystal flacons for perfumes and toiletries. Verreries Brosse was founded as a glass-makers in 1854, and in 1925 it became the first one to introduce automatic machinery for the mass production of bottles, mostly at that time for the pharmaceutical market. Its factory at Vieux-Rouen-sur-Bresle in Normandy now specializes in making high-quality perfume flacons, those of lead crystal being hand-finished by traditional methods. It operates another factory in the USA. Brosse provided the original flacons for many famous perfumes, such as 'Chanel No. 5' (1921), 'Shalimar' (1925) and 'Joy' (1935), and other distinguished perfumes for which Brosse bottles are currently used include: 'Amouage', 'Arpège', 'Cabochard', 'Coco', 'Giorgio Beverly Hills', 'L'Air du Temps', 'Mon Parfum', 'Obsession', 'Opium', 'Paris' 'Vicky Teal' and '1000'. See Perfume Containers.

'Brut'   A trend-setting men's fougere-type fragrance produced by Fabergé in 1964 for use in men's toiletries. Its main constituent fragrances are lavender and anise in the top note, geranium in the middle note and oak moss and vanilla in the base note. It is now marketed by Elida Gibbs.

Bruyere   An oil produced as an absolute which is extracted from the roots of a very large species of heather, *Erica arborea*; it grows up to 12 feet high and is found throughout the Mediterranean area. It has a mild, balsamic, spicy odour and is used in some chypre-type perfumes and in male fragrances. The roots of this plant, called Briar Roots, are also used for making the bowls of briar pipes.

Bucco   *see* Buchu Leaf Oil

Buchu Leaf Oil   An essential oil steam-distilled from the leaves of three species of the Buchu shrub (*Barosma venusta, B. betulina*, which is also called Bucco, and *B. crenulata*), native to S. Africa. The fragrance is mint and camphor-like, said to be reminiscent of blackcurrants, and very intense, so that only minute amounts are used.

Bulnesia sarmienti   *see* Champaca Wood Oil

Bulungu Resin   A resin extracted from the bark of a tree *Canarium edule*, which grows in tropical Africa. It is used locally as a perfume.

Burning Bush   *see* Dittany

Burning Oil An aromatic oil which is poured into a small bowl or ring-shaped trough and placed on a heat source such as an electric light bulb, the heat causing it to emit its aroma. Burning oil for perfuming a room is now produced by many fragrance firms. In earlier times such oil was placed in a Perfume Burner (French: *Brûle-parfum*), a bowl-shaped receptacle on a stand, heated by a candle or spirit burner and often very ornamental. See also Pastille Burner.

Bursera delpechiana *see* Linaloe

      gummifera *see* Tacamahac

Bush Apple A tree of tropical W. Africa (*Heinsia pulchella*). Its leaves are scented and are used locally to make a perfume.

But tree *see* Mattipaul

Butterfly Lily *see* Garland Flower

Buttons *see* Tansy

'Byzance' A semi-oriental–floral perfume created for Rochas in 1987 by Nicolas Mamounas. It is named after the Empire of Byzantium, from the theme of a fusing of East and West in a rich combination, and has some 200 ingredients. Fresh top notes, notably citrus and cardamom, lead into a spicy floral heart with rose, jasmine, tuberose and iris, underlined by a base containing sandalwood, musk and vanilla. The bottle is designed to reflect the colouring of Byzantine mozaics and the rounded shapes of its architecture.

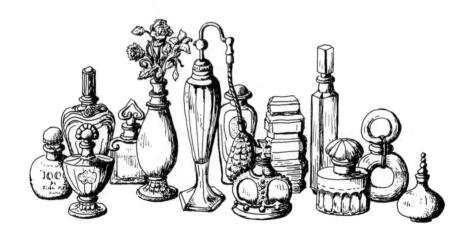

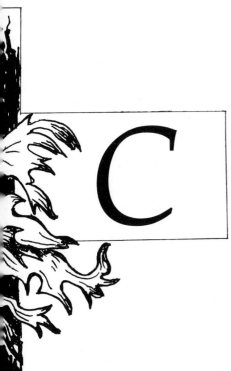

C

'Cabochard'   A trend-setting aldehydic chypre perfume created for Grès by IFF in 1958. Clary sage, tarragon and galbanum dominate the top notes, yielding to a floral bouquet in the middle notes based on jasmine, rose and ylang-ylang. The base notes include oak moss, sandalwood, vetivert and patchouli. The flacon, featuring a tied bow, is by Brosse.

Cabreu Oil   Also called Cabreuva Oil. A woody, rose-scented essential oil distilled from wood of species of the Cabreu tree (especially *Myrocarpus fastigiatus* and *M. frondosus*), which grows in Brazil, Argentina and Paraguay. It is used in low-cost perfumery. The trunk of *M. fastigiatus* also yields a balsam similar to Balsam of Peru.

Cacharel   A Paris fashion house instituted by Jean Bousquet in 1962 and now owned by L'Oréal. The company is named after a small wild duck found in Bousquet's native Provence. In 1979 Bousquet launched the wide-selling perfume 'Anais-Anais', followed by 'Cacharel pour l'Homme' in 1981 and 'Lou-Lou' in 1987.

Cacao   Also called Cocoa. An essential oil obtained by expression from the fruit and seeds of the Cacao (or Cocoa) tree (*Theobroma cacao*). The tree is native to central America but cultivated widely as the source of chocolate. (Cocoa was first introduced into Europe by Columbus, who found it being used by Aztecs as a beverage which they sweetened with Vanilla.) An absolute is prepared from the oil, mainly using Venezuelan cacao, for use in perfumery.

Cade, Oil of   *see* Cedar

Cajuput   Also written Cajaput and Cajeput. An essential oil which is steam-distilled from the leaves and twigs of the Cajuput tree, also called the Swamp Ti tree, Swamp Tea tree and White Ti tree (*Melaleuca leucadendron*), which grows in S.E. Asia from Malaysia to Australia. The name derives from Malaysian for 'white tree'. The oil has a penetrating odour of camphor and rosemary and is used in aromatherapy and for other medicinal purposes as well as in perfumery. It is very similar to Niaouli oil (from the Niaouli tree *M. viridiflora*, found in Indonesia), also sometimes called Gomenol, which has wider medical uses, and to Ti-tree Oil (or Tea-tree Oil), which has a eucalyptus-like odour and is used considerably in medicine and aromatherapy.

Calamint   Also called Mountain Mint, Mountain Balm, Bill Mountain and Basil Thyme. A bushy herb (*Calamintha officinalis* = *Satureja calamintha*), which grows up to 1 foot high and is found widely in Europe and Asia Minor. The name derives from the Greek meaning 'a good mint' (the Greeks believed it would drive away serpents). In Elizabethan times it was a remedy for 'sorrowfulness' and 'infirmities of the heart'. The essential oil, distilled from the leaves, has a minty, camphorous odour. The dried leaves, once infused as a tea, are used in pomander pastes, sachets and pot pourri. A sub-species, Lesser Calamine (*C. nepeta*), with a stronger fragrance resembling Pennyroyal, is used similarly.

Calamus   Also called Sweet Flag, Sweet Rush, Sweet Sedge, Myrtle Sedge, Myrtle Grass, Sweet Reed, Cinnamon Sedge and Sweet Root. A reed-like plant (*Acorus calamus*) which grows widely in Europe and elsewhere on the edges of lakes and streams. It was introduced into Europe from Asia Minor in the 16th century and may be of Indian origin. The word 'calamus' is from the Greek for a 'reed'. Calamus Oil is steam-distilled from the rhizomes and used in medicines and perfumes, and the dried rhizomes are used in sachets and pot pourri. Calamus was once used as a strewing herb in English churches. Its fragrance is earthy and slightly sweet and it is used particularly in spicy and herbal perfumes.

Calamus was a well known perfume material in ancient times, appearing in a fragrant oil in early Egypt and listed by Theophrastus as one of the principal fragrant plants of Greek perfumes. It is referred to in several places in the Bible, being an ingredient in the holy anointing oil of the Jews (see Bible Perfumes). Ancient South Arabian incense altars have been excavated inscribed with the name (as 'Qlm'), showing that it was one of the incenses used there. However, the Calamus of the ancients (sometimes called Sweet Calamus and Sweet Cane) was a different plant to that known as Calamus today. It grew, according to the classical authors, in Arabia, the best coming from north Arabia, and Syria as well as in Egypt, and was probably the plant now known as Lemon Grass.

Calamus draco   *see* Dragon's Blood

'Calandre'   A trend-setting green aldehydic perfume introduced by Paco Rabanne in 1968 and now regarded as a classic. It was created for Paco Rabanne by Roure perfumers. Floral middle notes, chiefly ylang-ylang, jasmine and geranium, take over from a first impression of green leaves provided by aldehydes with lemon and bergamot. The base notes are balsamic, with vetivert, cedar, amber and musk. Since 1980 this perfume has been sold in a Baccarat flacon and in bottles designed by Pierre Dinand.

'Calèche'   A floral–chypre aldehydic perfume created by Guy Robert and first marketed by Hermès in 1961. The heart, a combination mainly of jasmine, rose, orange flower, orris, gardenia and ylang-ylang, has fresh aldehydic top notes with touches of bergamot, lemon, neroli and cypress, and woody base notes mostly deriving from vetivert, oak moss and cedarwood. The flacon is designed by Jean Rene Guerrand Hermès and Joel Desgrippes.

Calendula Oil   *see* Marigold

'California'   A wide-selling floral–woody perfume launched in 1990 by Max Factor, for whom it was created by Firmenich perfumers. Floral top notes, with rose, muguet, geranium and bergamot, lead into a heart which includes sandalwood and vetivert, supported by carnation and orange flower. The base contains vanilla, amber, oak moss and musk.

Callitris quadrivalvis   *see* Sandarac
            rhomboides   *see* Oyster Oil

Calophyllum brasiliense   *see* Sandal Oil

Calvin Klein   The fragrance company of the Calvin Klein fashion organization launched its first perfume, 'Calvin Klein' in 1978. This has been followed by the immediately successful 'Obsession' (85), 'Eternity' (89) and 'Escape' (91), together with two men's fragrances, 'Calvin' (81) and 'Obsession for Men' (88). In 1990 the company was acquired by Unilever.

Calycanthus   An essential oil used in quality perfumery (e.g. 'Jardins de Bagatelles' and 'Nahema') which is distilled from the flowers of a species of Calycanthus tree (*Calycanthus occidentalis* – also the smaller *C. floridus*) also known as Carolina Allspice and the Sweet-scented Shrub. The tree grows to about 8 feet high and is native to N. America. The oil provides a fruity odour reminiscent of ripe apples. The bark of

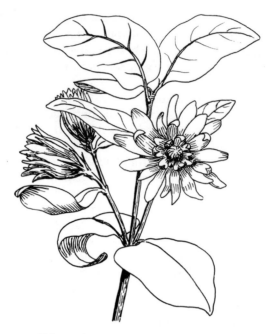

Calycanthus (*Calycanthus occidentalis*).

this tree has a fragrance like cinnamon, for which it is sometimes used as a substitute, hence the name Allspice (but not to be confused with pimento).

Camel Grass Oil   *see* Lemon Grass Oil

Camel Rush   *see* Lemon Grass Oil

Camellia   A shrub (*Camellia japonica*) growing to about 15 feet high and native to China and Japan. An essential oil, composed mainly of eugenol, is distilled from the leaves and used in quality perfumery (e.g. 'Arpège').

Camellia sinensis   *see* Tea Absolute

Camomile   Also spelled Chamomile and Chamomille. There are two sorts:

1. True Camomile (*Anthemis nobilis*), also called Roman Camomile, English Camomile, Common Camomile and Manzanilla, a small low-growing herb with a scent of apples (the name Camomile derives from the Greek 'ground apple' and Manzanilla means in Spanish 'little apple'). The plant is native to the Mediterranean area and also found growing in Iran, India and elsewhere. The apple-scented oil, usually called Oil of Roman Camomile, is steam-distilled from the flowers and used in liqueurs as well as in perfumes (examples of its use in modern quality perfumery are 'Giorgio

Beverly Hills', 'Ivoire' and 'Xia-Xiang'). The dried flowers are used in sachets and pot pourri. This plant has been grown for centuries in English gardens for its use as a general domestic medicine; in the Middle Ages it was used as a strewing herb. The ancient Egyptians used it to cure ague.

2. German Camomile (*Matricaria chamomilla*), also called Wild Camomile, Blue Camomile and Scented Mayweed, a small herb growing from Europe to Afghanistan and now cultivated widely, particularly in Egypt, Hungary and Germany, for its essential oil (Oil of German Camomile) obtained from the flowers. This oil, which is steam-distilled, has a very sweet apple fragrance and is used in perfumes and for scenting shampoos, liqueurs and tobaccos. A similar oil is derived from a closely related plant, *Matricaria discoidea*, also cultivated widely.

Campaif   *see* Balsam of Copaiba
Campernella   *see* Jonquil
Camphire   *see* Cyprinum and Camphor
Camphor   A highly aromatic white crystalline substance obtained from the balsamic crude oil found in the wood of the Camphor tree (*Cinnamonum camphora* = *Camphora officinarum* = *Laurus camphora*), also called Camphire (but see under Cyprinum), Gum Camphor and Laurel Camphor. The tree, which is closely related to cinnamon, is native to China and Japan and is now cultivated for this product in many countries, including India, Sri Lanka, Egypt, Taiwan, Madagascar, the Canary Islands, USA (California) and Argentina. The oil is distilled from the wood and allowed to settle until the camphor crystals emerge, the liquor then being redistilled to obtain other products, most importantly safrole, used for manufacturing heliotropin for the perfume trade. Camphor was once an important material in the manufacture of celluloid. A single tree can yield 3 tons of camphor. A synthetic camphor is made from pinene.

Camphor was one of the most popular of all perfume ingredients in the early Arab world. It features in more than a quarter of al-Kindi's perfume recipes and in many other medieval Arab works, including the *Arabian Nights Tales*. In Europe it was once a popular ingredient in pomanders, because it was thought to prevent infectious diseases.

The dry crystals are sometimes used in sachets and pot pourri.

A similar balsam is obtained from the Borneo Camphor tree (*Dryobalanops camphora* = *D. aromatica*), from which is produced East Indian Oil of Camphor, much prized by the Chinese for scenting soaps but little used in the West. This balsam is also used for manufacturing Borneol, occasionally used in soap perfumery. The balsam is also used locally as an incense.

Camphor Root   *see* Maudlin

Camphoraceous   A term used in perfumery to describe a fresh, clean medical fragrance. See Perfume Notes.

Canada Balsam   A balsam also called Canada Turpentine obtained from the Balsam Fir (*Abies balsamea*) and the Hemlock Spruce (*Abies canadensis*), which are found in N. America. It is used in perfumery and as a fixative in soaps.

Canadian Snake-root   A herb (*Asarum canadense*), also called American Wild Ginger and Coltsfoot, up to 12 inches high which grows in the East of N. America. A spicy and ginger-like essential oil is distilled from the roots and used in perfumery.

Cananga latifolia   *see* Ylang-Ylang
         odorata   *see* Ylang-Ylang

Cananga Oil   *see* Ylang-Ylang

Canarium commune   *see* Elemi
           edule   *see* Bulungu Resin
           luzonicum   see Elemi

Candleberry Myrtle   *see* Bog Myrtle

Candleberry Wax   A wax obtained from the berries of the Candleberry tree (*Myrica cerifera*), also called Wax Myrtle, of eastern USA. It was once used to make candles with a pleasing aroma.

Candle Plant   *see* Dittany

Candles, Scented   Scented candles have been made since the days of antiquity from various waxes with added perfume materials. The early Arabs were fond of candles perfumed with camphor. Some waxes obtained from plants burn with a pleasing natural aroma, notably Carnauba, Candleberry and Sweet Gale, which became popular materials for candlemakers during the 19th century.

Candlewood tree   *see* Sandalwood

Candlestick Bottle   *see* Tulip Bottle

Candy Rosemary   *see* Stoechas

Canella   Also called White Cinnamon, Wild Cinnamon, White Wood and Bahama White Wood. The fragrant bark of a tree (*Canella alba* = *C. winterama*), which grows up to 50 feet high and is native to Florida and the West Indies, though now cultivated more widely. The bark, first brought to Britain in about 1600, was initially thought by Spaniards in America to be a species of cinnamon. It has a spicy odour between cinnamon and clove and is exported in quills which can be powdered or broken up for use in sachets and pot pourri.

'Canoe'   An early fougere perfume for women, brought out by Dana in 1935 and the trend-setter for many masculine fragrances which have followed. Created by Jean Carles of Roure, the top note was principally lavender, with a floral, woody heart containing geranium, clove-pink, cedarwood and patchouli, and a sweet, powdery fougere effect obtained mainly from oak moss, tonka, musk, vanilla and heliotrope in the base note.

Capalaga   *see* Cardamom

Cape Jasmine   *see* Gardenia

Capon's Tail   *see* Valerian

'Capucci de Capucci'   A floral–oriental perfume launched in 1987 by Parfums Capucci, the perfume wing of Roberto Capucci's couture business. It was created for him by Firmenich perfumers. Hyacinth, lily of the valley, jasmine and rose in the top notes unfold to a heart containing ylang-ylang and iris, with nuances of patchouli, oak moss, sandalwood and vetivert. The sweet, powdery base includes frankincense, musk, amber and opoponax.

Caraway   A herb (*Carum carvi = Apium carvi = Seseli carvi*) growing up to 2 feet high, native to an area from the Mediterranean to the Himalayas, and cultivated in Europe and Morocco. An essential oil with a very intense, spicy odour (Oil of Caraway, also called Oleo Carvi) is steam-distilled from the fruits and leaves, mainly for flavouring but occasionally for use in perfumery (it appears, for example, in 'Tsar'). Some 6 lb of seeds will provide about 4 oz of oil. The seeds are used in sachets and pot pourri.

Caraway was well known in classical times. Pliny states that it was named after Caria, in Asia Minor, where it was first found. In early times it was believed that anything containing it would be safe from theft, also that it would prevent lovers from becoming fickle and pigeons from straying. Dioscorides advised that the oil was good for 'pale-faced girls'.

Cardamom   Also called Cardamon, Amomum, Capalanga and Ilachi. A tall, reed-like perennial shrub (*Elletaria cardamomum*) native to S. India and Sri Lanka, the seeds of which are valued as a flavouring, used in incenses and steam-distilled to provide an essential oil. The oil has a spicy, eucalyptus-like odour and is used in many perfumes, including quality ones (e.g. 'Diva' and 'Byzance') and eau de colognes. There are different varieties of cardamom from different species of the plant. It is cultivated for the seeds in S. India and Sri Lanka and also in Malaysia and Guatemala.

Cardamom was used in some of the unguents of ancient Egypt and was listed by Theophrastus in about 300 BC as one of the principal fragrant plants used in Greek perfumes. The Romans used it on a substantial scale, particularly as a flavouring, and Dioscorides mentioned its medicinal uses. It was among the raw materials of the early Arab perfume makers.

For Greater Cardamom see Grains of Paradise.

Cariophyllorum   *see* Clove Oil

Cardin   Pierre Cardin (b. 1922) opened his business in Paris selling theatrical masks and costumes after first working for Dior. By 1957 he had become a leading fashion designer, later extending his interests to include the designing of furniture, home accessories and cars. In 1977 he opened the first of a series of boutiques under the name 'Maxims de Paris', later acquiring the famous restaurant of that name. Cardin fragrances include 'Cardin' (1976), 'Choc' (81), 'Paradoxe' (83) and 'Maxims de Paris' (85), together with a fragrance for men 'Pour Homme'.

Carles, Jean One of Roure-Bertrand's most prominent perfumers and the founder of their School of Perfumery in Grasse. Known as 'the perfumer of Grasse' and, after insuring his nose for $1 million, as 'Mr Nose'. His creations included 'Shocking' and 'Canoe'.

Carmelite Water A toilet water first prepared in about 1380 by the nuns of the Carmelite abbey of St Just for the ageing King Charles V of France, which became popular throughout Europe. It was made of balm, lemon peel, orange flower water and various spices distilled in alcohol. (See Appendix B, recipes nos 53 and 54.)

Carnation An essential oil, often called Carnation, is obtained from the Carnation, or Clove-pink flower (see under Clove-pink). The name carnation is also used for compound perfumes with a carnation-like fragrance made from synthetics, mostly derived from eugenol.

Carnauba Wax A wax obtained from the leaves of the Carnauba Palm, or Wax Palm (*Copernicia cerifera*) of Brazil. During the 19th century it was imported into Europe on a substantial scale to be made into candles, which burned with the aroma of new-mown hay.

'Carnet du Bal' A classic oriental-type perfume launched in 1937 by Révillon whose first perfume it was. It was created by Maurice Shaller. Citrusy top notes introduce a floral heart built on cyclamen, with rose, jasmine, lily and ylang-ylang, and underlined by a warm, woody base note containing patchouli, amber, vanilla, civet and musk.

'Carolina Herrera' A perfume first launched in the USA in 1988 by Puig in conjunction with and to the formula of Carolina Herrera, the Venezuelan-born New York fashion designer and socialite. It is a 'linear fragrance' (i.e. without the classical three-layer structure) containing jasmine, tuberose and nard supported by amber, moss and sandalwood.

Caron Parfums Caron was established in Paris in 1904 by a perfumer, Ernest Daltroff. In 1910 he was joined by Félicie Bergaud, a fashion designer. In 1911 they launched 'Narcisse Noir', a world-wide success, to be followed, among others, by 'Tabac Blond' (19), 'Nuit de Noël' (22), 'Bellodgia' (27), 'Fleurs de Rocaille' (33), 'Fête des Roses' (36) (which appeared in a unique Baccarat gilded crystal bottle designed by Félicie Bergaud and now a rare collector's piece) and 'Rose de Noël' (in a flacon by Lalique also designed by Madame Bergaud). A men's fragrance, 'Pour un Homme' was issued in 1934. Daltroff died in 1940, and the company was then acquired by 'Révillon Fragrances launched subsequently include 'Infini' (70), 'Nocturnes' (81), 'Le 3e Homme de Caron' (85) and 'Parfum Sacré (90)'. The company now belongs to the Fine Fragrances and Cosmetics Group (see also Mary Chess).

Carophylli   *see* Clove Oil.

Carrot Oil   Also called Carrot Seed Oil. An oil with an orris-like fragrance steam-distilled from the seeds of the carrot plant (*Daucus carota*) and used in flavouring and liqueurs as well as in fougere and chypre-type perfumes. The carrot plant originated in Afghanistan but is now cultivated widely in temperate regions. The oil is produced in France, Hungary, Yugoslavia and the USSR. The carrot is mentioned in Greek literature from as early as 500 BC.

Carthamus lanatus   *see* Safflower
          tinctorius   *see* Safflower

Carum carvi   *see* Caraway
          copticum   *see* Ajowan

Carven   Opened in 1944 by Madame Carven as a fashion house catering for the 'petite', and now producing a variety of fashion wear and accessories, the house of Carven produced its classic perfume 'Ma Griffe' in 1944. This has since been followed by, among others, 'Robe d'un Soir' (47), 'Madame de Carven' (79), 'Guirlandes' (82) 'Intrigue' (86) and a men's fragrance 'Vetiver' (57).

Carvone   A chemical found in many essential oils which is used to provide perfumes with a clean, sweet, spearmint-like odour.

Caryophyllata   *see* Avens

Caryophyllene   A component of Clove Oil. Also the residue of Clove Oil after eugenol has been removed from it, which is sometimes used to perfume soaps. It is also found in many other essential oils.

Cascarilla   Also called Aromatic Quinquina, Bahama Cascarilla, Sweetwood Bark, Sweet Bark, Elutharia, False Quinquina. A fragrant bark from a small bush-like tree (*Croton eleutaria*) found in the Bahamas, particularly on the island of Eleutharia, and cultivated in Florida. The bark has a slight odour of musk. Introduced into Europe by the 17th century, it is used as an incense and in sachets and pot pourri, and an essential oil is distilled from the bark with a cinnamon-like fragrance and occasionally used in quality perfumes (e.g. 'Coco' and 'Oscar de la Renta').

Cassia   Also called Cassia Bark, Cassia Lignea, Chinese Cinnamon, Bastard Cinnamon and Canton Cassia. The fragrant bark of a small tree (*Cinnamomum cassia = C. obtusifolium* var. *cassia*) growing up to 30 feet high in S.E. China. The tree is cultivated in Japan, Sri Lanka, Indonesia, Mexico and S. America, where it is usually kept to about 10 feet high. The bark closely resembles cinnamon but is thicker and of a less delicate flavour. An essential oil (Oil of Cassia, but also called Oil of

Cinnamon), mainly consisting of cinnamic aldehyde, is obtained by steam-distillation of the buds, twigs and foliage and is used for flavouring and as a blender in soaps as well as in perfumery; it is also produced synthetically (see Perfume Creation); examples of its use in quality perfumes are 'Nina' and 'Lou-Lou'. About 80 lb of bark yield $2\frac{1}{2}$ oz of oil. The dried buds, known as Chinese Cassia Buds, have been used in Europe as a spice since the Middle Ages; since Victorian times both buds and bark have been used in sachets and pot pourri.

Cassia and cinnamon were among the most popular perfume materials of ancient times but were often confused in the classical texts. They are referred to in ancient Egyptian unguent recipes, and Theophrastus quotes them as ingredients of Megalaeion perfume. Their use in both Greece and Rome is well testified. The Bible contains a number of references to them and both were constituents of the Jewish holy anointing oil. But scholars do not believe that either product came in those times from the plants which provide them today. Herodotus said they both came from Arabia. Other classical authors described plants quite different from those of today, and a trade which, in around 300 BC, brought these materials to a S. Arabian Red Sea port on rafts from the nearby African coasts. It is now thought probable that the cinnamon of ancient times was a bark later called Qirfah in Arabic, which the Arabs of a later period regarded as an inferior sort of cinnamon coming from S. Arabia and Africa; but the tree which provided it has not yet been identified. Similarly the cassia of ancient times may have been a bark known to later Arabs as Salīkha, which also has not yet been identified further. Al-Kindi listed both these materials in his perfume recipes of the 8th century AD. By the 1st century AD it would appear that both Qirfah and Salīkha were beginning to be replaced by the superior forms of cinnamon and cassia available from the Far East which we know today and which assumed the names of the earlier materials. See also Cinnamon.

Cassidony   *see* Stoechas

Cassie Ancienne   An essential oil, also known as Cassie Farnese (and sometimes, incorrectly, as Cassia Oil), extracted from the flowers of the Sweet Acacia (*Acacia farnesiana*), also called Popinac, Opoponax (but see the entry under that name), and Huisache, a shrub-like tree growing to about 10 feet high in tropical and northern Africa. First cultivated for perfumery in Rome towards the end of the 16th century, the tree is now grown in the south of France, Lebanon and elsewhere for this oil, which is produced as a concrete or absolute. It appears in many modern perfumes (e.g. 'Bois des Isles' and 'Roma') and is used in fortifying a violet fragrance. It should not be confused with cassis or cassia.

Cassie Romaine   An oil extracted from the flowers of the Cavenia Acacia tree (*Acacia cavenia*), a small tree native to Chile which is cultivated for this perfume oil in the south of France.

Cassis   *see* Blackcurrant Bud Oil

Cassolette   Also known as Printanier. A small box made of ivory, silver or gold, with a perforated lid, into which was placed a perfumed paste. Cassolettes were popular in Europe, including Britain, during the 16th century. (See also under Pomander and Vinaigrette. See also Appendix B, recipes no. 30.)

Castanha de Cotia   *see* Sandal Oil

Castor Oil   Obtained from the seeds in the bean of the Castor Oil bush, also called Castor Bean and Palma Christi (*Ricinus communis*), native to India but now grown widely, including tropical areas of India, Brazil, China and Mexico. The oil is usually extracted by pressing. In the 5th century BC, Herodotus knew of it as *kiki*; at that time it was used by the ancient Egyptians as a base oil for perfumes, to absorb the scents of other plants (see Balanos). Early Arab perfumers soaked the wood in other fragrances to produce a solid perfume base. The oil is still used in a processed form in modern perfumery. Throughout history the oil has also been used as a lamp oil.

Castoreum   Also called Beaver Oil, Beaver Musk and Castor (not to be confused with Castor Oil). Castoreum is a secretion from the preputial follicles of both male and female Castor Beavers (*Castor fiber*), which is found in Canada and the USSR (CIS). As with musk and civet, it has a strong, disagreeable odour until it is considerably diluted, when it becomes highly fragrant; in early times the usual dilutant was wine. Castoreum was known to the early Arab perfume makers (9th century AD). It was once used in pomanders, but, being scarce and costly, not on any scale. In the 19th century it went out of fashion, but it is now used a lot in modern quality perfumes (e.g. 'Intimate' 'Oscar de la Renta' and 'Ysatis'). It is an excellent fixative and gives perfumes a spicy or oriental note. Ammoniacum, the fragrance of which is somewhat similar, is sometimes used as a substitute.

Cavenia Acacia   *see* Cassie Romaine

Cayenne Linaloe Oil   *see* Linaloe and Sandalwood

Cedar   A number of Cedar trees of the botanical species *Juniperus*, *Cedrus* and *Thuja* provide materials used in perfumery.

1. Red Cedar (*Juniperus virginiana*) native to N. America, provides Red Cedarwood Oil, also called Cedarwood Oil, which is the cedar oil mostly used today. This oil, which has to be employed very sparingly, is found among the main ingredients of some 14% of all modern quality perfumes (e.g. 'Blue Grass', 'Caleche', 'Calendre' and 'Ma Liberté') and in soaps; it is a good fixative and is a principal constituent of Extract of White Rose. N. American Indians burned the leaves as an incense.

2. Indian Juniper, also called Pencil Cedar and Appura (*Juniperus macropoda*), found in N. India and Malaysia, provides a Cedar Oil distilled from its sawdust and shavings.
3. Prickly Cedar (*Juniperus oxycedrus*), also called Prickly Juniper, yields Oil of Cade, distilled from the wood and nowadays used medicinally. It has a leathery, tar-like odour and was used by the early Arab perfume makers in many of their perfume recipes.
4. Cedar of Lebanon, also called Himalayan Cedar (*Cedrus libani*) provides a cedar oil sometimes used in perfumery.
5. Atlas Cedar, also called Atlantic Cedar (*Cedrus atlanticus*), which grows in N. Africa, provides an essential oil with a balsamic odour.
6. White Cedar (*Thuja occidentalis*) provides Arbor Vitae Oil.

In early times the twigs and roots of cedar were much used in incenses. The ancient Egyptians made coffins from the wood because of its durability and fragrance, and also used cedar oil in embalming. Dried cedarwood fragments are still used in sachets and pot pourri.

Cedar Leaf Oil   *see* Arbor Vitae Oil

Cedarwood Oil   *see* Cedar

Cedrat Oil   A name given to a mixture of Citrus oils.

Cedro Oil   *see* Lemon Oil

Cedronella tryphylla   *see* Balm of Gilead

Cedrus atlanticus   *see* Cedar
         libani   *see* Cedar

Celery Seed Oil   An oil obtained by steam distillation from the crushed seeds of the Wild Celery plant (*Apium graveolens*), also called Smallage, native to the Levant and southern Europe but cultivated widely. It has a spicy, sweet, celery-like odour and is used in creating perfumes with a sweet-pea or tuberose fragrance.

Celestial Water   A 16th century Italian concoction (originally known in the Latin as *aqua coloestis*) distilled from numerous fragrant herbs and flowers and used to purify the air and ward off disease. Its contents included calamus, cinnamon, citron peel, gith, sandalwood and zedoary.

Celtic Spikenard   *see* Spikenard

Cerutti   *see* Nino Cerutti

'C'Est La Vie'   A quality floral–amber perfume launched in 1990 which was created by Roure perfumers for the well-known Paris couturier house of Christian Lacroix (now a part of the Louis Vuitton–Moet–Hennessy group – see also Dior and Givenchy). The perfume, which is a linear fragrance, contains an unusual floral bouquet of seringa, orange blossom and osmanthus, underlined by sandalwood, vanilla and tonka bean. The bottle is shaped to suggest a heart, with a coral branch cap.

Ceylon Oak   *see* Macassar Oil

Ceylon Oil   *see* Citronella

'**Chamade**'   A floral–woody aldehyde perfume created by Jean-Paul Guerlain and brought out by Guerlain in 1970. In French the name means both 'wild heart beats' and 'the drum beats of surrender'. The top notes are green, principally from galbanum, with a floral heart which is based on rose, jasmine, muguet and lilac, made spicy by a touch of clove, and with sweet balsamic base notes founded mainly on benzoin, with vetivert, sandalwood, vanilla, balsam of Peru and balsam of Tolu. The flacon, heart-shaped with a spear-head stopper, is by Robert Granai.

Chamaerhodendron ferrugineum   *see* Alpine Rose

Chamomile   *see* Camomile

Champac   Also called Champaca Oil. A sweet-scented essential oil distilled from the flowers of species of the Champaca tree (*Michelia champaca, M. longifolia* and *M. montana*) growing in Nepal, India, Malaysia, Indonesia and the Philippines. The oil is usually produced as a concrete or absolute and is one of the principal attars used in perfumery, but is scarce and therefore expensive. In Thailand it is also used as a body oil and for scenting the hair. In India the flowers are used by women as a hair decoration.

An oil with the odour of Basil is also distilled from the leaves of this tree and is known as Champaca Leaf Oil.

Champaca Wood Oil   Also called Oil of Guaiac Wood. An essential oil with a soft rose-like fragrance steam-distilled from the wood of the Pao Santa tree (*Bulnesia sarmienti*), also called Palo Balsamo and Paraguay Lignum, found in Argentina and Paraguay. The oil is mostly used in soaps and household products, particularly to conceal the smell of harsh-scented aromatics. In Bulgaria it is sometimes used to adulterate rose oil. It also appears occasionally in high-class perfumes (e.g. 'Ricci Club').

Chanel   'Coco' Chanel (1883–1971), brought up in an orphanage, opened her first boutique in 1914. She quickly established herself as the leading figure in the move from the stiff fashion styles of the 19th century, combining her designs for clothes with complementary accessories to produce, in the 1920s, the 'Total Look', and launching, in 1924, the fashion of 'the little black dress'. By 1935 Mademoiselle Chanel employed some 4000 seamstresses and was a leading Parisian socialite and arts patron who could refuse an offer of marriage from the fabulously wealthy Duke of Westminster with the statement: 'There are many Duchesses but only one Chanel'. With the outbreak of war she closed her business for 15 years.

In 1921, having encouraged a perfume chemist Ernest Beaux with his experiments in the use of aldehydes, she became the first couturier to produce a perfume, 'Chanel No. 5', which met with resounding success. Other perfumes followed, including 'Chanel No. 22' (1921), 'Gardenia'

(25), 'Bois des Îles' (26), 'Cuir de Russie' (27) 'Sycamore' and 'Une Idée' (30), 'Ivoire' and 'Jasmine' (32), leading to 'Chanel No. 19' (70), 'Cristalle' (74), and 'Coco' (84), together with three men's fragrances – 'Pour Monsieur' (70), 'Antaeus' (82) and 'Boir Noir' (88), revised as 'L'Égoïste' (90). The company's 'nose' is at present Jacques Polge. The main factory is on the outskirts of Paris. All Chanel perfumes appear in a signature Chanel bottle, which follows the pattern of the original Sem bottle for Chanel No. 5 – plain and rectangular, with a stopper cut like an emerald.

'Chanel No. 5' One of the most famous perfumes ever made, setting a major new trend as the first of the aldehyde perfumes. It was created for Chanel by Ernest Beaux and first marketed in 1921. The aldehydic top note, fresh and floral, with ylang-ylang and neroli, gives way to a floral heart, mainly of blended jasmine and rose, and to woody base notes dominated by sandalwood and vetiver, but the perfume contains altogether about 130 ingredients. The bottle, designed by Sem, a French artist, was chosen by Mademoiselle Chanel to reflect the style of elegant simplicity found in her fashions. In 1986 the Eau de Toilette of this perfume was enriched in order to take advantage of the wider range of elements now available to perfumiers.

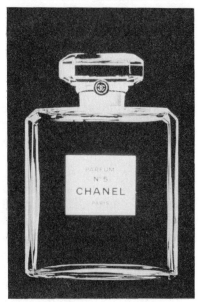

'Chanel No. 5'

'Chanel No. 19' A trend-setting floral–woody–chypre perfume created by Henri Robert and introduced by Chanel in 1970. It was called 'No. 19' because Coco Chanel was born on 19 August. The green top note is mainly obtained by galbanum, with neroli and orris predominating in the middle notes and cedar, oak moss and leathery notes in the base. The bottle is a Chanel design.

'Chanel No. 22' An intensely floral perfume created for Chanel by Ernest Beaux in 1926. A top note of orange blossom and citrus with a fruity touch from peach, heralds a floral bouquet in the heart, which is predominantly clove-pink, supported by rose, orchid, ylang ylang, iris and tuberose. The base includes amber, sandalwood, vetivert, frankincense, vanilla, tonka and musk.

'Chant D'Aromes'   An aldehydic floral perfume launched by Guerlain in 1962. It is said to have taken 7 years to compose. An aldehyde top note of mirabelle and gardenia heads a middle note containing jasmine, honeysuckle, clove buds and ylang-ylang, with a lower note which includes benzoin, musk, frankincense, vetivert, tree moss and heliotrope.

'Chantilly'   A classic quality perfume of the oriental family brought out by Houbigant in 1941; the creation of Houbigant's perfumer Marcel Billot, it is named after Chantilly lace, used in the bridal veils of royalty. Fresh top notes, which include orange blossom with spicy nuances, lead into a middle note in which rose and jasmine are joined by mossy, woody and chypre scents, with a base note containing sandalwood, vetivert, patchouli and amber.

Charabot, Eugene   French author of 'Les Parfums Artificiels', published in 1900, the first book devoted to the subject of synthetic perfumes.

Charles of the Ritz   Formed in the USA in 1934 by a French-born barber, Charles Jundt, who ran a fashionable salon at the Ritz Carlton Hotel in New York. The company initially sold skin care preparations and cosmetics, entering the fragrance market with 'Ritz' (1972), followed by 'Charivari', 'Enjoli' and 'Charles of the Ritz' (1978) and 'Senchal' (81). The company is now associated with the perfume houses of Gianni Versace (see 'V'E') and Claude Montana (see 'Montana') and forms a part of the Revlon group.

The quality perfume 'Charles of the Ritz' is a 'floriental' fragrance (see Perfume Families). Its top note, predominantly geranium, basil and tangerine, leads into a heart containing rose, jasmine, carnation and ylang-ylang, with a base note which includes amber, orange flower, sandalwood, tuberose, frankincense, vetivert and musk.

'Charlie'   A light floral–fresh type perfume by Revlon dating from 1973. It was created by Florasynth perfumers. A green top note, predominantly citrus, overlies a middle note of jasmine and other flower fragrances, with cedarwood the principal of the base notes.

Chassis   *see* Enfleurage

Chatelaine Bottle   A style of perfume bottle, popular in the late 19th and early 20th centuries, made to hang from a chatelaine (a set of fine chains attached to a belt to carry keys, scissors, etc.) or from a chain necklace.

Cheiranthus cheiri   *see* Wallflower

Chenopodium ambroisiodes   *see* Ambroisia

Cherry, Austrian   *see* Magalep

Cherry, Perfumed   *see* Magalep

Cherry Pie   *see* Heliotrope

Cherry, St Lucie   *see* Magalep

Chervil, Sweet   *see* Sweet Cicely

Chian Turpentine   *see* Terebinth Oil

Chimonanthus   A winter-flowering shrub, growing up to 10 feet high, native to China and Japan (*Chimonanthus fragrans* = *C. praecox*). A concrete is extraced from the flowers, which have a fragrance suggestive of jasmine, orange peel and jonquil.

China Root   *see* Galingale

Chinese Anise   *see* Star Anise

Chinese Cinnamon   *see* Cassia

Chio Turpentine   *see* Terebinth Oil

'Chique'   A floral chypre perfume first produced by Yardley in 1976 and relaunched in 1986. Aldehydic and spicy top notes lead into a heart which is predominantly rose and jasmine, blending with a base note mostly of patchouli, vetivert, sandalwood and oak moss.

'Chloe'   A sweet floral perfume by Lagerfeld first marketed in 1975. It was created by perfumers of IFF. Containing 178 ingredients, its principal middle note is tuberose, supported by other flower fragrances including jonquil, jasmine, rose, lily of the valley, iris and ylang-ylang. Heading this are fruity green top notes, while the main base note is musk. The spherical bottle, with a sculptured stopper representing a

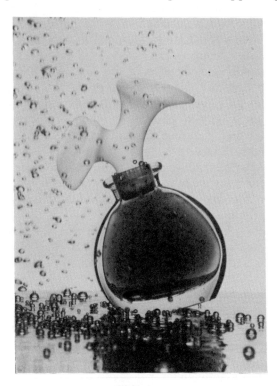

'Chloe'.

lily, was designed by Joe Messina and has won a Fragrance Foundation award.

Choisya ternata   *see* Orange Blossom

Chrysanthemum balsamita   see Costmary

perthenium   *see* Feverfew Chrysanthemum

Chua Oil   An oil used in perfumery which is distilled from Dammar Fat, yielded by the Sal tree (also called Salwa tree) (*Shorea robusta*) of India and the Himalaya region. Dammar itself is burnt as an incense.

Chucklusa   *see* Peucedan Gum

Chypre   An important perfume in Roman times (see Roman Perfumes) manufactured in Cyprus and made of storax, labdanum and calamus, which gave it a distinctively heady and oriental aroma. This style of perfume continued to be manufactured in Italy into the Middle Ages under a variety of formulas, retaining the name 'Chypre', and was also produced in France as Cyprus Powder, with oak moss as a base. In 17th and 18th century France there was a fashion for small models of birds, known as Oiselets de Chypre, moulded out of a Chypre perfume paste (one recipe required benjamin, cloves, cinnamon, calamus and gum tragacanth as ingredients) and contained in ornate hanging cages.

In modern times the term chypre is used to designate one of the main Perfume Families. Chypre perfumes are mostly based on oak moss, patchouli, labdanum or clary sage, with the addition of flowery notes such as rose or jasmine, and a sweet note such as bergamot or lemon.

The first of the 20th century chypre perfumes was issued by Coty in 1917 with the brand name 'Chypre'. It provided fresh top notes of bergamot, supported by traces of lemon, neroli and orange, with a floral middle note mainly of rose and jasmine, and a base note in which oak moss predominated, but with patchouli, labdanum, storax, civet and musk in the background.

'Ciao'   A quality semi-oriental–floral–chypre perfume created by Givaudan perfumers and launched by Houbigant in 1980. It is designed to reflect the excitement of the life of the 'international set'. The top note is created around osmanthus, with green and citrusy notes, leading into a heavily floral middle note in which osmanthus is joined by, among others, rose, jasmine, cassis and hyacinth. The base includes oak moss, sandalwood, patchouli, cedar and vetivert.

Cinnamon   Also known as Cinnamon Bark and Ceylon Cinnamon. The fragrant bark of the Cinnamon tree (*Cinnamomum Vera* = *C. zeylanicum* = *Laurus cinnamomum* and some related species) found in Indonesia, Malaysia, S. India and Sri Lanka and cultivated elsewhere. The trees, which reach a height of about 30 feet, grow best in sand. Only the inner bark of branches and young shoots is used to make cinnamon, appearing either as rolled quills or in powdered form. An essential oil is distilled from the bark, but the yield is very small. The oil, which is among those now synthesized for safety or environmental reasons (see Perfume Creation), is used in perfumery, particularly in oriental-type perfumes (examples of modern quality fragrances containing it are 'Dioressence', 'Mitsouko', 'Old Spice' and 'Xeryus'). Cinnamon can also be used in sachets and pot pourri, and was at one time used in pomanders and perfumed beads, but the main use of the dried materials now is in flavourings and medicines. Another oil, Cinnamon Leaf Oil, is distilled from the green leaves for use in perfumery and in flavourings.

Cinnamon has a very ancient history as an important perfume ingredient. It is mentioned in the Bible, notably as an ingredient of the holy anointing oil (see Bible Perfumes) and by many Greek and Roman authors (see Greek Perfumes and Roman Perfumes), usually in conjunction with cassia. Pliny described a cinnamon unguent which also contained Xylobalsam and which 'fetches enormous prices'. However, the cinnamon of very early times would appear to have come from a different plant, growing in areas of Africa opposite the coasts of S. Arabia, which has not yet been identified. On this subject see Cassia. The true cinnamon of today seems unlikely to have appeared in Europe on any scale until Roman trade with the Far East began to develop around the end of the 1st century BC. At this time the Romans also began to import malabathrum from northern India. Cinnamon brought from China was well known to Arab perfume makers by the 9th century AD. In the 17th and 18th centuries the cinnamon trade was a monopoly of the Dutch, who only handled wild produce and would not permit the tree to be cultivated.

Cinnamon, Oil of   *see* Cassia
Cinnamon Sedge   *see* Calamus
Cinnamon Wood   *see* Sassafras
Cinnamonum camphora   *see* Camphor
　　　　　　cassia   *see* Cassia
　　　　　　cecicodaphne   *see* Storax
　　　　　　iners   *see* Cinnamon
　　　　　　laureirii   *see* Nikkel Oil
　　　　　　obtusifolium   *see* Cassia
　　　　　　tamala   *see* Cinnamon and Malabathrum
　　　　　　zeylanicum   *see* Cinnamon
Cistus creticus   *see* Labdanum
　　　cyprius   *see* Labdanum
　　　incanus   *see* Labdanum
　　　ladanifer   *see* Labdanum
　　　monsplensis   *see* Labdanum
　　　villosus   *see* Labdanum

Citral An aldehyde found in oils such as lemon, lime, verbena and lemon grass and, importantly, Litsea Cubeba Oil, and also made synthetically. It is used to give perfumes a fresh, lemon odour. In its pure commercial form it is so powerful that the nose can be paralysed by it and unable to smell anything else for some hours (see Perfume Creation).

Citron A lemon-like essential oil used in perfumery, which is distilled from the rind of the Citron tree (*Citrus medica*), sometimes called Jewish Citron. The tree is native to subtropical Asia and mainly cultivated for the oil in S. Italy and Corsica. Under the name Etrog Citron the oil is used in Jewish festivals. The Arabs, who first introduced the tree into the Mediterranean area from India, call the tree *Utruj*, which is of Persian origin, although in Iran that word now means an 'orange'. Early Arab perfume makers used oils obtained from the flowers, pips, leaves and peel.

Citronella A pungent, lemon-scented essential oil distilled from the leaves of a grass known as Winter's Grass (*Cymbopogon nardus* − *Andropogon nardus*, and also the species *Cymbopogon winterianus*). This grass, which is native to tropical Asia, is cultivated in Indonesia, Burma, Sri Lanka, Taiwan and Guatemala. The oil is used on a substantial scale in perfumes, soaps and aerosols. It also provides Geraniol, Citronellal and Citronellol, used in many synthetic fragrances. In perfumery the oil produced in Sri Lanka, which comes from a different variety of the plant and is inferior, is termed Ceylon Oil, that produced in other parts of the Far East being known as Java Oil.

Citronellal An aldehyde manufactured synthetically from pinene or obtained from citronella and certain eucalyptus oils. It has a powerful herbaceous odour, and is used in synthetic perfumes.

Citronellol A constituent of Oil of Citronella with a sweet rose-like fragrance which is extracted as an alcohol and used in making synthetic perfumes imitating fragrances such as lily of the valley, hyacinth, narcissus and sweet pea. It is also found in geranium and rose oils.

Citronnier *see* Petitgrain

Citron Myrtle *see* Backhousia

Citron Scented Gum *see* Eucalyptus

Citrus aurantium *see* Bitter Orange, Neroli, Petitgrain and Cravo Oil

    aurantium **var.** *bergamia* *see* Bergamot Oil

    bergamia *see* Bergamot Oil

    bigaradia *see* Neroli

    hystrix *see* Colobot

    limonum *see* Citron

    madurensis *see* Mandarin Oil

    medica *see* Citron

    medica **var.** *cimonum* *see* Lemon Oil

nobilis   *see* Mandarin

Citrus Note   In perfumery this term is used to describe the fresh, light fragrance characteristic of citrus fruits, but also imitated synthetically. See Perfume Notes.

Citrus paradisi   *see* Grapefruit

reticulata   *see* Mandarin

sinensis   *see* Sweet Orange

Civet   Also called Zibetha (from the Arabic *Zibād*), civet is one of the few perfume materials obtained from an animal and also one of the most important. It is a soft, paste-like glandular secretion, yellow and butter-like when fresh but turning brown on exposure to the air, and is taken from a pouch under the tails of both male and female civet cats (*Viverra civetta* and certain other species). These are wild animals native to Ethiopia and nearby parts of Africa, and, in respect of the other species (notably *V. rasse* and *V. tangalunga*), also found in Burma, Thailand and Indonesia. In its original and concentrated form, civet has a very strong and most obnoxious smell, but when minute quantities are diluted they become highly fragrant. It is an excellent fixative and a constituent of many top-quality perfumes of today, being shown as a principal ingredient in nearly 10% of them (e.g. 'Bal à Versailles', 'Boucheron', 'Shocking' and 'Parfum d'Hermès').

Civet was not known in classical times nor, from its absence in the perfume recipes of al-Kindi, does it appear to have been known in the early days of the Arab perfume makers. It seems to have been discovered by the Arabs in about the 10th century AD, when it quickly established itself as one of the most desirable of all perfume ingredients. It was well known in Shakespearean England and was for long used for scenting gloves. It is now mostly used in an 'absolute' form (but highly diluted).

There have been various attempts, sometimes successful, to keep civet cats in captivity, in England and elsewhere, for the perfume material, but Africa has continued to provide the main supply. 'Civetone' (or 'Zibethone'), the principal odorous constituent in civet, is now made synthetically, and there are many artificially made substitutes.

Clary Oil   Also called Clary Sage Oil. An oil extracted from the Clary plant (*Salvia sclarea*), also called Clary Sage, Musky Sage, Clear-eye, See-bright, Eye-bright, Clay Wort and Muscatel Sage, native to Syria, southern Europe and N. Africa, but now found widely. This plant, which grows up to 3 feet high and has many varieties, was introduced into Britain in 1562. The name comes from Latin *clarus*, meaning 'clear', because of its use during the Middle Ages to treat eye complaints. The oil is variously described as having a fragrance between balsam of Tolu and Muscatel grapes, or as akin to a mixture of musk, ambergris, neroli and lavender. It is a valuable additive in eau de cologne, is often used in perfumes in a floral concrete form, and makes an excellent fixative. It is also used to improve the quality of artificial musks. Examples of its use in modern quality fragrances are 'Antaeus', 'Cabochard' and 'L'Heure Bleue'. The dried leaves can be used in sachets and pot pourri. The oil is also used in flavouring wines. See also Sage Oil.

'Climat'   An aldehydic floral perfume first marketed by Lancome in 1967. It was created by Robertet perfumers. The middle note, a bouquet principally based on lily of the valley, is topped by aldehyde notes with suggestions of bergamot, violet and peach, while the base notes, chiefly vetiver and amber, contain hints of sandalwood, tonka, musk and civet. The bottle was designed by Serge Mansau.

Clove Oil   Also called Clove Bud Oil. An oil made from cloves, the dried flower buds of the Clove tree (*Eugenia caryophyllata* = *E. aromatica* = *Caryophyllus aromaticus* = *Syzygium aromaticum*), also called Antofle, Cariophyllorum and Caryophylli. The tree, which grows up to 50 feet high, is native to the Molucca Islands but cultivated widely elsewhere, most notably in Zanzibar since early in the 19th century. The fragrance resembles that of clove-pink (carnation). The oil, which consists of 85% of eugenol, is used in perfumes, especially floral ones, and soaps, and also in medicines as a pain killer. Examples of quality perfumes containing it include 'Fidji' and 'Ysatis'. Cloves were used in medicines and as a flavouring spice in Europe from the 4th century BC and in China from the 3rd century BC (when court officials were required to hold cloves in their mouths when addressing the Emperor). Clove oil was one of the ingredients of the early Arab perfume makers. A similar oil is also distilled from the roots of the Clove tree. See also Caryophyllene.

Clove Leaf Oil   An oil steam-distilled from the leaves and twigs of the Clove tree (see above). It is used in perfumery to provide a spicy, herbaceous tone.

Clove-pink Oil   Also called Carnation Oil. An essential oil extracted by volatile solvents from the flowers of the Clove-pink (*Dianthus caryophyllus*), the old-fashioned carnation, which was one of the earliest flowers to be cultivated in British gardens, being known in Chaucer's time (14th century). The plant, native to southern Europe, is also called Gilliflower, Clove July Flower, Carnation and Picotee. The odour of Clove-pink Oil is rich and of a clove-like spiciness, so that it is much used to add a spicy piquancy to floral middle notes. Most flower production for use in perfumery is now in southern France and Italy. Some 500 kg of flowers provide only about 1 kg of concrete and about one-tenth of that amount of absolute, making the latter extremely costly, so that it is found only in very high-quality perfumes (e.g. 'Je Reviens' and 'L'Air du Temps'), but the oil is used in some 14% of all modern quality perfumes and 20% of all men's fragrances. The flowers were used in medieval Arab perfumes. In Tudor times the oil was used both in perfumes and cordial waters, and the plant was being cultivated in Britain for perfumery in the 18th century. It was once believed that the scent of this plant could be improved by burying real cloves under the roots; it appears to be a fact that the fragrance has improved with cultivation. Dried flower petals are used in sachets and pot pourri. See also Carnation.

Clove Root   *see* Avens

Clover   Also called Trèfle. A plant of the genus *Trifolium*, of which there are many species. The honey-like fragrance of clover blossoms is easily imitated synthetically and no attempt is made to extract it from the plants for commercial use. See also Melilot.

Coarse Myrrh   *see* Opoponax

'Coco'   An innovative 'spicy–floral–amber' perfume created by Jacques Polge for Chanel in 1984 and named after Mademoiselle Chanel. Floral–fruity top notes, including jasmine and frangipani, introduce middle notes of cascarilla, orange flower and rose, and overlie a base which includes labdanum, sandalwood and tonka. The bottle is in the traditional Chanel style, designed by Jacques Helleu and made by Brosse.

Cocoa   *see* Cacao

Cocograss   *see* Cyperus

Coffin Wood Oil   *see* Bois de Siam

Cognac, Oil of   An oil obtained by distillation during the fermentation of grape juice by yeast, usually from the residue of wine used for brandy. It is occasionally used in perfumery. See also Wine.

Colewort   *see* Avens

Colic Root   *see* Galingale

Colobot   An oil distilled from the peel of the fruit of the Colobot tree (*Citrus hystrix* var. *torosa*), which grows to about 20 feet high in the Philippines. Mostly used as a flavouring, it is occasionally used in perfumes, having a lime-like fragrance.

Colocai   *see* Balsam of Copaiba

Coltsfoot   *see* Canadian Snakeroot

Columback Wood   *see* Aloewood

Combretum hartemannianum   *see* Mumuye Gum

Commiphora abyssinica   *see* Myrrh

        africana   *see* Bdellium

        erythraea   *see* Opoponax and Bdellium

        foliacea   *see* Myrrh

        gileadensis   *see* Balsam of Makkah

        habessinica   *see* Myrrh

        hildebrandtii   *see* Bdellium

>*kataf*   *see* Myrrh and Opoponax
>*mukul*   *see* Bdellium
>*myrrha*   *see* Myrrh
>*opobalsamum*   *see* Balsam of Makkah and Myrrh
>*roxburghi*   *see* Bdellium
>*wighti*   *see* Bdellium

Communelle   A term used in the perfume industry to describe an oil produced from a mixture of flowers of the same species but obtained from different growers or different areas.

Compass Plant   *see* Rosemary

Compass Weed   *see* Rosemary

Comptonia asplenifolia   *see* Sweet Fern Oil

Concrete   A semi-solid product obtained by the process of extraction of essential oils by volatile solvents. It consists of the absolute together with stearoptene, an odourless waxy substance, and has the advantage of being a very good fixative. In French perfumery it is known as *Essence Concrète*. Many natural perfume materials are preferred by perfumers in their concrete form, particularly when the perfume is used in soap. The concretes of essential oils obtained from flowers are sometimes called Floral Concretes.

Coniferous Note   A term used in perfumery to describe the fragrance of pine, spruce, juniper and similar such trees, often used in men's fragrances. See Perfume Notes.

Convallaria   *see* Lily of the Valley

Convallaria majalis   *see* Lily of the Valley

Convolvulus floridus   *see* Rhodium Oil

>*scoparius*   *see* Rhodium Oil

Copaiba   *see* Balsam of Copaiba

Copaifera guyanensis   *see* Balsam of Copaiba

>*lansdorfii*   *see* Balsam of Copaiba
>*officinalis*   *see* Balsam of Copaiba
>*reticulata*   *see* Balsam of Copaiba and Bois d'Olhio

Copernica cerifera   *see* Carnauba Wax

Coriander   A small (1–3 feet high) annual (*Coriandrum sativum*) originating in southern Europe and Asia and now cultivated widely, especially in India, N. Africa and Italy. Oil of Coriander, steam-distilled from the dried seeds, has a pungent, spicy aroma and is used in quality perfumery (e.g. 'Coriandre', Gucci No. 1' and 'Le Jardin d'Amour') and soaps, especially to provide a masculine note. It is also much used in flavouring. Coriander is an excellent fixative and contains a large proportion of linaloe. The dried seeds, used in sachets and pot pourri, are sometimes called Dizzycorn, because when freshly crushed the odour can promote dizziness.

Coriander seeds were found in the tomb of King Tutankhamun.

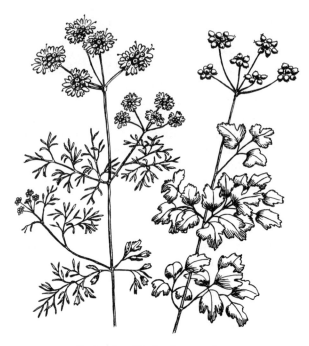

Coriander (*Coriandrum sativum*).

Mentioned in the Bible, it was introduced into Britain by the Romans, being valuable both in medicines and cooking. Pliny noted that in his time the best coriander came from Egypt, observing that it was, among other things, an antidote for 'the poison of the two-headed serpent'. In medieval times it was used in love potions.

'Coriandre'   A popular chypre perfume, created by Roure perfumers and brought out by Jean Coutourier in 1973, with an unusual spicy top note achieved mainly by coriander. The middle note is floral, principally rose and geranium, and the base note is built on patchouli, with other ingredients which include traces of vetiver, sandalwood, civet and musk.

Coronation Oil   The anointing oil used at the coronation of the British sovereign. It is based on a 17th century formula, and consists of a sesame oil base to which has been added essences of rose, orange blossom, jasmine and cinnamon, together with benzoin, musk, civet and ambergris.

Corylopsis   A plant (*Corylopsis spicata* and other species) native to China and Japan, with cowslip-scented flowers. The name is given to a type of perfume which imitates the scent. It usually contains ylang-ylang and patchouli.

Corylus avellana   *see* Hazel Nut Oil

Costmary Also called Alecost, Alespice, Balsam Herb, Balsamita, Bible Leaf, Coursemary, English Mace and Mint Geranium. A medium sized perennial (*Chrysanthemum balsamita* = *Balsamita major* = *Pyrethrum balsamita* = *Tanacetum balsamita*) belonging to the daisy family, native to W. Asia but grown in Europe for centuries. The plant is closely related to Tansy. It has a strong scent of mint, and the dried leaves, which retain their odour for years, are used in sachets and pot pourri to intensify other fragrances. The plant was introduced into Britain by the Romans. The name signifies 'Costus of St Mary' (in France it is still known as Herbe Sainte-Marie), being associated with Our Lady in the Middle Ages. The name Alecost derives from a time when it was used to give ale a sharper flavour. The name Bible Leaf comes from an old custom of using it in a Bible as a book-marker. Bundles of the dried leaves were once placed in linen presses and on beds 'for sweet scent and savour'.

Costus Also called Sweet Costus and Indian Orris. A perennial thistle-like herb (*Saussurea lappa* = *Aplotaxis lappa* = *Auklandia costus*) growing up to 6 feet high and found chiefly in the Himalayas around Kashmir. Its many local names include Koosht, Ouplate and Pachak. A heavy oil with a violet-like scent, Costus Root Oil or Oil of Costus, is steam-distilled from the dried roots and used in perfumes and incenses, especially in China, India, Iran and the Middle East. It is a good fixative and needs to be used only in minute quantities. In India it is employed, like patchouli, to protect expensive clothes from insects. The dried roots are sometimes used in pot pourri and sachets. In western perfumery the fragrance of costus oil is now largely replaced by synthetics (see Perfume Creation).

Costus was known in ancient times and Theophrastus listed it as one of the principal plants used in Greek perfumery, noting that is was very long-lasting. Some commentators believe it was the cassia of the Bible. There is uncertainty whether the costus of ancient times was the same species as the plant known as costus today. Pliny referred to a white and a black variety of costus, and other writers have noted a white Arabian variety (*Costus arabicus* = *C. speciosus*), described as the most fragrant. The early Arab perfume makers used costus of one species or another in a variety of perfume oils and unguents.

Cotton Lavender *see* Lavender Cotton Oil

Coty The House of Coty was founded in 1905, as a two-roomed perfume shop in Paris, by Francois Spoturno (1873–1934), a Corsican, who is often regarded as the first of the great perfumers of modern times. He adopted the name Coty because of its simplicity. Coty had spent two years in Grasse learning the details of his trade. His first perfume, 'La Rose Jacqueminot', was immediately successful following the famous incident when one of the Baccarat bottles containing it, which he was delivering to a Paris department store, slipped through his fingers and shattered, filling the store with its aroma. From then until his death 29 years later Coty produced over 50 perfumes, including famous classics such as 'L'Origan' (1905), 'Chypre' (17) and 'L'Aimant' (27), which is still marketed. The company passed from the Coty family to the Pfizer Corporation in the 1960s, then to Colgate–Palmolive in 1980, and it is now run by Beauty International, a division of European Brands Group Ltd.

House of Coty's later perfumes have included 'Muguet des Bois' (41), 'Muse' (46), 'Accomplice' (54), 'Imprévu' (65), 'Masumi' (68), 'Wild Musk' (68), 'L'Aimant Éternelle' (87), 'Fatale' (88) and 'Exclamation!' (90). Coty believed that his perfumes should be supplied in containers of impeccable taste, and his early perfumes were sold in flacons by Baccarat and Lalique.

Coumarin   An important constituent of many fragrant herbs and fruits which occurs as a white crystalline substance once they have begun to wither and which carries the odour of new-mown hay. Certain plants, such as melilot, tonka bean and woodruff, are rich in coumarin and are used in perfumery both for their fragrance and because the coumarin content makes them good fixatives. But most coumarin used in perfumery today is manufactured synthetically from coal tar.

Coumarouna odorata   *see* Tonka Bean

Courrèges   A fashion house founded in 1961 by Andre Courrèges, who has since become involved in the designing of accessories, interiors and automobiles. The company's first perfume was 'Empreinte' (71), followed by 'Amerique' (74) and 'Courrèges in Blue' (83). It is now owned by L'Oréal.

'Courrèges in Blue'   A spicy–floral perfume introduced by Courrèges in 1983. Created by Roure perfumers, it has aldehydic top notes, with bergamot, coriander and basil, which evolve into a strong floral heart, including rose, violet and tuberose, and a woody, powdery base note dominated by vetivert. The cylindrical bottle is an in-house design, with bevelled squares capped by a gilded dome.

Crab Apple   The fragrance of the fruit of certain species of Crab Apple tree (*Pyrus coronaria* and others) is not extracted for use in perfumery but is instead made synthetically.

Crabtree & Evelyn   Founded in 1970, this company is now a leading producer of high class toiletries based on the products of the old manor house still-room of earlier centuries. Fragrances in the form of toilet waters and colognes include a version of Hungary Water, a floral fragrance, 'L'Elisir d'Amore' (1989), 'Millefleurs' (80) and fragrances based on rosewater, lily of the valley, gardenia, violet, lavender, carnation, vetiver and sandalwood.

Crataegus oxycantha   *see* Hawthorn

Cravo Oil   An oil obtained by expression from the fruit peel of a hybrid tangerine known in Brazil as Laranja Cravo (*Citrus aurantium* × *C. reticulata*). It has a very fresh orange/mandarin odour and is used in perfumes with fruity notes and in Eau de Colognes.

Creeping Tuberose   *see* Stephanotis

'Crêpe de Chine'   One of the earliest of the modern chypre perfumes, first marketed by F. Millot in 1925. The top note is bergamot, with traces of lemon, orange, neroli and fruity fragrance in support. The middle note is floral, including jasmine and rose, but given a spicy tang by clove-pink. The base note is mostly oak moss and vetiver, modified by benzoin, labdanum, patchouli and musk.

'Cristalle'   A fresh–floral fruity perfume created for Chanel in 1974 by Henri Robert. Its principal ingredients are lemon in the top note, honeysuckle in the middle note and vetiver in the base note.

Crocus sativus   *see* Saffron

Croton eleutharia   *see* Cascarilla

Crystal Tea Ledum   *see* Marsh Rosemary

Cubeb   Also called Tailed Pepper. Cubebs are the dried fruits of a climbing perennial (*Piper cubeba*) native to Indonesia, where it is cultivated in coffee plantations. They have a spicy aroma. Oil of Cubeb, extracted from them for use in flavouring, medicine and, occasionally, in perfumery, was known to the early Arab perfume makers; it is very volatile and hence evaporates very quickly. The dried fruits are also powdered and used in sachets, pot pourri and incenses. Another form of Oil of Cubeb is obtained from the fruits of the Ashanti Pepper tree (*Piper clusii*) of W. Africa.

Cucumber Juice   The juice of the cucumber, from a trailing annual (*Cucumis sativus*), is extracted and distilled into a concentrated form for use in blending certain bouquet perfumes.

Cucumis sativus   *see* Cucumber

'Cuir de Russie'   A distinctively original perfume created by Ernest Beaux and produced by Chanel in 1924. For the first time among feminine fragrances it contained a pronounced leathery note, providing a new perfume type from which many men's fragrances were subsequently developed. The top note was dry and fresh, deriving mainly from orange blossom, the middle note a floral combination with rose, jasmine and ylang-ylang predominating. The leather note came from balsamic ingredients in the base, including labdanum and birch tar.

Cumin   An oil once used extensively in perfumery which is steam-distilled from the dried seeds of the Cumin plant (*Cuminum cyminum*), a small herb native to the Mediterranean area and Arabia, but cultivated widely, especially in Morocco, the Mediterranean region and India, since ancient times. It has a bitter, musky aroma, with a resemblance to aniseed. For safety reasons it is now used in commercial perfumery only in synthetic form (see Perfume Creation). The plant is mentioned in the Old and New Testaments and in the works of Hippocrates, Dioscorides and Pliny for its medical and flavouring uses. Among the ancient Greeks it symbolized cupidity – misers were said to have 'eaten cumin'.

Cupressus hodgsinii   *see* Bois de Siam

   sempervivens   *see* Cypress

Curcuma Oil   An oil steam-distilled from the rhizomes of the perennial turmeric plant (*Curcuma longa*), native to southern parts of Asia and cultivated in India, China, Indonesia and the West Indies. The plant, which no longer grows wild, was cultivated over 2000 years ago in Assyria, China and India. The oil, which has an earthy fragrance, is a vivid yellow and used as a dye, particularly in the manufacture of curry powders, but has also been used in perfumes and, in Egypt, for scenting new slippers. It is little used in perfumery today.

Curcuma zeodoaria   *see* Zedoary Oil

   zerumbet   *see* Kuchoora

Curry Plant   *see* Everlasting Flower

Cyclamen   There are many species of the cyclamen plant, but the fragrance, which recalls a blending of lily, lilac, violet and hyacinth, is not extracted commercially. Cyclamen fragrances used in perfumery are made from various combinations of synthetic and natural materials. They appear in quality perfumes (e.g. 'Nocturnes' and 'Carnet du Bal').

Cydonia oblonga   *see* Quince

Cymbopogon caesius   *see* Kachi Grass

   citratus   *see* Lemon Grass de Cochin

   flexuosus   *see* Lemon Grass de Cochin

   martinii   *see* Ginger Grass Oil and Palma Rosa Oil

   nardus   *see* Citronella

   schoenanthus   *see* Lemon Grass Oil

   winterianus   *see* Citronella

Cyperus   A number of species of the Sedge family of plants yield aromatic materials used in perfumery.

1. *Cyperus longus*. Called Cyperus, Long Cyperus, Sweet Cyperus and English Galingale. Native to central Europe, Italy and Sicily, but also found in English marshes, where it grows up to 4 feet high. The rhizomes, sometimes called Cypress Roots, which have a violet-like fragrance, are used (and were formerly much used) in perfumery, especially as an addition to Lavender Water. This may be one of the materials listed in ancient Egyptian recipes for Kyphi.

2. *C. articulatus*. Found in the Old and New World. The fragrant rhizomes have been used dried to perfume clothing.

3. *C. pertenuis*. Grows in India, where it is called *Nagar Motha* or *Koriak*.

The roots, dried and powdered, are used locally for powdering the hair.

4. *C. maculatus*. Grows in tropical Africa, where the tubers are a source of local perfume.
5. *C. scarious*. Grows in India, where the rhizomes are employed in Indian perfumery.
6. *C. rotundus*. Called Cocograss and Nut Grass. A weed throughout the tropics. The dried rhizomes are used in India to perfume the hair and clothes. This may have been the *Radix Junci* of the Romans.

A species of cyperus was used by the early Arab perfume makers. The dried rhizomes of cyperus are, in perfumery, often known by the French name for them, *Souchet*.

Cypress, Oil of   A yellowish oil with a pleasingly smoky, woody smell, also described as labdanum-like and amber-like, which is distilled from the leaves and twigs of the Cypress tree (*Cupressus sempervivens*). This tall tree, which grows from southern Europe to western Asia, is associated with cemeteries, probably because the Romans regarded it as a tree of death and the underworld. Oil of cypress is mostly produced in the south of France; it is much used in men's fragrances, but is also found in feminine ones (e.g. 'Rumba' and 'Salvador Dali').

Cyprinum   A sweetly-scented and very long-lasting essential oil obtained from the flowers of Henna (*Lawsonia inermis* = *L. alba*), a shrub growing up to 10 feet high, indigenous from Egypt and Syria to India and now grown widely. The plant is also known as al-Khanna, Smooth Lawsonia, Egyptian Privet and Jamaica Mignonette. The oil is also called Gulhina and Mehndi and is used in many eastern perfumes. Henna dye is extracted from the leaves of this plant, which has been cultivated since ancient times. It was formerly called the Cyprus tree and is the Camphire of the Bible. The ancient Egyptians believed that the scent of henna flowers could bring the dead back to life, and used the oil to keep limbs supple. Pliny noted that Cyprinum was made by boiling the flower seeds in olive oil, and listed it as one of the many ingredients of the famous Royal Unguent.

Cyprus Powder   Also called Cyprian Powder and Alexandria Powder. An aromatic powder formerly used in sachets, as a toilet powder and for powdering wigs. It was made of dried oak moss or tree moss fumigated with burning resin or mixed with other aromatic substances including, in one 16th century recipe, rosewater, musk, civet and sandalwood.

Cytisus lanigerus   *see* Aspalathus

Czech & Speake   A London firm established in 1979 by Frank Sawkins, a designer, in partnership with Shirley Brody, a perfumer, to produce high quality bathroom fittings and accessories and aromatic toiletries.

The company's fragrances, marketed at cologne strength and also in soaps, bath oils, burning oils and incense sticks, include 'Frankincense and Myrrh' (83), 'Mimosa' (82), 'Neroli' (84), 'Rose' (85) and 'Grapefruit' (91), together with a men's fragrance 'No. 88' (81).

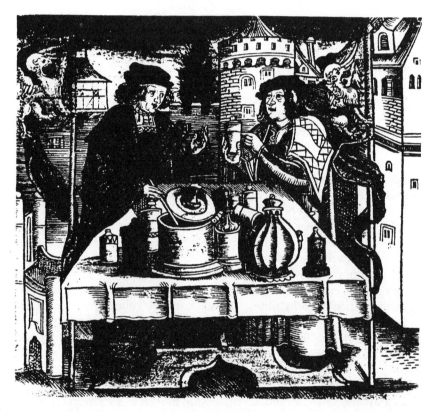

16th century perfumers (*Source* Lancelot Andrews, *The Small Boke of Distillacyon*, 1527, a translation of a German perfume handbook by Hieronymus Braunschweig (1500)).

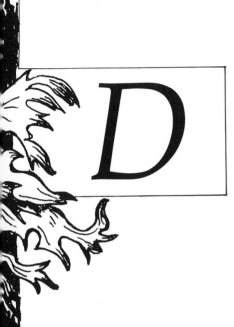

Dacrydium franklinii   *see* Huon Pine

Dagaganthum   *see* Tragacanth

Dai-ui-Kio   *see* Japanese Star Anise

Dalbergia junghuhnii   *see* Akar Laka

Daffodil   The fragrance called Daffodil in Perfumery is usually obtained from a variation of the fragrance of Narcissus made synthetically.

Damask   *see* Honesty Oil

Damask Water   A compound perfume popular in England in the 16th century which was based on rosewater ('Damask' relating to the Damask Rose, or Rose of Damascus) but contained a variety of other ingredients. One early 16th century recipe for Damask Water required lavender, thyme, rosemary, bay leaves, marjoram and other materials to be distilled in a mixture of rosewater and wine, various spices being added afterwards together with spikenard, ambergris, musk and camphor. Sometimes the Damask Water, in effect a thick oil, was dried and used in sachets as a perfumed powder.

Dame's Violet   *see* Honesty Oil

Dammar   *see* Chua Oil

Damor   *see* Star Anise

Daniella thurifera   *see* Balsam of Copaiba

'Dans la Nuit'   The first perfume to be launched by Worth. It was created by Maurice Blanchet in 1924, initially as a gift for distinguished lady clients of the fashion house. With a heart of jasmine, rose, tuberose and orris, the top notes include blackcurrant and the base contains labdanum. It is sold in a blue Art Deco-style orb-shaped flacon by Lalique.

Daphne *see* Bay

Darwinia Oil An oil (Oleum Darwinii aetherum) with a geranium-like odour which is used in perfumes. It is distilled from the wood, twigs and leaves of three species of Darwinia (*Darwinia fascicularis*, *D. grandiflora* and *D. taxifolia*), a small tree, growing to about 15 feet high, which is found in south eastern Australia.

Date Palm Among fragrant flowers used in perfumes in India are those of Kurna, the date palm (*Phoenix dactilifera*). The tree is native to Asia Minor, but now grows widely.

Daucus carota *see* Carrot Oil.

Davana Oil An oil obtained by steam-distillation from Davana, a flowering herb (*Artemisia pallens*), native to India and cultivated there for this oil; the whole plant is distilled. The oil has a sweet, tea-like odour reminiscent of dried fruit and is used in eastern perfumes and also occasionally in western ones (e.g. 'Knowing').

Deer's Tongue *see* Lacinaria

'Demi-Jour' A floral-chypre perfume introduced by Houbigant in 1987. Flowers, spices and fruity nuances in the top note include violet, hyacinth and orange flower. The floral middle notes contain rose, jasmine, ylang-ylang, mimosa and tuberose, and the base, which is woody, mossy and musky, includes sandalwood. The perfume is sold in a lead crystal flacon based on an early Houbigant design.

De Mourgues, Alain A leading designer of perfume bottles. His works include bottles for, among others, Gianni Versace (see 'V'E'), Giorgio Armani, Houbigant, Van Gils and Yves St Laurent. See Perfume Containers.

Desprez A perfume house established in Paris by Jean Desprez (1898–1973), a perfumer by profession. Aiming for very high quality products, he employed an artist, Paul Mergier, to design his packaging and a sculptor, Leon Leyritz, to design his flacons. Three perfumes, 'Grande Dame', 'Votre Main' and 'Etourdissant', were launched in 1939, the former in a bottle of Sevres porcelain and the latter in a startling, cut-crystal flacon made by Baccarat, both to Leyritz designs. Subsequent perfumes included 'Bal à Versailles' (62), 'Jardanel' (73) and 'Sheherazade' (83), together with a men's fragrance 'Versailles pour Homme' (80). The firm is still run by the Desprez family.

'Detchema' A quality aldehyde perfume created by the perfumers of IFF and Révillon in 1953. Fresh aldehydic top notes open up a floral middle note, principally of rose, jasmine, ylang-ylang, lily of the valley and carnation, with a base note mainly composed of orris, sandalwood and vetivert.

Devardari Oil   An essential oil distilled from the wood of the Bastard Sandalwood tree (*Erythroxylon monogynum*) found in India. It has a sandalwood odour and is used in low grade perfumes.

Devil's Dung   *see* Asafoetida

Devil's Gum   *see* Asafoetida

Devil's Nettle   *see* Milfoil

'Devin'   A trend-setting 'green' men's fragrance issued by Aramis in 1978 as a light, sporting Eau de Cologne. It followed the style of the feminine perfume 'Alliage'. Principal ingredients are galbanum and bergamot in the top notes, jasmine, clove-pink and cinnamon in the heart, and cedarwood, frankincense and a leather fragrance in the base.

Dianthus barbatus   *see* Sweet William

       caryophyllus   *see* Clove-pink

Dictamo/Dictame   *see* Dittany

Dictamus albus   *see* Dittany

       fraxonella   *see* Dittany

Digestion   *see* Maceration

Dill   A fennel-like herb (*Anethum graveolens*) growing up to $2\frac{1}{2}$ feet high, indigenous from the Mediterranean area to India, and cultivated in Hungary, Rumania, Germany, Britain and the USA. From it is steam-distilled Oil of Dill, used principally as a flavouring but also in perfumes and soaps. The oil has a caraway or mint-like fragrance.

Dill was used in ancient Egypt, mainly as a flavouring and in medicines, and Theophrastus listed it among the principal plants used in Greek perfumery in his time. It is mentioned by other classical writers, and in the Middle Ages was used by magicians in spells and charms against witchcraft.

A similar oil, Dill Oil, is distilled from the ripe fruits of East Indian Dill (*Peucedanon graveolens* = *P. sowa*), found in tropical Asia.

Dinand, Pierre   (b. 1932). A prominent designer of contemporary scent bottles and head of a company, 'Atelier Dinand', with studios in Milan, New York, Tokyo, Amsterdam, Paris and Moscow. Since his first work, for Rochas, in 1959, he has designed bottles for, among others, Azzaro, Balenciaga, Balmain, Cardin, Caron, Desprez, Givenchy, Léonard, Molyneux, Paco Rabanne and Yves St Laurent. See Perfume Containers.

Dior, Christian   Parfums Christian Dior was established in Paris by the prominent couturier Christian Dior (1905–1957) in 1947 at the same time that he set up his *haute couture* business and introduced the 'New Look' into fashion. Its first perfume was 'Miss Dior', launched that year. The company's subsequent perfumes have been 'Diorama' (49), 'Eau Fraiche' (55), a 'unisex' fragrance, 'Diorissimo' (56), 'Diorella' (72),

'Dioressence' (79), 'Poison' (85) and 'Dune' (91), together with four fragrances for men – 'Eau Sauvage' (66), 'Jules' (80), 'Eau Sauvage Extreme' (84) and 'Fahrenheit' (88). The company was acquired in 1968 by what has now become the Louis Vuitton–Moet–Hennessy (LVMH) group (see also under Givenchy). The main Dior factory is at St Jean de Braye.

'Diorella'   A floral–fruity chypre perfume created by Edmond Roudnitska and launched by Christian Dior in 1972. Designed for the outdoor woman, it set a trend in floral perfumes with a fresh, cool feeling to them. The dominant fragrances are lemon, bergamot and peach in the top note, honeysuckle and jasmine in the heart, and oak moss and patchouli in the base. The bottle was designed by Serge Mansau.

'Dioressence'   A quality oriental-type perfume created by the perfumers of IFF for Christian Dior, who launched it in 1979. The top note, aldehydic with green and fruity tones, includes rose. Floral notes in the heart contain jasmine and geranium, given a spicy touch by cinnamon and vanilla, and lead into a base which includes patchouli, oak moss, musk and vetivert.

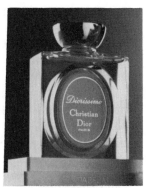

'Diorissimo'.

'Diorissimo'   A classic, trend-setting floral perfume created by Guy Robert for Christian Dior, who launched it in 1956. It set a fashion for floral perfumes with a spring-like green note, achieved in this case by, among other fragrances, boronia and calycanthus. The heart is built on lily of the valley (Dior's favourite flower) with jasmine, amaryllis and ylang-ylang included in the support. In the base note rosewood predominates. The perfume was originally sold in a flacon made by Baccarat in a design of faceted tear drop form with a gilt metal stopper (one fetching £410 at auction in 1990). The present bottle was designed by Guericolas.

Dioscorides   A Greek from Asia Minor who travelled widely as a military surgeon in the Roman army. In about 78 AD he produced his celebrated 'Materia Medica', a very detailed account of natural materials used in medicines and the formulas for their use; this included some information about perfumes. See Greek Perfumes.

Dipteracarpus tuberculatus   see Gurjun Balsam
            turbinatus   see Gurjun Balsam
Dipteryx odorata   see Tonka Bean
          oppositifolia   see Tonka Bean
Diserneston gummifera   see Ammoniacum

Distillation   The main method of obtaining essential oils from plants, other methods being enfleurage, maceration, expression and extraction by volatile solvents. Distillation is based on the principal that when plant material is placed in boiling water the essential oil in it will evaporate with the steam; once the steam and oil have then condensed back, the oil will separate from the water, floating on the water's surface, from which it can be collected. Sometimes this process is repeated to obtain a purer essence. A primitive form of this technique was used by the ancient Egyptians and Mesopotamians, and in ancient India, from as early as 3500 BC (crude distillation vessels of that period have been found both in Nineveh and in Mohenjodaro). The Arabs greatly improved the technique in the 7th or 8th centuries AD, inventing the alembic for the purpose. Late in the 19th century steam-distillation was introduced, under which the evaporated oils were condensed in narrow pipes passing through cold water, sometimes in a partial vacuum ('vacuum distillation'). In the case of certain essential oils with aromatic constituents which are unusually soluble in water, the distilled water retains traces of the aromatic material, providing what is known as Distilled Water or Floral Water, which can be used as a toilet water; rosewater and orange flower water are produced in this way.

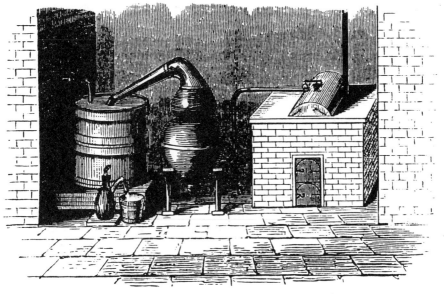

Distillation – a 19th century steam still (from Rimmel: *Book of Perfumes*, 1895).

Dittany   Two different plants bear the name Dittany and both are used in perfumery.

1. White Dittany (*Dictamus albus* = *D. fraxonella* = *Fraxonella dictamnus*), also called False Dittany, Candle Plant and Burning Bush, a herb growing up to 3 feet high and found widely in temperate areas of Europe and Asia. A fragrant essential oil is obtained from the leaves and flowers. In strong heat the oil in this plant can vaporize and catch fire, though without harming it.
2. True Dittany (*Origanum dictamnus* = *Amaracus dictamnus*) also called Dittany of Crete, Dictame and Hop Plant, an aromatic dwarf shrub native to Crete but cultivated elsewhere, including in Britain. The leaves, which have a thyme-like odour, are dried for use in pot pourri, sachets and incenses. The plant was used in ancient Greece for medicinal purposes.

'Diva'   An innovative floral–amber perfume launched in 1984 by Parfums Ungaro, the perfume branch of the couture house opened in Paris in 1965 by Emanuel Ungaro. It was created for Ungaro by Jacques Polge. The heart is principally rose (both Damask and Centifolia), orris, narcissus and jasmine, with tuberose, cardamom, mandarin and ylang-ylang in the top note, and ambergris, supported by woody notes from sandalwood, patchouli and oak moss, in the base. An eau de toilette containing a revised version of the Diva formula was launched in 1989 under the name 'Eau de Seduction'. The perfume flacon was designed by Emanuel Ungaro and Jacques Helleu to suggest the folds of a woman's dress.

Dizzycorn   *see* Coriander

Dolloff   *see* Meadowsweet

Dorema ammoniacum   *see* Ammoniacum

Doryphora sassafras   *see* Sassafras

Double Scent Bottle   A type of perfume bottle, popular in Victorian times from about 1850, which opened at both ends. Made by fusing two ordinary glass bottles together, one end contained perfume and the other held smelling salts. Double scent bottles were usually made of coloured glass with metal caps. See Perfume Containers.

Douglas Fir Oil   An essential oil distilled from the leaves of the Douglas Fir tree (*Pseudostuga menziesii* = *P. douglasii* = *P. mucronata* = *P. taxifolia*), also called Douglas Spruce and Red Fir, which is found widely in N. America. It has a pineapple-like fragrance. The oil from firs growing in Oregon, also called Oregano Oil, is reputed to be particularly fragrant.

Dracaena cinnabari   *see* Dragon's Blood

      draco   *see* Dragon's Blood

      schizantha   *see* Dragon's Blood

Dragon Flower   *see* Iris, Yellow

Dragon's Blood   The cinnabar of classical times, a red resin drawn from a number of different trees and plants, more particulary *Dracaena cinnabari* (Soqotra), *D. draco* (Canary Islands), *D. schizantha* (S. Arabia, Somalia and E. Africa) and *Calamus draco* (India and the Far East). It was known to Pliny and Dioscorides, the principal source in classical times being Soqotra. The Arabs call it 'Blood of the Two Brothers'. Its principal use was and still is in medicines and as a varnish, but early Arab perfume makers used it to give perfumes an attractive red colour. The cinnabar of modern times is red sulphur of mercury (which the ancients called 'Minium').

Droga de Jara   *see* Labdanum

Dropwort   A plant native to northern Europe and Asia Minor, *Filipendula hexapetalex* (= *Spiraea filipendula* = *Ulmaria filipendula*) used in Europe throughout history for medicinal purposes. Theophrastus quoted Dropwort as an example of a plant from which a perfume was made from the leaves, but this may have been a reference to Meadowsweet.

Dry Note   A term used in perfumery to describe the aromatic effect of perfume ingredients such as woods and mosses in contrast to sweet and warm fragrances. See Perfume Notes.

Dryobalanops aromatica   *see* Camphor
               camphora   *see* Camphor

'Dune'   An innovative floral–'oceanic' perfume designed to invoke the feeling of an open beach. Created for Dior in 1991 by Jean-Louis Sieuzac under the direction of Maurice Roger, it is a linear fragrance, with floral notes which feature peony and lily, underscored by 'Oceanic' notes principally obtained from amber, broom and lichen. The bottle is an in-house Dior design. See Perfume Notes.

Dunkal tree   *see* Bdellium

Dwarf Pine Oil   *see* Pine Needle Oil

Dyer's Saffron   *see* Safflower

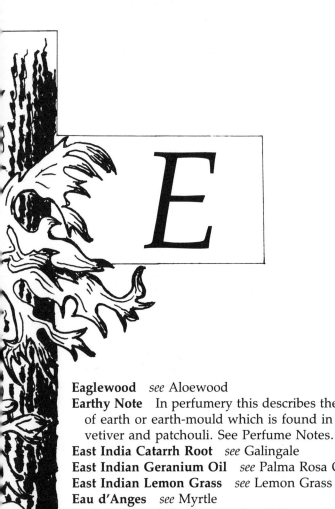

Eaglewood   *see* Aloewood

Earthy Note   In perfumery this describes the subtle fragrance impression of earth or earth-mould which is found in certain essential oils such as vetiver and patchouli. See Perfume Notes.

East India Catarrh Root   *see* Galingale

East Indian Geranium Oil   *see* Palma Rosa Oil

East Indian Lemon Grass   *see* Lemon Grass de Cochin

Eau d'Anges   *see* Myrtle

'Eau de Bonpoint'   An eau de toilette created and sold by Annick Goutal which is notable as the first quality fragrance designed for babies and young children. It is produced with or without an alcohol base and contains orange flower, bitter orange, tangerine and lemon leaf oils.

Eau de Brout   An absolute obtained by extraction from the distillation waters of many essential oils, the most important being neroli and petigrain. It has a harsh, herbaceous orange blossom odour and is used in small amounts in colognes and some perfumes.

Eau de Cologne   A toilet water first developed early in the 18th century by an Italian, Paul Feminis, living in Cologne, who called it L'Eau Admirable'; it was based on citrus, neroli, lemon, bergamot and lavender. At the beginning of the 19th century the product was modified by Jean Farina, a descendent of Feminis, under the name Eau de Cologne and became immensely popular. Napoleon is said to have used 60 bottles a month. The formula was acquired in 1862 by Roger et Gallet of Paris, who made a revised version of the product called 'Jean Marie Farina'. Very many different eau de colognes have subsequently been marketed, using a variety of further ingredients such as rosemary and honeywater. The original formula is still basically adhered to by the 4711 Mullhens company of Cologne, providing a top note of bergamot, mint, lemon and orange, with traces of petitgrain and neroli, a middle note of rosemary and rose, and a base note of musk. Modern eau de colognes are toilet waters containing 3–5% of perfume oil in a 70% alcohol/water mix. See also under Perfume, Splash Cologne and Eau Fraiche. See also Appendix B, recipes nos 59, 60 and 61.

'Eau de Cologne Imperiale' A famous early eau de cologne, first issued by Guerlain in 1850. It was created by Pierre Guerlain for the Empress Eugenie and led to his appointment as perfumer to the Imperial Court, the bottle then being decorated with the Napoleonic bees. Made for use by both men and women, it contains bergamot, lemon, neroli, verbena, orange blossom, rosemary and various floral fragrances. It is now sold in a flacon by Baccarat.

Eau de Cologne Mint *see* Mint

'Eau de Givenchy' A fruity–floral quality fragrance brought out as an eau de toilette by Givenchy in 1980. It was created by the perfumers of Givaudan and designed to invoke the excitement of youth. Top notes of bergamot, mandarin, grapefruit and basil lead to a floral heart with honeysuckle, jasmine, rose, ylang-ylang, tuberose and narcissus, on a base which is predominantly sandalwood.

Eau de Parfum In modern perfumery this is the highest grade of Eau, being a perfumed toilet preparation containing substantially more perfume oil than either eau de cologne or eau de toilette. It usually contains 15–18% of perfume oil mixed with an 80–90% grade alcohol. See Perfume.

Eau de Portugal A toilet water popular in Europe during the 19th century. It was similar to eau de cologne. (See Appendix B, recipe no. 69.)

Eau de Toilette In modern perfumery this signifies a perfumed toilet preparation with a perfume oil content of 4–8% in an alcohol, thus stronger than eau de cologne and weaker than eau de parfum.

Eau de Vie A weak alcohol developed in France late in the 16th century for use as a solvent in extracting fragrance from gum resins.

Eau Fraiche A toilet water similar to eau de cologne, but made with a higher grade (around 80% pure) of alcohol. The name is also used as a brand name for fragrances by Dior and Léonard.

'Eau Sauvage' A trend-setting masculine eau de toilette, classified as a citrus fragrance, first brought out by Dior in 1966. It was created by Edmond Roudnitska. Principal constituents are bergamot, lemon and basil in the top note, jasmine and patchouli in the heart, and oak moss in the base. The bottle was designed by Pierre Camin.

Ecuelle   A method, formerly practiced in Italy but now only rarely used, for obtaining essential oil from the peel of citrus fruit by expression. The fruits were rolled about in a hollow vessel, the walls of which were covered in spikes which pricked the rinds, allowing the oil to escape.

'Edwardian Bouquet'   A quality floral perfume first issued by Floris in 1901 as a celebration of the Edwardian era. It was reintroduced in 1984 with a revised formula created by Douglas Cope. Its principal ingredients are hyacinth and bergamot in the top note, leading into a heart which is predominantly jasmine, and with base notes containing sandalwood and musk.

Egyptian Perfumes   The perfumes of Egypt were famous in the ancient world, and in the later periods of the Egyptian civilization they were exported both to Greece and Rome. Perfume recipes have survived from as early as 1600 BC and perfume artefacts have been found from as early as 3500 BC. Egyptian fashions in perfume changed over the centuries, but their general preference was for heavily scented perfumes and unguents. Food was often scented. Incense was used both in religious ceremonies and in the home. Aromatics were important in the processes of embalming and mummification (see Pissasphalt). The Egyptians set the fashion followed by both Greeks and Romans for rubbing perfumed oils and unguents into the body after a bath. Scented flowers were popular in the form of wreaths and garlands. Perfumed oils were generally made by steeping flower heads or other plant parts into an oil which was then strained through a cloth, the process being repeated several times until the oil was fragrant. Oil of moringa (oil of Ben), castor, linseed, safflower, olive, sesame and bitter almond were available for this purpose, but the most desirable of these base oils was Balanos, from a plant which grew only in Egypt. The wide range of fragrant substances used by the Egyptians included aloe, calamus, cardamom, cedar, citron, ginger-grass, heliotrope, henna (see Cyprinum), lily, myrtle, peppermint, rose and rosemary, together with resins such as galbanum, juniper, labdanum, myrrh, opoponax and storax; some of these resins were imported from the regions bordering the south of the Red Sea, known to the Egyptians as the Land of Punt, from as early as 1500 BC. The composition of a number of compound perfumes is known from inscriptions, surviving papyri and Greek writings; the most famous was Kyphi, a heady incense of many fragrant ingredients added to a base of raisins, honey and wine; other known compound perfumes include Kypros, Mendesian perfume, Metopian perfume and Sampsuchinon. An unusual way of applying perfume in ancient Egypt was the Unguent

Cone, made of perfumed fat and placed on the head to drip down as it melted. See also Herodotus.

Egyptian Plum Tree   *see* Balanos

Egyptian Privet   *see* Cyprinum

Elaphrium simarusa   *see* Tacamahac

Elder Flower Oil   An oil distilled from the fragrant blossom of a species of Elder (*Sambucus nigra*), a small shrub-like tree native to Europe. The oil has a very sweet, honey-like fragrance, but is present only in minute traces, so that its use is very limited. It is imitated synthetically.

The name Elder derives from Anglo-Saxon 'aeld', meaning 'fire', because the stems of the branches were easily hollowed out and were used to blow up fires. Hence also other names such as Pipe tree. The plant is surrounded by much tradition, partly deriving from the legend that Judas Escariot hanged himself from an Elder tree. It has been used in medicines and foods (and the berries to make a wine) since ancient times. The flowers have for long provided Elder Flower Water, which is used for cosmetic purposes and is mildly fragrant.

Elecampane Oil   An essential oil distilled from the roots of a herb Elecampane (*Inula helenium* = *Helenium grandiflorum*), also called Alant, Horseheal, Scabwort, Yellow Starwort, Velvet Dock, Wild Sunflower and Elf Dock. The plant, which grows up to 4 feet high, is found throughout Europe, the Balkans and central Asia, and is cultivated widely. The oil has a minty, violet-like odour and is used in flavouring and medicinally as well as in perfumery. The dried roots are used in sachets and pot pourri. The plant is mentioned in classical literature; Horace recorded its use in making a sauce and Pliny noted medicinal uses which included 'fastening the teeth'.

Elemi   A fragrant gum, yielding both a resinoid and an oil, which is obtained from species of *Canarium* and *Protium* trees: (1) from the Manila Elemi tree (*Canarium luzonicum*), also called the Elemi Canary tree, native to the Phillipines; both resinoid and oil have a fresh, spicy, lemon-like fragrance. The gum, also called Manila Elemi, is powdered and used in pomander pastes and as a fixative in sachets; (2) from the Java Almond tree (*Canarium communi*) of the Moluccas, cultivated in Malaysia. The resin, sometimes called Manila Resin, is used both as a perfume fixative and in incenses; (3) from the Incense Gum tree (*Protium attenuatum*) of the W. Indies; from *P. chapelieri* of Madagascar (the resin also being known as Ramy); from *P. guianese* of tropical America (the resin being called Elemi of Guiana); and from *P. heptaphyllum* of tropical America (the resin also being called Hyawa Gum or Ronima Resin). All the Elemi resins are used in incenses.

Elemi, West Indian   *see* Tacamahac

Elf Dock   *see* Elecampane

Elizabeth Arden   Founded by Florence Graham, an American of British parentage who opened her first salon on Fifth Avenue, New York, in 1910 to provide beauty treatment with natural products. The name was derived from a book 'Elizabeth and Her German Garden'. The company's first perfume, 'Blue Grass', was brought out in 1936 and was immensely successful. It was followed by other perfumes which include 'On Dit' (46), 'Mémoire Chérie' (57), 'Cabriole' (77) and the recently launched 'Red Door', but the firm's main business lies in cosmetics. In 1989 the company was acquired by Unilever.

Elletaria cardamomum   *see* Cardamom

Elqueme   *see* Tacamahac

Elutharia   *see* Cascarilla

Emblic   Also called Myrobalan. A shrub (*Phyllanthus emblica*) native to India and tropical Asia and cultivated for its fruits. Pliny noted that it was grown in Arabia, India and the Horn of Africa 'for its scent', which was obtained from its oil, the best being that from N. Arabia. The perfume recipes of al-Kindi show that the early Arab perfume makers used the fruit in their concoctions in conjunction with musk.

Emilio Pucci   Founded in 1947 by the fashion designer the Marquis Emilio Pucci (b. 1915), an Italian skiing champion and later an MP, to produce fashions and fashion accessories. The company entered the perfume market with 'Vivara' in 1967, subsequently producing 'Zadig' (72) and, for men, 'Signor Vivara' (70).

Encapsulation   In perfumery this describes the technique of enclosing perfume oils in minute gelatine capsules which are applied to the skin in an alcoholic mix and break whenever the skin is rubbed, thereby releasing further fragrance. *See also* Micro-fragrance.

Enebro   *see* Juniper

Enfleurage   A process first used by the ancient Egyptians, by which the petals or other fragrant parts of a plant are steeped in fat or a non-evaporating oil which will absorb their fragrance. In early times, balanos, almond, olive, sesame and mastic oils were used for this purpose; later oil of ben came into favour. Fats used included pork, lard and beef suet. The process has continued in use, with improved techniques, into modern times, with an increasing use of mineral oils, which do not become rancid. It enables perfume makers to take advantage of the fact that some flower heads continue to produce essential oil over a period of time, even after they have been picked; it therefore obtains a considerably greater amount of essential oil than other techniques. It is particularly appropriate for jasmine, tuberose, violet, jonquil, mignonette and rose. From the 17th century the French perfume industry carried out enfleurage on a commercial scale by laying the flower heads on sheets of glass coated with fat (the fat being treated with benzoin, styrax or musk to prevent it becoming rancid);

the frames of glass were pressed one upon the other; the process was repeated several times with fresh flower heads until the fat was totally absorbed with essential oil, the resultant substance being known as 'pomade'; the oil was then retrieved from the fat by dissolving in an alcoholic solvent, such oil being known as 'chassis'. This method is still in use. Sometimes enfleurage is now carried out with cloth soaked in olive oil or liquid paraffin, which is laid over the frames instead of fat, the resultant perfumed oil being then known as 'huile antique'.

English Galingale   *see* Cyperus

'English Lavender'   An early masculine eau de toilette, introduced by Atkinsons in 1910. It was the first brand name fragrance manufactured for male use to feature lavender. Its principal constituents are lavender and rosemary, which are apparent in the top note; the middle and lower notes are also fresh and herbaceous.

English Mace   A perennial herb *Achillea decolorens*. The dried leaves are used in sachets and pot pourri.

Erica arborea   *see* Bruyere

Eriocephalus   A shrubby plant, *Eriocephalus africanus*, native to East Africa and cultivated in the south of France. An essential oil extracted from the leaves and stems has a herbaceous balsamic odour.

Erodium moschatum   *see* Musk Geranium

Eryngium maritimum   *see* Sea Holly

Erythroxylon monogynum   *see* Devadari Oil

'Escada'   A floral perfume launched in 1990 by the German fashion house Escada, owned by Margaretha Ley, for whom it was created by perfumers of Créations Aromatiques. A top note containing bergamot, hyacinth, peach and coconut introduces a heart which includes jasmine, ylang-ylang, orris and orange flower, underlined by a base in which sandalwood, musk and vanilla predominate. The perfume comes in a hand-blown, heart-shaped bottle designed by Ben Kotyuk and Margaretha Ley.

Essence   A word often used loosely to mean Essential Oil. More strictly it signifies an alcoholic or aqueous plant extract; such extracts are seldom employed in modern perfumery but are widely used in cosmetics and flavourings.

Essence d'Amali   *see* Galingale

Essence d'Aspice   *see* Lavender

Essence de Bois Rose   *see* Linaloe

Essence Concrète   *see* Concrete

'Essence Rare'   A quality floral aldehyde perfume first brought out by Houbigant in 1930 and relaunched in 1976. Aldehydes in the top note, which contains bergamot, provide a cool, green effect. Rose predominates in the floral heart, which also includes geranium, lily of the valley and orris. The base note is principally vetivert, supported by oak moss, tonka, civet and musk. The perfume was originally marketed in a flacon by Baccarat.

Essential Oil   Also called volatile oil, ethereal oil and essence. The odorous oil contained in the flowers, buds, leaves, stems, wood, fruit, seeds, bark, gum, roots or rhizomes of a plant and sometimes in more than one of these parts. In some cases the whole plant contains essential oil and is therefore entirely fragrant. In some cases different essential oils, and therefore different fragrances, are obtained from different parts of the same plant (e.g. neroli, orange flower oil, oil of bigarade and oil of petitgrain, all from the Bitter Orange tree). Among flowers, those with the thickest petals contain most essential oil and white flowers tend to be the most fragrant (the rose being an exception). The oil distilled from flowers is known as attar. Essential oils have been obtained from about 57 different plant families, comprising several hundred different plants. There are several methods of obtaining the essential oil from plant material – see under Distillation.

In the 14th century it was recognized that, although insoluble in water, essential oils could be dissolved in alcohol, the alcoholic solution being known as an 'essence' (in French: *esprit*). Essential oils are composed of numerous organic compounds which chemists can now isolate and reproduce, enabling synthetic perfumes to be produced.

Estée Lauder   A New York perfume and cosmetics company established in 1946 by Mrs Estée Lauder, who entered the cosmetics business working for her uncle, a dermatologist. The company's first and highly successful perfume 'Youth Dew' was launched in 1952. It was followed by 'Estée Super' (68), 'Azurée' (69), 'Alliage' (72), 'Private Collection' (73), 'Cinnabar' and 'White Linen' (78), 'Beautiful' (86), 'Knowing' (89) and 'Spellbound' (91). Mrs Lauder has been closely involved in the creation of all her perfumes. The company now also owns Aramis.

'Estée Super'   A classic perfume of floral–sweet fragrance introduced by Estée Lauder in 1968. The top notes are aldehydic with a spicy touch from coriander, and give way to a heart mainly comprising rose, lily of the valley and jasmine, supported by tuberose and carnation, with base notes mostly of sandalwood and tree moss. The bottle was designed by Ira Levy.

Estragon Oil   *see* Tarragon

'Eternity'   A Calvin Klein perfume created by Sophia Grojsman of IFF and launched in 1989, which uses some ingredients made by living flower technology. It has floral top notes from lily, freesia and narcissus, leading into a fruity middle note in which apricot and peach predominate, with woody and musky base notes. The bottle was designed by Pierre Dinand.

Ethereal Oil   *see* Essential Oil

Ethyl Cinnamate   A natural component of storax and some other plants which has a sweet amber odour. For commercial use, however, it is manufactured artificially. It is used in oriental-type bouquets, in making amber colognes and in scenting soaps.

Eucalyptus   A fragrant oil is distilled from the leaves of several species of Eucalyptus tree, native to Australia. They include the Lemon-scented Gum tree, also called Citron-scented Gum tree or Spotted Gum tree (*Eucalyptus citriodora*) and the Lemon-scented Ironbark tree (*E. staigeriana* var. Muell.). The former, found in eastern parts of Australia, is now cultivated widely, including Europe, S. America, Indonesia, S. Africa and the Seychelles. The latter is cultivated in Brazil. The essential oil of these two trees, which is much used in perfumery for its lemony fragrance, contains up to 98% of citronellol. In addition are included *E. stuartiana*, the oil of which has an apple fragrance; *E. odorata*, which provides an oil used in scenting soaps; *E. macarthurii* (the Paddy River Box tree), the fragrant oil of which is rose-scented and valuable as a source of geraniol; and *E. globulus*, cultivated in Spain and Portugal, which provides an oil with a camphor-like fragrance used in scenting soaps. The name Eucalyptus derives from Greek meaning 'well-covered', from the cup-like membrane which covers the buds before they open.

Eucarya acuminata   *see* Sandalwood
      spicata   *see* Sandalwood
Eugenia aromatica   *see* Clove Oil
      caryophyllata   *see* Clove Oil

Eugenol   The principal chemical constituent of Oil of Cloves. It is also found in a number of other plants, including allspice, bay, cinnamon leaf, clove-pink, patchouli and pimento, providing a clove-like element in their fragrance. Eugenol is used in many synthetic perfumes. Isoeugenol is extracted from it by a further chemical process.

Eurangium   *see* Sumbul

European Bugle   *see* Ground Pine

Evaluator   A person employed in the perfume industry to locate and select fragrant materials suitable for the requirements of a perfume creator and manufacturer.

Everlasting Flower   Also called Italian Everlasting Flower, Curry Plant and Herb of St John (*Helichrysum augustifolium* and also *H. stoechas*). Small herbs native to southern Europe and cultivated there. An essential oil (Everlasting Flower Oil) with a fragrance between rose and camomile is extracted from the fresh flowers and used to give perfumes a flowery sweetness. The main production area is in Yugoslavia. This plant was not used in perfumery before the 19th century.

Evernia furfuracea   *see* Tree Moss
      prunastri   *see* Oak Moss

'Exclamation' ('Ex'cla-ma'tion')   A wide-selling fruity–floral perfume created by IFF perfumers for Coty, who launched it in the UK in 1990. In the USA it was voted the Best New Fragrance of 1988 and headed the mass-market best sellers list for 1989. The bottle is in the shape of an exclamation mark.

Expression   A method of extracting oil from plants or parts of plants by applying pressure. The ancient Egyptians gathered flowers in a cloth bag which was twisted until the oil dripped out; expression by similar means was practiced widely until the discovery of distillation. In modern perfumery the technique is mainly used to extract the fragrant oils of citrus fruit rinds, which are mostly crushed between rollers, the oil being separated from the resultant pulp by centrifuge. By this method essential oils, known as Agrumen Oils, are obtained from bergamot, citron, colobat, grapefruit, lemon, lime, mandarin and orange. Lemon and orange peel are also sometimes expressed by a process using sponges. In Italy lemon oil is also occasionally expressed by a process called ecuelle (q.v.).

Extraction   A process known more fully as extraction by volatile solvents. Volatile solvents, i.e. various substances such as ether or high-grade petroleum which evaporate rapidly, are used in modern perfumery to dissolve essential oils from fragrant plant and animal materials. The usual method involves placing the fragrant material on perforated metal plates in a container (the extractor); the solvent is passed over them and led into a still, where it evaporates, leaving a semi-solid mass known as concrete (q.v.), which contains the essential oil together with stearoptene. The essential oil can then be separated from the stearoptene by extraction with alcohol in a 'batteuse', producing the substance called absolute (q.v.), which is the purest and most concentrated form of essential oil known. Floral fragrances obtained by this method include carnation (clove-pink), cassie, jonquil, mimosa, narcissus, orange flower and ylang-ylang. See also Distillation and Enfleurage.

Extrait   The most concentrated form of perfume sold over the counter, consisting of 15–30% perfume oil in a high-grade alcohol. See Perfume.

Eye-bright   *see* Clary

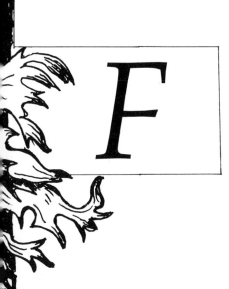

Factor *see* Max Factor

Fagara chalybea *see* Igugu

'Fahrenheit' A floral–woody–balsamic fragrance for men created for Dior by Jean-Louis Sieuzac and launched in 1988. The floral notes come mainly from hawthorn and honeysuckle, being built on to a base which includes sandalwood, cedar, storax and mastic (lentisk).

False Acacia Oil An essence, also called Robinia Oil, which is derived from the fragrant flowers of the False Acacia tree (*Robinia pseudoacacia*), also known as the Robinia tree and Locust tree, native to S. America but now grown widely. The oil is produced as a floral absolute by extracting the flowers with volatile solvents.

False Myrrh *see* Opoponax

False Quinquina *see* Cascarilla

Fan Stopper A flamboyantly ornate, fan-shaped perfume bottle stopper, often bigger than the bottle itself. Fan stopper bottles were introduced by Czechoslovakian glass makers in the 1930s. The style was adopted by American glass manufacturers, notably the Imperial Glass Company and the US Glass Company, in the 1940s, when war prevented further imports from Czechoslovakia, and is still used occasionally in commercial perfume bottle designs. See Perfume Containers.

Fargeon, J.H. A famous 18th century Parisian perfume maker who was appointed 'glover–perfumer' to the King (see under Gloves, scented).

He had a widespread business with other French cities and with other countries including Britain, but was forced into bankruptcy in 1788 because of unpaid bills, including one for over £20 000 worth of perfumes and cosmetics supplied to King Louis XV. His name appears on many perfume pots now collected as antiques.

Farnesol   A colourless, oily liquid which is found in musk, ambrette seed, cabreuva and some other oils. It is manufactured synthetically for use in perfumery, providing a delicate fragrance reminiscent of lily of the valley.

'Fatale'   A quality 'floriental' perfume created for Coty by IFF and launched in 1988. Osmanthus and rose mix with green tones in the top note, leading to a heart which includes jasmine, honeysuckle, orange flower, gardenia, tuberose, muguet, rose, carnation, narcissus and hyacinth, together with origanum and clove. In the base note sandalwood and oak moss are underlined by musk and amber.

Fath   *see* Jacques Fath

Featherfew   *see* Feverfew

Featherfool   *see* Feverfew

Female Frankincense   *see* Opoponax

'Femme'   The first of the Rochas perfumes, created by Edmond Roudnitska and launched by Marcel Rochas in 1944 as a tribute to his wife. 'Femme' is a trend-setting classic chypre perfume and is said to be the favourite perfume of Margaret Thatcher. Fruity top notes, dominated by peach, plum and apricot, give way to a floral middle note, chiefly jasmine and rose, underlined by patchouli and amber, with a backing of oak moss and vanilla, in the base notes. The flacon, in the form of a stylized female torso, was designed by Rochas himself in conjunction with Lalique.

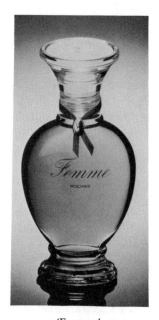
'Femme'.

Fendi   Parfums Fendi is a subsidiary of the Fendi International fashion house (itself now a part of the Sanofi group), which commenced in Rome in 1925 as a small fur and leather shop owned by Adele Fendi and is now run by her five daughters. Their perfume 'Fendi', created by Firmenich and launched in 1988, is a linear fragrance containing a floral bouquet, chiefly of rose, jasmine and ylang-ylang, on a base of patchouli, sandalwood, musk and amber, with hints of spice and leather. It is sold in a bottle designed by Pierre Dinand. A men's fragrance, 'Fendi Uomo', was put on the market in 1989.

Fennel   An essential oil used in perfumery is steam-distilled from the seeds of both Wild (or Common) Fennel (*Foeniculum vulgare*) and Garden Fennel (*F. officinale* = *F. capillaceum*). These plants, indigenous to the Mediterranean area, now grow from Europe to India and are cultivated for the oil in France, Germany, India, Iran, China, the USSR and elsewhere. Some other species (*F. azoricum*, *F. dulce*, *F. sativum* and *F. piperatum*) also provide aromatic oils. Fennel Oil is used in herbaceous-type perfumes. The name fennel derives from Latin *foenum*, meaning 'hay'; the oil contains coumarin and has an aroma resembling aniseed. Fennel has been cultivated in the Middle East, India and China for thousands of years, particularly for its culinary and medical properties. In medieval times it was hung over doors on Midsummer's Eve to ward off witches and evil spirits.

Fennel Flower   *see* Gith

Fenugreek   A clover-like annual (*Trigonella foenum-graecum* = *Follicugera graveolens* = *Foenumgraecum officinale*), also called Bird's Foot and Greek Hayseed, growing up to 2 feet high and cultivated, principally for fodder, in S. Europe, the Middle East, N. Africa and India. The name *foenum-graecum* means 'Greek hay', because it was once used by the Greeks to give a scent to inferior hay. The aromatic seeds, which contain coumarin, have been used since ancient times in cooking and medicines and provide the 'helba' of modern Egyptian dishes. Pliny described a Roman 'unguent of fenugreek', made with a number of other ingredients. The roots were sometimes used in the perfumes of the early Arabs. Today the dried seeds are used in sachets and pot pourri, while an oil extracted from them with volatile solvents is used to give tone in several types of perfume; it has a walnut-like fragrance.

Fern   The principal fern used in perfumery is the Common Male Fern (*Dryopteris felixmas*), abundant in Britain and found in Europe, temperate Asia, India and Africa. An essential oil, Oil of Male Fern, is extracted with volatile solvents from the rhizomes, mainly for medical and veterinary uses, but it is also used in fougere-type perfumes. The medicinal values of Oil of Male Fern have been recognized since the time of Theophrastus. See also Scented Maidenhair and Sweet Fern Oil.

Ferula asafoetida   *see* Asafoetida
       communis   *see* Ammoniacum
       galbanifera   *see* Galbanum
       marmarica   *see* Ammoniacum
       narthax   *see* Asafoetida
       persica   *see* Sagapenum
       sumbul   *see* Sumbul

Feverfew   Chrysanthemum   Also called Featherfew, Featherfool, Flintwort and Bachelor's Buttons. A perennial plant (*Chrysanthemum parthenium* = *Matricaria parthenium*) growing to about 28 inches high, native to the Mediterranean area and the Caucasus, but now widely grown in Europe, where it has been highly regarded for its medicinal properties. An essence, extracted from the leaves and flower heads, is used in medicines and liqueurs and occasionally in perfumes.

'Fidji' A quality floral perfume with fresh notes, created for Guy Laroche in 1966 by Josephine Catapano of IFF. Top notes of rose, ylang-ylang, jasmine, iris, tuberose and galbanum give way to heart notes of spices, clove and aldehydes, with an underlying base of sandalwood, patchouli and balsam of Peru. The bottle was designed by Serge Mansau.

Field Mint *see* Peppermint

Filipendula hexapetala *see* Dropwort

ulmaria *see* Meadowsweet Oil

Firmenich One of the world's leading wholesale fragrance and flavouring manufacturers (see Perfume Manufacture). Established in Switzerland in 1895 by two brothers-in-law named Chuit and Naes, the Firmenich Group's headquarters is in Geneva, where its main factory complex is situated. It has associated companies all over the world; the British company, Firmenich UK Ltd, was set up in 1949 and is based in Southall, Middlesex, while the US headquarters has been in Princeton since 1936. Firmenich established its scientific research department as early as 1902 and its chemists have won many international research awards, including a Nobel Prize. Besides making fragrances for a wide variety of purposes ranging from detergents and fabric softeners to hair shampoos and cosmetics, the company creates and manufactures over 10% of all the quality perfumes now on the market.

'First' A quality floral perfume which was the first fragrance issued by Van Cleef & Arpels. Created by Jean-Claude Ellena of Givaudan and launched in 1976, it contains fruity aldehydic top notes, heralding a floral heart led by jasmine, rose, lily of the valley, orris and tuberose. The base notes include vetivert, oak moss, sandalwood, amber and musk. The bottle was designed by Jacques Llorente.

Fixative A perfume ingredient which prolongs the retention of fragrance on the skin and makes other fragrant ingredients mixed with it last longer. It does this by prolonging the rate of evaporation of other ingredients, so that the aroma of the perfume mixture changes only gradually as the ingredients in it fade away. Fixatives, also known as 'fixators', are mostly plant materials containing gum, resin, balsam or slow-evaporating essential oil. Thus in ancient times myrrh, a gum resin, was highly valued because of its fixative qualities, while sandalwood oil has been an important fixative in Indian perfumes from ancient times until the present day. But the fragrant substances derived from animal sources (musk, ambergris, civet, castoreum and propolis) are also excellent fixatives. Among many other resinous materials which are valuable as fixatives may be listed: balsams of Copaiba, Peru and Tolu, frankincense, galbanum, labdanum, opoponax, storax and tacamahac. Essential oils with a fixative property include: basil, cedarwood, clove, costus, guaiacwood, mace, myrtle, orris, patchouli, saffron, spikenard, thyme, vetivert and ylang-ylang. Some plants, or parts of plants, are so rich in oils or resins with strong fixative properties that they are valuable as fixatives in themselves; these include aloewood, camomile flowers, cistus leaves, cloves, costus roots, orris roots, sassafras bark, tarragon leaves and verbena leaves. Synthetic fixatives, now much used, include musk ambrette, musk ketone, coumarin, isoeugenol and vanillin.

'Flair' A light chypre fragrance launched by Yardley in 1957 and now marketed as a cologne. Aldehydic in the top note, with bergamot predominating, the heart is principally jasmine, rose and gardenia, while the base contains oak moss and patchouli.

Flax *see* Linseed Oil

'Fleur de Fleurs' A quality floral–aldehyde all-purpose perfume introduced by Nina Ricci in 1980 which is based on a bouquet of white flowers. Created by the perfumers of Créations Aromatiques, it contains jasmine and rose (both from Grasse), hyacinth, ylang-ylang and iris. It is sold in a distinctive crystal flacon featuring a flower head made by Lalique.

Fleur de Lys *see* Iris (Yellow)

'Fleurs de Rocaille' A classic floral perfume created by Ernest Daltroff and brought out by Caron in 1933. Top notes led by rosewood and bergamot herald a middle note which includes jasmine, carnation, rose, orris and jonquil, with a woody base dominated by sandalwood with traces of musk and civet. The flacons were designed by Felicie Bergaud and Michel Morsetti.

Flirtwort *see* Feverfew

Floral Absolute *see* Absolute

Floral Concrete *see* Concrete

Floral Note Also Flower Note or Flowery Note. A term used in perfumery to describe the general fragrance of flowers. Almost all perfumes contain some proportion of floral notes. See Perfume Notes.

Floral–Fruity Note A term used in perfumery to describe a floral fragrance containing an extra element of fruit fragrance. Such effect is usually introduced into the top notes of a perfume which is predominantly floral. See Perfume Notes.

Floral Perfume A perfume with a predominantly floral (or flowery) note. About half of all the brand name perfumes now sold over the counter fall into this category, which forms one of the main 'families' into which perfumes are conventionally classified. See Perfume Families.

Floral Water   *see* Distillation

Florida Water   A toilet water which became very popular in the USA in the 19th century. It was regarded as combining the fragrances of lavender water and eau de cologne and was usually rounded off with cassia, clove or lemongrass oil. (See Appendix B, recipes nos 57 and 58.)

Floris   Founded in 1730 as a barber's shop in Jermyn Street, London, by a young Spaniard from Minorca, Juan Floris, who soon turned to making and selling fragrances. Floris is the oldest perfume house in the world. At the beginning of this century the business of J. Floris Ltd passed by marriage to the Bodenham family, who still run it from the original premises. The company's chief perfumer ('nose') is Douglas Cope and its factory is in Horsham. Floris have been perfumers to the monarch from 1820 onwards and currently hold royal warrants to supply both the Queen and the Prince of Wales. 'Lavender' was first sold in 1730 and the Floris list of some 18 current men's and women's fragrances also includes 'Jasmine', 'Lily of the Valley', 'Stephanotis' and 'Rose Geranium', all first sold in the 18th century, together with 'Malmaison', 'Sandalwood', 'Red Rose' and 'Special No 127' from the 19th century. Other fragrances include 'Edwardian Bouquet' (1901), 'Ormonde' (57), 'Florissa' (78) and 'Zinnia' (90).

'Florissa'   A quality floral perfume launched by Floris in 1978. Top notes of syringa and orange oil introduce a floral bouquet which includes a blending of rose, lily of the valley, jasmine and orris, with woody, ambery base notes mostly obtained from amber and sandalwood.

Flouve Oil   An oil obtained by steam-distillation from a dried grass, Spring Grass (*Anthoxanthum odoratum*), known in France as *flouve odorante* and grown for forage all over the world. Containing coumarin, it has a hay-like odour which is reminiscent of mimosa. It is used in many different types of perfume.

Flower de Luce   *see* Iris (Yellow)

Flower de Luce (White)   *see* Orris

Flower Note   *see* Floral Note

Flussiger Amber   *see* Storax

Foeniculum azoricum   *see* Fennel

       capillaceum   *see* Fennel

       dulce   *see* Fennel

       officinale   *see* Fennel

       piperatum   *see* Fennel

       vulgare   *see* Fennel

Foenumgraecum officinale   *see* Fenugreek

Foin-coupe (New-Mown Hay)   A type of perfume popular in the early 19th century which reproduced the odour of new-mown hay. It was based on coumarin with added lavender, bergamot and other fragrances.

Fokiena hodginsii *see* Bois de Siam

Follicugera graveolens *see* Fenugreek

Food of the Gods *see* Asafoetida

'Forever' A floral–oriental perfume launched by Yardley in 1991. Created by Roure perfumers, it contains ylang-ylang, marigold and citrus in the top notes, opening into a heart dominated by jasmine, orange flower and 'white florals', with sandalwood and sweet and musky undertones in the base. The bottle was designed by Coley Porter Bell.

Fougère In perfumery the term fougere (French for 'fern') describes a fragrance of fresh, herbaceous notes on a moss and fern-like base. It is especially popular in masculine fragrances. Fougère perfumes now form one of the main 'families' into which perfumes are conventionally classified. See Perfume Notes, Perfume Families and Fern.

'Fougère Royale' The first modern perfume marketed with a pronounced fougere-type fragrance. Created for Houbigant by Paul Parquet, the company's owner and principal perfumer, in 1882, it set a trend for a very large number of masculine fragrances devised later. The top notes, aromatic and fresh, with a preponderance of lavender and 'new-mown hay', yielded to a floral middle note based principally on rose and orange flower. The base note obtained the fougere effect from oak moss and musk with support which included tonka and vanilla. Houbigant issued a modified version of this perfume in 1959 in a flacon designed by Enrico Donati.

Fragonard Parfumerie Fragonard was established in Grasse by Eugene Fuchs after the Great War and is still run by his grandsons. It was named after the painter Fragonard, who lived in Grasse and whose father was a 'glover and perfumer' (see Gloves, scented). It creates and manufactures high-class perfumes and other fragrances for well-known perfume houses (e.g. 'Blue Grass', created for Elizabeth Arden in 1936), selling its products to tourists in Grasse (and from a factory in Eze, near Nice) under its own brand names. The company's first factory, in the centre of Grasse and originally owned by a perfume makers called Mottet, was built in 1783; it is now mostly a shop and museum, containing one of the finest collection of perfume items in the world.

Fragrance Blotter Also called Smelling Strip and Mouillette. A small strip or wand of absorbent paper which perfume makers dip into their mixtures, allow to dry and then sniff in order to test the perfume being created. See also Organ.

Fragrance Components The technical term in perfumery for the ingredients of a perfume. An average perfume may have some 30–50 components; some may have many more: 200–300 components is not uncommon in a modern quality perfume. The recently launched perfume 'Red' is claimed to contain 692 ingredients. See Perfume.

Fragrant Moss   An odorous lichen which grows on trees and is also known as Tree Moss (*Alectoria usnesides*). It was listed by Dioscorides, who noted its fragrant smell. This and a number of other species of odorous lichens were known to medieval Arabs under the single name *Ushna* and used by them in perfumery. See also under Oak Moss and Tree Moss.

Frangipani   Frangipani was originally a powdered perfume created in Rome by an aristocratic Renaissance family called Frangipani. It was made of orris and an equal amount of mixed spices, together with civet and musk. During the 15th century a member of the family developed this into a long-lasting liquid perfume by digesting it in wine alcohol. Perfumed gloves using the scent were known as 'Frangipani gloves'. Subsequently French colonists in the West Indies found a tree with a flower having a similar fragrance, *Plumiera alba*, and gave it the name Frangipani – a rare case of a plant being named after a perfume. (See Appendix B, recipe no. 64.)

The trees called Frangipani now embrace several species of *Plumiera*.

1. *Plumiera rubra*, also called Red Jasmine. This tree, native to Mexico, grows to a height of some 20 feet and is now cultivated in all tropical countries, its blossoms being used in vast quantities for garlands throughout the Orient and Africa.
2. *P. acutifolia*. The Pagoda tree of the Orient, as it is planted close to temples. Native to Mexico, Guatemala and the West Indies, but now grown on a substantial scale from Burma to China, Indonesia and the Philippines; the scent has been described as a mixture of tuberose and gardenia.
3. *P. alba*. Called White Frangipani, as that is the colour of its flowers, which have a jasmine-like fragrance.
4. *P. bicolor*. The flowers are said to have a scent between tuberose and jonquil.

Essential oil from all these flowers is used in modern quality perfumes (e.g. 'Coco' and 'Mystere').

Frankincense   Also called Olibanum, Gum Thus and, in both early and modern perfumery, Incense. A fragrant gum resin exuded from the trunks and branches of several species of small trees of the botanical classification *Boswellia*. The Arabian species, *Boswellia sacra*, which

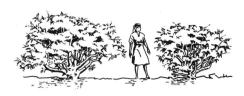

Frankincense (*Boswellia sacra*).

provides the best-quality frankincense, is found in south Arabia between Dhofar and, on a much lesser scale, Hadramawt. Three species grow in Somalia – *B. carteri*, *B. bhau-dajiana* and *B. frereana*. Frankincense of lesser quality is obtained from *B. serrata* (= *B. thurifera* = *B. glabra*), found in India, and from a larger tree, *B. papyrifera*, which grows in Ethiopia and neighbouring parts of Somalia. Other species of frankincense-producing *Boswellia* grow on the island of Soqotra. The gum is produced in small drops, known as tears, after incisions have been made in the bark.

Frankincense was a major perfume material in ancient times, used principally as an incense, either on its own or as an ingredient. There is record of Egyptian ships collecting it (with myrrh) in 1500 AD (see Egyptian Perfumes). Herodotus mentioned it as an import into Europe from Arabia c. 450 BC. From this time for about a thousand years substantial quantities were carried by highly organized camel caravans (which Pliny has described) from a collecting point at Shabwa, in south Arabia, along the 'incense road' to Petra and thence into Europe and the Levant. Under the Roman Empire this trade was supplemented by imports by sea from Qana, on the south Arabian coast, to Egyptian Red Sea ports, from where it was taken, together with spices brought from India, overland to the Nile, down the Nile by boat to Alexandria for sorting and processing, and thence by ship to Rome. The Romans burned frankincense on its own as the sacred incense for all religious and state ceremonies (see Roman Perfumes), in addition to which it was used domestically and had considerable value in medicines.

Frankincense is still burned in incenses, and the essential oil is used in fumigants and in perfumery; it is valuable as a fixative, though needing to be used in very small quantities because of the strength of its fragrance. It is one of the main ingredients in about 13% of all modern quality perfumes and 3% of all men's fragrances (for example, 'Amouage', 'Beautiful', 'Charles of the Ritz' and 'Jazz'). A purified form of resin called Kiou-nouk is also obtained from frankincense and used occasionally in perfumery.

Fraxmella dictamus   *see* Dittany

Freesia   Although the flowering plant (*Freesia refracta* and other species) is highly popular because of its fragrance, attempts at extraction have never been successful and the fragrance is reproduced synthetically. It appears in modern quality perfumes (e.g. 'Red Door' and 'Eternity').

French Lavender   *see* Lavender Cotton Oil

Fuming Pot   An earthenware pot with perforated sides used in Europe from the 15th to the 17th century to perfume or fumigate rooms and clothes.

Fusanus spicatus   *see* Sandalwood

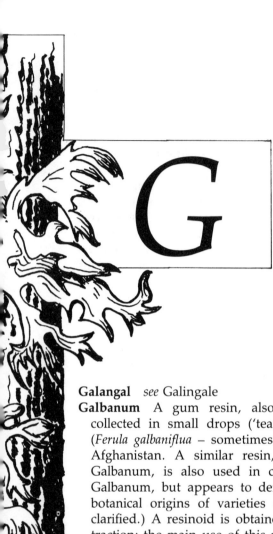

G

Galangal *see* Galingale

Galbanum A gum resin, also called Persian Galbanum, which is collected in small drops ('tears') from the stems of a giant fennel (*Ferula galbaniflua* – sometimes written *galbaniflora*) found in Iran and Afghanistan. A similar resin, of softer texture and called Levant Galbanum, is also used in commerce under the general name of Galbanum, but appears to derive from other species of *Ferula*. (The botanical origins of varieties of galbanum have never been exactly clarified.) A resinoid is obtained from galbanum resin by solvent extraction; the main use of this resinoid is in medicine. An essential oil steam-distilled from the resinoid is used in perfumery in a strong alcoholic extract, usually in combination with opoponax and ammoniacum. The odour has been described as spicy-green and leaf-like, and having a suggestion of musk. Galbanum Oil is valuable as a fixative but is also found in the top notes of quality perfumes (for example, in 'Chanel No. 19', 'Cabochard', 'Ysatis' and 'Xeryus'). The resin is also used as a fixative in sachet powders.

A resin from the stem of a herb *Laretia acaulis*, which grows in mountainous areas of Chile, is sometimes used as a substitute for galbanum.

Galbanum appears in the Old Testament as an ingredient of the holy incense (Exodus) and 'a pleasant odour' (Ecclesiasticus). It is also mentioned by Pliny as an ingredient of the Egyptian perfume called Metopian. As the odour of *F. galbaniflua* resin is unremarkable and, when burned, even disagreeable, it seems probable that in ancient times the name referred to the product of a different plant, either another species of *Ferula* or, as some believe more probably, *Peucedan galbaniflora* (see Peucedan Gum).

Galimard   Parfumerie Galimard, based in Grasse, was established in 1747 by Jean Galimard, founder of the French 'Corporation of Glovers and Perfumers' (see Gloves, scented), and originally supplied the French court with 'olive oil, pomades and perfumes'. It now manufactures perfumes and other fragrant products for prominent perfume houses, selling them under its own brand names to tourists visiting its premises in Grasse (and Eze, near Nice), where it also has a museum of perfume artefacts.

Galingale   A rose-like essential oil called Galingale, Galangal or Galanga is extracted from the rhizomes of the Lesser Galangal plant (*Alpinia officinarum = Languas officinarum*), also called China Root, India Root, Colic Root, East India Catarrh Root and Gargant, indigenous to S.E. Asia and cultivated in Thailand and China. The resin from the root relieves indigestion and the roots were once used by the Arabs 'to make their horses fiery'. Galanga perfume, which is particularly popular in India, was being widely used as early as the 15th century. The dried roots were once much used as a spice and today they are added to sachets and pot pourri.

A fragrant essential oil, known as Essence d'Amali, is extracted from the roots of the Greater Galangal plant (*Alpinia galanga = Languas galanga*) also called Langwas, a considerably larger plant, native to tropical Asia, which is cultivated for this purpose. Essence d'Amali is also obtained from the rhizomes of another, related species, *A. malaccensis*, found in N. India and Malaysia.

Gallium odorata   *see* Woodruff

Gallnut   The gallnut, or oakapple, formed by an insect on the leaves of oak trees (*Quercus infectoria* and other species), was an ingredient in a solid, fragrant mixture called Sukk (q.v.), which was a popular perfume among the Arabs of early medieval times.

Gamelo   *see* Balsam of Copaiba

Gardenia   Essential oils used in perfumery are extracted from the flowers of species of gardenia, trees or shrubs native to India, China, Japan and Indo-China but cultivated elsewhere. They include Cape Jasmine, or Garden Gardenia (*Gardenia jasminoides = G. florida*), of Chinese origin (where it is used to scent tea), with flowers having a fragrance reminiscent of jasmine; *G. citriodora*, with flowers having a distinct scent of orange flower; and *G. deroniana*, found in the W. Indies, with flowers of a fragrance suggesting jasmine. The yield of concrete from *G. jasminoides* is about 1 kilo from 3 to 4 thousand kilos of flowers, the concrete providing 500 g of absolute; the product is therefore extremely expensive. Synthetic gardenia perfumes are usually based on jasmine, tuberose and orange blossom. Gardenia is used in modern high-quality perfumes (e.g. 'Jolie Madame', 'L'Air du Temps' and 'Ma Griffe').

'Gardenia-Passion'   A high-quality single-note perfume created and launched by Annick Goutal in 1989. It is composed entirely of natural elements, synthesizing the aroma of the gardenia flower by a combination which includes jasmine, tuberose, orange blossom and mosses. It is sold in a ball-shaped flacon with a stopper featuring a butterfly.

Gargant   *see* Galingale

Garland Flower   Also called Butterfly Lily. A flowering plant growing up to 5 feet high (*Hedychium flavum*) of Indian origin. A concrete is extracted from the flower heads for use in perfumery.

Gaultheria   Oil of Gaultheria, also called Wintergreen Oil, is distilled from the leaves of a small N. American evergreen shrub, growing up to 6 inches high underneath trees and other shrubs, called Gaultheria (*Gaultheria procumbens*), also known as Wintergreen, Winter-berry, Tea Berry and Box Berry. The oil, which is very powerful and has a fresh, medicinal odour, is used in flavourings and medicines as well as in perfumes. Its principal constituent is methyl salicylate. A similar oil is also obtained by steam-distillation from the leaves of the Indian Wintergreen (*G. fragrantissima*) of N. America, and also from *G. fragrantissima* var. *punctata* and *G. leucocarpa*, both found in Indonesia, where they are used locally in perfumes and as hair oils.

'Gem'   A quality floral–oriental perfume brought out by Van Cleef & Arpels in 1987. It was created by the perfumers of Firmenich. Marigold and camomile in the top notes herald a heart which includes jasmine, tuberose and ylang-ylang, together with spicy elements from coriander, clove, sage and cardamom. The base notes are dominated by cypress, patchouli and vanilla. The bottle was designed by Joel Desgrippes and is made by Brosse.

Genêt perfume   *see* Broom

Genévrier   *see* Juniper

Geoffrey Beene   *see* Sanofi

Geraniol   An odorous chemical found in the rose and also obtainable from citronella, geranium, ginger grass, palma rosa, one species of eucalyptus and some other plants. It is also manufactured synthetically from pinene. It is used at the present time in a large number of synthetic perfumes.

Geranium   The Geranium, or Pelargonium, which originates from S. Africa, numbers over 300 species, of which many are scented, providing essential oils by steam-distillation of the leaves and stems. The oils have a range of fragrances resembling, among others, apple, camphor, citronella, eucalyptus, lemon, lime, mint, nutmeg, orange, pennyroyal, pine, pineapple, rose, sage and wormwood. Species with a rose fragrance are particularly in demand; rose–geranium oil is made from the Rose–Geranium (*Pelargonium graveolens*), first introduced into Europe in 1690, by a process of distillation with rose petals – see Geranium sur Rose. Other popular rose-scented species include *P. roseum* and *P. odoratissimum*. One of the most commonly cultivated species is *P. capitatum*, the oak-leaved geranium, which provides an oil with a musky lemon odour. Other species cultivated for their fragrant oil include: *P. citriodorum* (citrus); *P. cristum-minus* (melissa); *P. extipulatum* (pennyroyal); *P. fragrans* (pine-nutmeg); *P. radula* (balsam); and *P. tomentosum* (peppermint). The principal chemical substance contained in geranium oil is geraniol. Cultivation of this plant for the oil now extends to France, Spain, Algeria, Morocco, the USSR, Madagascar, Sri Lanka, East Africa, Réunion and the USA. See also Mawah Oil. Geranium Oil is an ingredient in many modern quality perfumes (e.g. 'Gucci No. 1', 'L'Aimant' and 'Paris'). The plant should not be confused with musk geranium.

Geranium macrorhizum   see Zdravets

Geranium Moschatum   see Musk Geranium

Geranium Oil, Indian   see Gingergrass Oil

Geranium sur Rose   A fragrant oil prepared in Grasse on a large scale from 1847 onwards by distilling geranium oil with rose petals. See Geranium.

German Jasmine   see Mock Orange Blossom

Geum urbanum   see Avens

Ghaliya   The most luxurious of all the standard compound perfumes of the early Arabs. The principal fragrance was musk, with added ingredients such as ambergris and camphor, on a base of ben oil. The name itself means, in Arabic, 'expensive', being derived, it is said, from the comment of the Caliph of Baghdad on being told what the ingredients were.

Giant Hyssop   The name of two species of a herb (*Agastache pallidiflora* and *A. anethiodora*) native to the S.W. region of the USA. An essential oil (Oil of Giant Hyssop) is distilled from the leaves; it has a fragrance halfway between peppermint and thyme. See also Hyssop.

Gillyflower   The name Gillyflower is applied to several species of flowering plants which have in common a fragrance reminiscent of cloves and are therefore all used in perfumery. These are Wallflower, Stock and Clove-pink (Carnation). The name is also used for Sea Pink (Thrift) (*Armeria maritima* = *A. elongata* = *A. vulgaris* = *Statice armeria*), which grows in Europe and Asia.

Ginepro   see Juniper

Ginger   Ginger (*Zingiber officinale* = *Amomum zingiber*) is a tall, perennial, reed-like plant, native to western Asia. The rhizomes provide the substance ginger, for which the plant is cultivated in India, the Far East, Africa, the West Indies and other tropical parts of the Old and New World. Ginger has been produced in India and the Far East since ancient times and was one of the spices imported by the Romans. The rhizomes are used in sachets and pot pourri, and Oil of Ginger is steam-distilled from them and used in perfumery as a toner (e.g. in 'Montana').

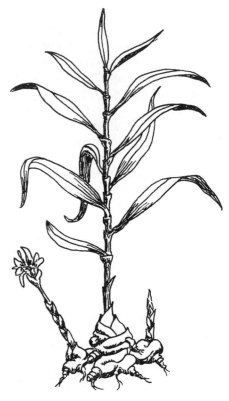

Ginger (*Zingiber officinale*)

Ginger, American Wild   *see* Canadian Snakeroot

Ginger, Green   *see* Wormwood

Ginger Grass Oil   A spicy-scented oil distilled from a variety of Rosha (Rusa) Grass (*Cymbopogon martinii*) called Sofia growing in moist areas of India and Indonesia. It is used in soaps and low-grade perfumes. Another variety of Rosha Grass produces the superior Palma Rosa Oil. A similar oil is obtained from a similar plant, also called Ginger Grass (*Andropogon odoratus* = *A. aromaticus*) found in the Far East.

Gingle Oil   *see* Sesame

Ginny Grains   *see* Grains of Paradise

Giorgio Armani   A fashion tailor, born 1936, who founded the firm which bears his name in 1975. In 1982 he launched his first perfume for women, 'Armani', in an octagonal bottle designed by Pierre Dinand, followed in 1984 by a fragrance for men 'Armani Eau pour Homme'. The company is now owned by L'Oreal.

Giorgio Beverly Hills   Originally a well-known fashion boutique which opened in Beverly Hills, California, in 1961 under the ownership of Fred and Gale Hayman. In 1981 they launched their first perfume, 'Giorgio Beverly Hills', using the boutique's yellow and white awnings in the packaging design. Created by the perfumers of Florasynth, this perfume, which is floral and made to give an instant and very strong effect, was the first of the so-called linear fragrances. It includes rose, jasmine, gardenia and orange flower in its main body, with a base note principally comprising sandalwood, patchouli and camomile. It comes in a bottle made by Brosse. One of the top-selling perfumes of the 1980s, it was followed in 1984 by 'Giorgio Beverly Hills for Men' and in 1986 by 'VIP Special Reserve for Men'. In 1987 the company was bought up by Avon, under which it launched 'Red' in 1989.

Giroflee   *see* Wallflower

Giroflier   *see* Wallflower

Gith   Also called Git, Black Cumin, Melanthion, Fennel Flower, Roman Coriander and Nutmeg Flower. A small annual (*Nigella sativa*) related to 'Love-in-the-Mist', growing up to 12 inches high and native to Syria, but now found from central Europe to N. Africa and western Asia. It is not related to Fennel. The plant is cultivated on a large scale in the eastern Mediterranean area, where the seeds are sprinkled on bread. In perfumery, the seeds, which have a coriander-like odour, are used in sachets and pot pourri, and in India they are placed in linen to deter insects. They were used for flavouring and in medicines in ancient Egypt and Rome, hence the name Roman Coriander, and are said to have been introduced into temperate Europe by returning crusaders. See also Nigella Oil.

Givaudan   The Givaudan Group, based in Switzerland, is one of the world's leading wholesale producers of fragrances and flavours (see Perfume Manufacture). The company was founded in 1895 by two French brothers, Leon and Xavier Givaudan, both chemists, to supply the French perfume houses from a factory at Vernier, near Geneva, where its headquarters are still located. In 1963 it became a part of the Hoffmann-La Roche group of companies.

Givaudan is now represented by subsidiary companies all over the world, the British subsidiary, Givaudan & Co Ltd, being based at Whyteleafe, in Surrey. About 10% of all the quality perfumes now sold by the major perfume houses are Givaudan creations, in addition to which it manufactures fragrances for clients for a wide range of products from hair lotions, cosmetics and soaps to detergents and aerosols. Its production of flavourings for the wholesale food market is equally substantial. It also undertakes considerable research activity (its laboratories developed, for example, Parsols to protect the skin from sunburn). Its Vernier headquarters includes a training school for perfumers.

Givenchy   Parfums Givenchy was founded in 1957 as a branch of the Paris fashion house established five years earlier by Hubert de Givenchy (b. 1927), a close colleague of Balenciaga. It is now part of the Louis Vuitton–Moet–Hennessey group (together with Dior and Christian Lacroix – see 'C'est la Vie'). Its factory complex at Beauvais was opened in 1969. Its main perfumes and fragrances include:

'L'Interdit' (1957), 'Le de Givenchy' (57), 'Monsieur de Givenchy' (59), 'Givenchy III' (70), 'Givenchy Gentleman' (75), 'Eau de Givenchy' (80), 'Ysatis' (84), 'Xeryus' (86) and 'Amarige' (91).

'Givenchy III' An innovative chypre–green perfume created by the perfumers of IFF for Givenchy, who launched it in 1970. Designed for the career woman, it has mainly bergamot and mandarin top notes, which lead into a floral heart of lily of the valley, hyacinth, rose and jasmine. The principal base notes are oak moss, sandalwood and patchouli. The flacon was designed by Pierre Dinand.

Gladden *see* Calamus

Glechoma hederacea *see* Ground Ivy

Gloves, scented Also called Perfumed Gloves. A fashion among women for wearing scented leather gloves developed early in the 16th century in Spain and Portugal and spread among all the nobility of Europe (see Grasse). In England, Queen Elizabeth started to wear them after the Earl of Oxford had brought her a pair from Italy (c. 1575) and by the time of Charles I they were used so widely that glove-makers were usually also perfumers. In France, perfume makers were 'Glovers and Perfumers' until the 18th century. It was believed that scented gloves kept the skin of the hands white and soft, and for this reason they were even worn in bed. The perfumes used to scent Queen Elizabeth's gloves contained ambergris, civet and orange flower butter, but musk and many other long-lasting fragrances were also used, the very strong scents having to survive frequent washings. (See Appendix B, recipe no. 35.)

Glycine An alternative name for Wisteria as used in perfumery. The Wisteria plant (*Wisteria sinensis*) is a climbing shrub native to China and now grown widely, bearing flowers with a 'peppery and rosy' or 'honey-like' fragrance. The natural oil is not much used in perfumery, but the fragrance is imitated synthetically. The name Glycine is also given to some perfume 'bouquets' made from violet, lilac and jasmine.

Goatnut tree *see* Jojoba Oil

Golden Rod *see* Sweet Golden Rod Oil

Goldy Star *see* Avens

Gomenol *see* Cajuput

Gonostylus miquelianus *see* Ramin Oil

Goutal *see* Annick Goutal

Grains of Paradise Also called Ginny Grains, Guinea Pepper, Meleguata Pepper, Greater Cardamom and Maniguette. The seeds of a perennial, reed-like plant (*Aframomum meleguata*), found in W. Africa, and a similar plant (*Ampelopsis grana paradisi*), also called Habzeli, found in Ethiopia (these plants may be identical). When crushed, the seeds release a sharp, spicy fragrance suggesting ginger and eucalyptus. Grains of Paradise were popular in Britain in medieval times both as a flavouring and to add a spicy note to pomanders and sachets. They are still used in sachets and pot pourri and also in incenses.

Grape   *see* Oil of Cognac

Grapefruit Oil   An oil obtained by expression from the fruit peel of the grapefruit tree (*Citrus paradisi*), which probably originated in the W. Indies but is now cultivated widely. It is largely used in flavouring, but is sometimes found in colognes and quality perfumes (e.g. 'White Satin' and 'Ricci Club'). The dried peel is used in sachets and pot pourri.

Grasse   The town in Provence, in the south of France, which has been the centre of the French perfume industry since the 16th century (see also Montpellier). Originally well known for their leather goods, Grasse tanneries took a leading part in the 16th century in making perfumed leather articles and especially in catering for the fashion, introduced by Catherine de Medici from Italy, for wearing fine-quality scented gloves (see under Gloves, scented); at the same time, Catherine de Medici had a laboratory established in Grasse to study perfume so that French perfumers could compete with the Arabs (see Arab Pefumes). The location and unusually even climate of the Grasse region was particularly well suited for growing plants for perfumery; by the end of the 17th century Grasse was already producing oils of cassie, hyacinth, jasmine, jonquil, narcissus, orange blossom, rose, tuberose and violet. In the present century the range and quantity of fragrant plants growing in the region was enormous. At one time Grasse was handling 2000 tons of jasmine flowers a year, and until recently its factories were processing 370 tons of roses and 270 tons of violet leaves annually. The only other comparable centre growing flowers for perfumes is Kazanluk, in Bulgaria. During the 1980s the rising value of land and the high cost of labour have considerably reduced the scale of cultivation around Grasse, with Morocco and Egypt, for example, taking over much of the rose and jasmine production. But Grasse remains the perfume capital of the world, with some 30 factories processing perfume materials, including those of Roure, Molinard, Fragonard, Galimard, Houbigant, Chanel and Quest.

   In 1989 the Musée International de la Parfumerie was opened in Grasse to provide a permanent exhibition of the history of perfumery; the museum has a conservatory containing a display of the more important plants cultivated for perfume materials, and it possesses many rare and valuable pieces, from ancient Egyptian, Greek and Roman scent bottles to the travelling toilet case which belonged to Queen Marie-Antoinette.

Greek Perfumes   Perfume was used by the ancient Greeks from earliest days, being mentioned frequently by Homer (10th century BC). It was offered to the gods, used to provide fragrance in cooking, and employed for medicinal purposes and personal hygiene, as well as being enjoyed simply for the pleasure it gave. Sometimes different perfumes were used for different parts of the body, as is satirized by Antipanes: 'He really bathes in a large gilded tub, and steeps his feet and legs in rich Egyptian unguents; his jaws and breasts he rubs with thick palm oil, and both his arms with extract of sweet mint, his eyebrows and his hair with marjoram, his knees and neck with essence of ground thyme.'

The Greeks were particularly fond of perfume made from flowers, but used a wide variety of other ingredients. As early as 450 BC, Herodotus recorded that frankincense, myrrh, and other aromatic gums, were imported from Arabia. Our most detailed knowledge of Greek perfumes comes from the botanist Theophrastus, who wrote both on botany and on perfumes. He observed that in his time (which encompassed the conquests of Alexander the Great) spikenard, cardamom and other materials were brought to Greece from India. Theophrastus described several compound perfumes popular with the Greeks, including Mendesian (called in Greece 'the Egyptian'), Kypros, Megalaeion, Rose Perfume and Susinon. Another favourite compound perfume was Metopian. Theophrastus also mentioned several important perfumes based on single plants, including gilliflower, bergamot, thyme, saffron, myrtle, quince, and a perfume based on marjoram which also contained costus. Balanos and sesame oil were recommended as base oils. Besides the plants mentioned above, he recorded a number of others used by the Greeks in perfume making, including: cassia, cinnamon, a balsam, storax, iris, all-heal, camel-grass, sweet-flag and dill. A perfume called Oenanthe was made from vine leaves. Scented powders made from dried aromatic plants, and used by sprinkling over clothes, were sometimes fortified with Magma. Most of the Greek perfume makers were women.

Green Ginger   *see* Wormwood Oil

Green Notes   The term 'green' is used in perfumery to denote the general fragrance of grasses and green plant parts. Green fragrances are much used in modern perfumery to give a special touch to Top Notes. Green Perfumes, i.e. perfumes with a predominantly green effect, form one of the principal 'families' into which perfumes are conventionally divided. See Perfume Notes and Perfume Families.

Grès   A company formed in the 1930s by a sculptor/painter, Madame Alix Grès (b. 1910). Forced to close during the war, she resumed her business in Paris in 1945. Her first perfume, 'Cabochard' was launched in 1958, followed by 'Alix' (82), 'Cabotine' (90) and three men's fragrances.

Grey-backed Acacia   *see* Gum Arabic

Grojsman, Sophia   An American perfumer of Russian origin, now senior perfumer for IFF in the USA. She is one of the few prominent women 'noses'. Her creations include 'Eternity', 'Paris', 'Trésor', 'Vanderbilt', 'Escape', 'Spellbound' and 'White Diamonds'.

Ground Ivy Also called Alehoof, Aleroot and known by many other local names, including Candlesticks, Catsfoot, Creeping Jenny, Devil's Candlesticks, Gill-go-by-the-Hedge, Haymaids, Hedge Haymaids, Lizzy-run-up-the-Hedge, Robin-run-in-the-Hedge and Tun-hoof. A perennial evergreen plant (*Glechoma hederacea* = *Nepeta glechoma* = *N. lederacea*) with blue to purple flowers, closely related to Catmint. It grows widely in Europe, Asia and Japan. The steam-distilled essential oil, known in perfumery as Ivy Oil, has a balsamic odour and is occasionally used in quality perfumes. Small quantities of the dried leaves are used in sachets and pot pourri. Ground Ivy Oil was once used to clarify beer.

Ground Needle *see* Musk Geranium

Ground Pine Also called Yellow Bugle and European Bugle. A small aromatic herb (*Ajuga chamaepitys*) which grows up to 8 inches high. It is a native of Europe but is now found widely in the Levant and N. Africa. When crushed, all parts of the plant have a strong pine-like odour. The dried leaves are used in sachets and pot pourri.

Guaiac, Oil of *see* Champaca Wood Oil

Guadil Oil *see* Rhodium Oil

Gucci Founded in Florence in 1904 as a leather factory by Guccio Gucci, a saddle maker, who turned to producing canvas luggage when leather was in short supply after the Great War. The House of Gucci now produces a wide range of high-quality goods. It is still run by the Gucci family. House of Gucci perfumes commenced in 1974 with the launching of 'Gucci No. 1'. Subsequent fragrances have been 'Gucci pour Homme' (76), 'Eau de Gucci' (82), 'Gucci No. 3' (85) and 'Nobile' (88).

'Gucci No. 1' Gucci's first perfume, created for him by Guy Robert in 1974. This classic floral perfume with a spicy touch is composed with an emphasis on natural products. It is predominantly bergamot in the top note, with rose, geranium, neroli, iris, ylang-ylang and jasmine in a floral bouquet in the middle note, and coriander, patchouli and oak moss in the base note.

'Gucci No. 3' A floral–aldehyde perfume created by the perfumers of Firminich for Gucci in 1985. Aldehyde top notes introduce a floral bouquet in the heart of rose, jasmine, narcissus and iris on a base which includes patchouli, vetivert and amber. The flacon, in a style reminiscent of architectural columns, was designed by Peter Schmidt.

Guerlain One of the earliest of the great French perfume houses, Guerlain was founded in 1828 when Pierre Guerlain, a chemist, opened a shop in Paris to sell scents and toiletries; his first perfume, 'Lotion de Guerlain' was produced in 1850. The company is still run by the Guerlain family and now has a world-wide business, with factories at

Courbevoie and Chartres manufacturing perfumes, beauty preparations and cosmetics. Since it was founded it has created more than 120 different fragrances; currently it makes more quality perfumes than any other perfume house. Its fragrances have all been created by members of the Guerlain family, notably Jacques Guerlain, the 'nose' for fragrances brought out between 1912 and 1933, and Jean-Paul Guerlain, for those from 1960 onwards. Fragrances currently marketed include: 'E de C Imperiale' (1850), 'Jicky' (1889), 'Après l'Ondée' (1906), 'L'Heure Bleue' (12), 'Mitsouko' (19), 'Shalimar' (25), 'Liu' (29), 'Vol de Nuit' (33), 'Vetiver' (60), 'Chant d'Aromes' (62), 'Habit Rouge' (64), 'Chamade' (70), 'Parure' (75), 'Nahema' (79), 'Jardins de Bagatelle' (84), 'Derby' (85), 'Samsara' (89). Many of the early Guerlain perfumes are sold in flacons designed by Baccarat, the later ones in flacons by Robert Granai.

Guaiacwood Oil   *see* Champaca Wood Oil

Guinea Pepper   *see* Grains of Paradise

Gulhina   *see* Cyprinum

Gum Acacia   *see* Gum Arabic

Gum Ammoniack   *see* Ammoniacum

Gum Arabic   Also called Gum Acacia, Gum Senegal, Gum Turick, Picked Turkey and Acacia Sorts. The dried gum obtained from a thorny tree, the Gum Arabic Acacia, or Grey-backed Acacia (*Acacia senegal*) and some ten other species of Acacia found in Africa, Arabia and India. The gum is tapped, when it exudes in honey-coloured tears or lumps. It is used in perfumery as a bonding agent, particularly for incense pastes, sometimes in combination with Gum Tragacanth. It appears in recipes of the early Arab perfume makers. See Perfume Making at Home (under 'Pomanders') and Appendix B, recipe no. 27.

Gum Benjamin   *see* Benzoin

Gum Draganth   *see* Tragacanth

Gum Dragon   *see* Tragacanth

Gum Mastic   *see* Mastic

Gum Senegal   *see* Gum Arabic

Gum Thus   *see* Frankincense

Gum Tragacanth   *see* Gum Arabic

Gum Turick   *see* Gum Arabic

Gurjun Balsam   A balsam obtained from the wood of species of Gurjun trees (*Dipteracarpus turbinatus, D. tuberculatus* and some others) found in India and throughout S.E. Asia. An oil is steam-distilled from the balsam. It has a weak odour of warm wood with a hint of patchouli and is occasionally used in perfumery as a fixative.

Gutta Ammoniaca   *see* Ammoniacum

Guy Laroche   A fashion firm opened in Paris by the clothes designer Guy Laroche (b. 1923) in 1957. His first perfume, 'Fidji', was launched in 1966. In 1977 he produced 'J'ai Osé' (bottle designed by Serge

Mansau) and in 1982 the men's fragrance 'Drakkar Noir' (bottle designed by Pierre Dinand). The company is now owned by L'Oréal.

Gymnocladus chinensis   *see* Pingshe-Feitsao

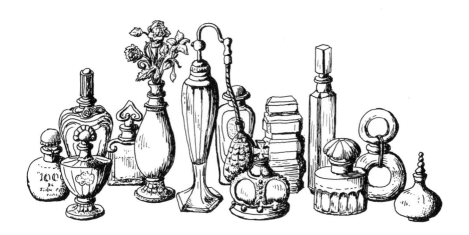

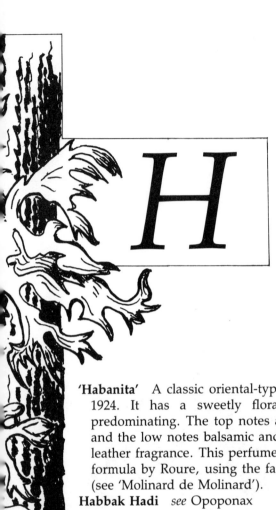

H

'Habanita' A classic oriental-type perfume brought out by Molinard in 1924. It has a sweetly floral heart, with rose and ylang-ylang predominating. The top notes are fruity, mostly bergamot and peach, and the low notes balsamic and powdery, dominated by vanilla and a leather fragrance. This perfume was relaunched in 1988 with a revised formula by Roure, using the famous Lalique flacon known as 'Beauty' (see 'Molinard de Molinard').

Habbak Hadi *see* Opoponax

Habzeli *see* Grains of Paradise

Hair Powder In 17th and 18th century Europe there was a widespread demand for hair powders, used for cleaning wigs and giving them a fashionable grey–white appearance. Such powders were supplied by perfumers, often being scented with musk, rose and other fragrances.

'Halston Z-14' A trend-setting chypre-type fragrance for men produced by Halston in 1976 for use in men's toiletries. Its main ingredients are bergamot and lemon in the top note, jasmine and patchouli in the middle note and amber and leather fragrance in the lower note.

Handflower *see* Wallflower

Hang Kan A woody vine (*Hanghomia marseillei*) native to Indonesia and Malaysia. The aromatic roots are burnt as incense in local pagodas and a liquid and a powder made from the roots are used locally in religious ceremonies.

Hardwickia Balsam   *see* Balsam of Copaiba
Hardwickia pinnata   *see* Balsam of Copaiba
Hart's Tree   *see* Melilot
Hawthorn   Also called May Blossom. A hedge tree (*Crataegus oxycantha*) native to northern Europe and Asia with flowers having a spicy, almond-like fragrance. The hawthorn was regarded by the Greeks as a tree of fortune and by the Romans as a symbol of marriage. It is not used as a natural material in perfumery; the Hawthorn or May Blossom fragrances of the present day are made synthetically, being used in particular to provide freshness and 'sparkle'. The fragrance appears in many modern quality perfumes (e.g. 'Paris' and 'Fahrenheit').
Hay Plant   *see* Woodruff
Hayfield Notes   A term used in perfumery to describe fragrances, usually based on coumarin, which have an odour of new-mown hay. See Perfume Notes.
Hazelcrottle   A lichen, also called Hazelraw, Lungwort and Rage (*Lobaria pulmonaria*), found in sub-alpine woods of Europe. It yields an essential oil found in perfumery.
Hazel Nut Oil   Also called Filbert Oil. An oil extracted from the fruits of the European Hazel tree (*Corylus avellana*), found in Europe and temperate Asia and cultivated widely. The oil has many uses, including its use in perfumery.
Hazelwort   *see* Asarabacca
Head   *see* Perfume Notes
Heart   *see* Middle Note
Heavy Notes   In perfumery the term 'heavy' denotes a fragrance in which the least volatile ingredients, such as mossy or animalic ones, are dominant, giving a very strong effect. Such fragrances are mostly used in chypre and oriental-type perfumes. See Perfume Notes.
Hedychium flavum   *see* Longosa Oil
        spicatum   *see* Kapur-kachri
Heinsea pulchella   *see* Bush Apple
Helenium grandiflorum   *see* Elecampane
Helichrysum augustifolium   *see* Everlasting Flower
        stoechas   *see* Everlasting Flower
Heliotrope   A fragrant oil used in perfumery which is obtained from the flowers of the Heliotrope (*Heliotropium peruvianum* and related species), also called (because of its aroma) Cherry Pie. The plant is an annual growing up to 2 feet high which originated in Peru but was introduced into Europe in the mid-18th century and is now cultivated widely in both tropical and temperate regions. A species of the Heliotrope was used in the perfumes of ancient Egypt (see Egyptian Perfumes). Today the dried flowers are used in pot pourri, but the fragrance called Heliotrope, of which there are different varieties, is mostly produced

synthetically using heliotropin, vanillin and other ingredients. Heliotrope appears in many modern quality perfumes (e.g. 'Lou-Lou' and 'Chant d'Aromes').

Heliotropin A chemically produced aldehyde discovered in 1885. It is made from safrole, has the fragrance of the Heliotrope flower and is used in synthetic Heliotrope fragrances in perfumes and toiletries.

Heliotropium peruviana *see* Heliotrope

Helleu, Jacques A prominent contemporary designer of perfume bottles and packaging, head of design for Parfums Chanel, who has provided designs for, among others, Bourjois, Chanel ('Coco') and Ungaro ('Diva').

Henna *see* Cyprinum

Herb Bennet *see* Avens

Herb Louisa *see* Verbena

Herb Walter *see* Woodruff

Herbaceous Note A term used in perfumery to describe the characteristic general fragrance of herbs and herbal medicines. Sage, rosemary and lavender are examples. Such fragrances are widely used in masculine perfumes. See Perfume Notes.

Hermès A distinguished French fashion house particularly associated with sporting wear and accessories. The company was originally established in 1837 by Thierry Hermès as a harness-making business, a fact now reflected in the names of some of its perfumes. The perfume division (Hermès Parfums) was set up in 1950, marketing the first Hermès perfume, the classic 'Calèche', in 1961. Since then it has produced 'Équipage' (70), 'Amazone' (74, relaunched 89), 'Hermès Eau de Cologne' (79), 'Parfum d'Hermès' (84) and 'Bel Ami' (86). Since 1979 the company's fragrances have been prepared from a factory complex at Le Vaudreuil, near Rouen.

Herodotus A Greek, born in Asia Minor in about 485 BC (died 425 BC), who wrote the earliest book on the history and geography of the ancient world which is still extant. Known as 'The Histories' and produced in about 446 BC, the work contains information about the use of perfumes at the time and in particular about the trade in cinnamon, cassia, labdanum, frankincense and myrrh from Arabia. See Egyptian Perfumes and Greek Perfumes.

Hesperides A term used in perfumery to describe the fragrances obtained from citrus fruits. See also Agrumen Oils.

Hesperis matronalis *see* Honesty Oil

Hibiscus abelmoschus *see* Ambrette

Hibiscus, Target-leaved *see* Ambrette

Hierichloe odorata *see* Sweet Grass

Hoar Strong *see* Peucedan Gum

Hogweed *see* Knot Grass

Holcus odoratus   *see* Sweet Grass

Holy Wort   *see* Verbena

Homoranthus Oil   An oil used in perfumes which is distilled from an Australian (New South Wales) shrub *Homoranthus virgatus* (= *H. flavescens*).

Honduras Balsam   *see* Storax

Honesty Oil   Also called Huile de Julienne and Rotrops Oil. An oil obtained from the seeds of the Damask plant (*Hesperis matronalis*), also called Garden Rocket, Dames' Rocket, White Rocket, Sweet Rocket, Purple Rocket, Ruchette, Roquette, Dames' Violet and Vesper Flower. The plant, native to central Europe but now found as far as central Asia, is a biennial growing up to 3 feet high. It emits its fragrance in the evenings, and as it has no fragrance during the daytime it is held to represent deceit. The oil is sometimes used in perfumery and the dried flowers are used in sachets and pot pourri.

Honey   Honey was used as an ingredient in early Arab perfumes and appears in later European ones (see, for example, Honey Water). In modern perfumery a substance providing the sweet aromatic effect of honey and known as Honey (or Miel) is manufactured synthetically. See also Beeswax and Propolis.

Honeysuckle   Essential oils are extracted from the flowers of many species and hybrids of honeysuckle (*Lonicera*), including *Lonicera periclymenon*, the English wild honeysuckle, *L. caprifolium* (Europe) and *L. fragrantissima* (China). They have a warm, jasmine-like odour with a suggestion of vanilla, but the yield of essential oil is extremely low. Most fragrances called Honeysuckle used in perfumes are therefore compounded synthetically using a mixture of natural and chemical substances. Examples of Honeysuckle used in high-quality modern perfumes include 'Madame Rochas' and 'Cristalle'. The dried flowers of honeysuckle are used in sachets and pot pourri.

Honey Water   A toilet water popular in France and England from the 18th century as a face lotion and known to apothecaries as Aqua Mellis. The recipe varied, but at one time the ingredients included brandy, honey, coriander, cloves, benzoin, storax, rosewater, neroli, musk and ambergris. Lemon peel, nutmeg, orange flower and saffron were also sometimes employed. The preparation was also sometimes used as a medicine. (See Appendix B, recipe no. 42.)

Hop Oil   An essential oil obtained by steam-distillation from the flower tops of the Hop plant (*Humulus lupulus*). It has a bitter, herbaceous odour and is occasionally used in perfumes with a herbal fragrance.

Hop Plant   *see* Dittany

Horsefieldia irya   *see* Kalapa Tijoong

Horsehair Lichen   A lichen, *Alectoria jujuba*, which grows widely in temperate areas. It provides a dye and has occasionally been used in perfumery.

Horseheal   *see* Elecampane

Horsemint   *see* Mint

Horse Radish tree/oil   *see* Ben Oil

Hoslundia opposita   *see* Kamyuye Oil

Houbigant   Oldest of the great French perfume houses, and pre-dated among the existing perfume houses of the world only by Floris, the firm of Houbigant was established in Paris in 1775, as 'glovers and perfumers' (see Gloves, scented) by Jean-Francois Houbigant, then aged 23. By 1782 the clientele of the House of Houbigant included Queen Marie Antoinette and the royal court and nobility, to whom it supplied toilet waters (such as Eau de Mousseline, Eau de Millefleurs and Eau de Chypre), powders and scented gloves. The firm survived the difficult years of the French Revolution and soon began to prosper again. In 1807 it passed to Houbigant's son, and then to his partner Chardin, who became personal perfumer to Napoleon. It is recorded that Napoleon ordered perfumes, toiletries and gloves from Houbigant shortly before Waterloo, and that when he lay dying 'two of Houbigant's perfumed pastilles were burning in his room'. Houbigant were appointed perfumers to King Louis Phillipe's sister, Princess Adelaide, in 1829, to Queen Victoria in 1838, to Emperor Napoleon III in 1870, and to the Tsar of Russia in 1890 (when they created a special perfume called 'The Czarina's Bouquet'). In 1880 the company passed into the hands of a prominent perfumer, Paul Parquet, one of the first to use synthetics and the creator of 'Fougère Royale' (1882). At the turn of the century it was joined by another distinguished perfumer, Robert Bienaimé, the creator of 'Quelques Fleurs' (1912).

Among the many other perfumes produced by Houbigant may be cited: 'Idéal' (1900) (sometimes described as the first true composite perfume), 'Parfum d'Argeville' (13), 'Ambre' (19), 'Un Parfum Précieux' (27), 'Essence Rare' (30, relaunched 76) and 'Étude' (31), all of which appeared in notable flacons made by Baccarat. In addition to 'Fougère Royale' and 'Quelques Fleurs', recent and current Houbigant perfumes include: 'Chantilly' (41), 'Ciao' (80), 'Raffinée' (82), 'Les Fleurs' (83), 'Lutèce' (86), 'Demi Jour' (87) and two men's fragrances 'Monsieur Houbigant' (69) and 'Musk Monsieur' (77).

The company still compounds its fragrances at Grasse, and since 1880 has operated its main factory at Neuilly-sur-Seine, a suburb of Paris.

Houmiri   Also called Umari. A scented oil obtained from a fungus which attacks the bark of the Bastard Bullet tree (*Houmiri floribunda*) of Brazil and Guyana. It is used locally for scenting the hair and body.

Hound's Tongue   *see* Lacinaria

Hudnut, Richard   One of the founders of the American perfume industry. The son of a chemist and druggist, he set up a highly successful perfumery in New York, marketing his first perfume, 'Violet Sec', in 1896. Other well-known Hudnut perfumes included 'Aimee' (1902), 'Vanity' (10) and 'Three Flowers' (15). Hudnut sold his business in 1916, but it continued to manufacture perfumes until 1946.

Huile Antique   *see* Enfleurage

Huile de Julienne   *see* Honesty Oil

Huisache   *see* Cassie

Humulus lupulus   *see* Hop Oil

Hungary Water   One of the earliest toilet waters made by distilling aromatic plants with wine alcohol. It was first produced in about 1370 AD for the Queen of Hungary and became very popular throughout Europe. It was made from the flowers of rosemary, with smaller portions of marjoram and pennyroyal, to which in later years were added citron, lavender and orris. In later times some other recipes for it also came into use. A modern version, made of rosemary with mint, lemon balm and orange peel, is marketed by Crabtree & Evelyn. (See Appendix B, recipe no. 55.)

Huon Pine   A tall tree (*Dacrydium franklinii*) growing in Malaysia, Borneo, New Caledonia, Tasmania, Australia and New Zealand. Huon Pine Oil, which has a clove-like smell, is distilled from the wood for use in toilet waters and soaps.

Hurtleberry   *see* Magalep

Hyacinth   The flowers of the Hyacinth (*Hyacinthus orientalis*), which is of Syrian origin but is now cultivated widely and with innumerable varieties, provide by extraction an essential oil of considerable value in perfumery. The oil is usually used as an absolute or concrete, but the yield of concrete is only about 0.01–0.02%, making it extremely expensive. The odour is powerfully floral with a suggestion of storax. A less powerful, though fresher and more flowery, perfume is obtained from the wild Blue Hyacinth (*H. non scriptus = Scilla nutans*). However, most of the Hyacinth oils now sold are prepared artificially. Examples of modern quality perfumes containing Hyacinth are 'Nino Cerutti', 'Givenchy III' and 'White Linen'. Scholars now believe that *H. orientalis* was the plant referred to in the Bible as Lily of the Valleys. Greek legend holds that the flower grew from the blood of Hyacinthus, a youth accidentally killed by Apollo; in Greece it now signifies remembrance.

Hyacinthus tuberosus   *see* Tuberose Flower Oil

Hyawa Gum   *see* Elemi

Hypericum androsaemum   *see* St John's Wort

Hyraceum   The product of the Hyrax (the Coney of the Bible), a small rabbit-like vegetarian animal of the genus *Procavia* which lives in rock clefts in Arabia and the Middle East. It is a digestive excretion and is found in irregular, amorphous masses which are plastic when kneaded. The odour is somewhat musky and recalls that of castoreum, for which it is sometimes used as a substitute. It has little part in western perfumery. It is probably the substance called in Arabic *Ba'r tibbi* ('fragrant dung') used as an ingredient in one of al-Kindi's early Arab perfume recipes.

Hyssop   Hyssop Oil is obtained by steam-distillation from the leaves, stem and flowers of hyssop, a small shrubby aromatic herb (*Hyssopus officinalis*) native from the Mediterranean area to Iran. Hyssop is cultivated for this oil, mainly in France and Germany, the yield being about 0.5%. The oil has a fine, warm, spicy, slightly camphorous odour and is mostly used in eau de colognes and as a flavouring (notably for liqueurs). The dried leaves are used in sachets and pot pourri.

The name Hyssop derives from the Greek *azab*, meaning a holy herb, because the Old Testament notes its use in cleansing temples. It was also used from early times in medicines, and is so recorded by Dioscorides. However, it is now believed that the Hyssop of the Old Testament was a different plant, a species of marjoram (*Origanum maru*) common in the Middle East. *O. maru* is also thought to have been the fragrant material used by the early Arab perfume makers under the name *Marmakhuz*. See also Giant Hyssop.

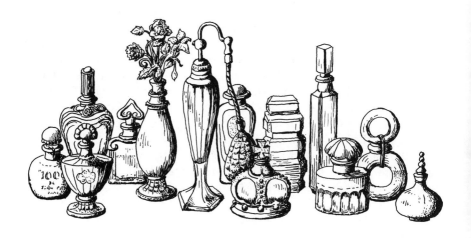

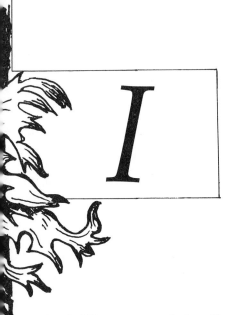

Iceland Wintergreen A handkerchief perfume popular in the USA during the late 19th century. It was made from rose, lavender, neroli, vanilla, cassie and wintergreen.

IFF *see* International Flavours and Fragrances.

Iguga A tree native to tropical Africa and known also as Mpopwa and Popioe (*Fagara chalybea*) from the seeds of which an oil used in local perfumes is obtained.

Ilachi *see* Cardamom

Ilex paraguensis *see* Mate

Illicium anisatum *see* Japanese Star Anise

     religiosum *see* Japanese Star Anise

     verum *see* Star Anise

'Imperial Leather' A famous fragrance now used by Cussons in their toiletries. In 1768 Count Orloff, visiting Bayleys, the court perfumers, in London, challenged them to create a perfume which reproduced the aroma of the leather worn and favoured by the Russian nobility. The result was a new perfume, 'Eau de Cologne Imperiale Russe', which became the favourite fragrance of the Empress Catherine the Great. After Cussons absorbed Bayleys early in this century they adopted this fragrance, under the name 'Imperial Russian Leather', for their new soaps, the word 'Russian' being dropped in 1989.

Incense A fragrant smoke produced by burning aromatic substances;

also substances burned to create such smoke. Incense has been burned since earliest times in all parts of the world in religious rites, as a fumigant, and simply for the pleasure of its perfume. Fragrant plant materials such as frankincense and storax are used on their own, or incenses are compounded from a number of different resins, herbs and spices mixed together. Under the Roman Empire frankincense was the principal incense used, and enormous quantities of it were imported from South Arabia and the Horn of Africa for the purpose. The 'holy incense' of the Jews was compounded in the time of Exodus, and incense was burned in Christian churches from the 5th century AD. Incense tablets were used in wealthy homes in Europe to sweeten the air in the 18th century. In modern times Indian joss sticks, formed by binding a mixture of powdered resins and other aromatic materials into a paste with a gum and rolling it on to sticks, have continued to be used in Europe, while most of the great religions, except Islam, continue to use incense in their ceremonies, and it is still burned for domestic purposes in many parts of the world. In modern western perfumery the term 'incense' is sometimes used to signify frankincense as a perfume ingredient. See also Bible Perfumes and Roman Perfumes; also Perfume Making at Home; also Appendix B, recipes nos 25–29.

Incense Gum tree   *see* Elemi

Incensier   *see* Rosemary

Incenso Macho   The local name for a resin obtained in Peru, probably from a tree *Styrax ovatum*, which is used as an incense and also in perfumery. Its fragrance recalls Siam benzoin or vanilla.

Inchi Grass   *see* Kachi Grass Oil

Inchy, Oil of   *see* Lemon Grass de Cochin

Indian Carnation   *see* Marigold

Indian Geranium Oil   *see* Ginger Grass Oil

Indian Nard   *see* Spikenard

Indian Orris   *see* Costus

Indole   A chemical which occurs naturally in many essential oils, including jasmine, neroli, orange blossom, robinia, wallflower and some species of citrus, and is also manufactured synthetically. It is a crystalline substance with an odour which is unpleasant until greatly diluted, when it becomes agreeably fragrant with a distinct floral note of an orange blossom and jasmine type. It is used in preparing artificial jasmine and neroli perfumes.

'Infini'   An intensely aldehydic floral perfume created by IFF perfumers for Caron, who launched it in 1970. The name was first chosen for a perfume issued in 1912 and was re-used to celebrate the advent of space flight. Green aldehydic top notes introduce a floral heart containing jasmine, jonquil, rose, lily of the valley and tuberose, on a base which is principally sandalwood. The fragrance is said to have taken 15 years to develop. The bottle was designed by Serge Mansau.

Infusion   A term used in perfumery to describe the process for producing attars by extraction with a solvent solution under heat. It is also used to denote the substance so derived.

Ink Root   *see* Marsh Rosemary

International Flavours and Fragrances   Generally abbreviated to IFF. An American company which is the largest wholesale manufacturer of flavourings and fragrances in the world (see Perfume Manufacture). Formed in the USA in the 1930s by Hank van Amerigen and a colleague, Haebler, the company was originally called Van Amerigen–Haebler and developed rapidly. In 1958 it amalgamated with Van Amerigen's former employers, the Dutch fragrance firm Polak & Schwarz, founded at the end of the 19th century, and became IFF, with its headquarters in New York. The company sells its fragrances to makers of perfumes and cosmetics, hair and other personal care products, soaps and detergents, household and other cleaning products and area fresheners. Fragrances account for 62% (and flavours for 38%) of its sales. It has created about 16% of all the quality perfumes now on the market.

IFF operates some 57 sales offices in 38 countries throughout the world, with 30 factories and about the same number of creative laboratories. It has major installations in New York, New Jersey and Hilversum, Holland and its main complex in Britain is at Haverhill, Suffolk. It has a substantial investment in research and development, maintaining a computerized 'library' which records over 30 000 different fragrance and flavour molecules; recent developments include 'living flower technology' (q.v.).

'Intimate'   A classic chypre perfume brought out in 1955 by Revlon, for whom it was created by IFF perfumers. The heart is floral, chiefly jasmine and rose, with woody undertones from sandalwood and cedarwood, among others. The top notes are aldehydic, with bergamot and rose among the underlying fragrances. Amber and castoreum provide the main base notes, with hints of oak moss, civet and musk.

Inula helenium   *see* Elecampane

Ionone   An important synthetic perfume ingredient with the scent of violets discovered by Tiemann and Kruger in 1893. It is made chemically from citral, a substance found in the oils of citrus fruits and some other plants, and by other chemical processes.

Iris   *see* Orris

Iris florentina   *see* Orris

   germanica   *see* Orris

   pallida   *see* Orris

   pseudoacorus   *see* Iris, Yellow

Iris, Yellow   The Yellow Iris (*Iris pseudoacorus*), also called Yellow Flag,

Dragon Flower, Myrtle Flower, Flower de Luce (Fleur de Lys) and Myrtle Grass, grows in watery areas such as on river banks throughout Europe and N. Africa and as far as Siberia. The powdered roots were once used to perfume linen and clothes.

Isoeugenol A substance with the fragrance of carnations which is found naturally in the essential oils of nutmeg and ylang-ylang and is obtained from eugenol. It provides perfume makers with a good fixative.

Iva An intensely musky essential oil distilled from the leaves and flowers of the Musk Yarrow plant (*Achillea moschata*), which grows in Italy and Switzerland. It is principally used to manufacture liqueurs (e.g. Esprit d'Iva) but is occasionally used in perfumery.

'Ivoire' A quality floral perfume created for Balmain in 1979 by the perfumers of Florasynth. The top notes are green with a touch of spice, containing marigold, bergamot, galbanum, wormwood and camomile. The heart is intensely floral and includes jasmine, lily of the valley, rose, orris, jonquil and neroli. Warm, woody lower notes are based on frankincense, vetivert, sandalwood and amber. The square-shaped flacon, sealed inside an ivory covering, was designed by Pierre Dinand.

Ivy Oil *see* Ground Ivy

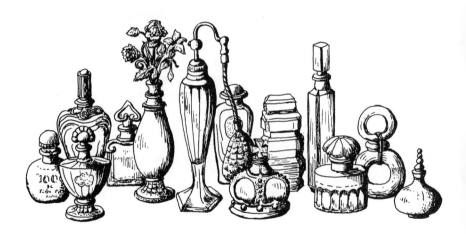

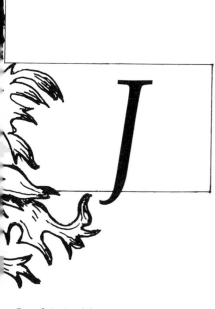

Jacob's Ladder *see* Lily of the Valley

Jacques Fath A celebrated Paris fashion house set up in 1937 by the couturier Jacques Fath (1912–1954) and closed three years after his death from leukaemia. His fragrance business still survives. Jacques Fath perfumes include 'Ellipse' and 'Expression' (1977), both coming in bottles designed by Serge Mansau, and a men's fragrance 'Green Water' (53).

Jamaica Mignonette *see* Cyprinum

Jamaican Pepper Tree *see* Pimento

Japan Flowers A name given to certain types of floral bouquet perfumes which were popular early in this century.

Japanese Star Anise A tree (*Illicium anisatum = I. religiosum*) native to China (where it is called *Mang-tsao*, meaning 'the mad herb') and Japan (where it is called *Shikimi* and *Dai-ui-Kio*). In Japan the aromatic branches are used to scent tombs, while the bark is burned in Japanese homes and in Buddhist temples as an incense. An essential oil obtained from the leaves provides a fragrance resembling lemon oil and nutmeg.

'Jardins de Bagatelle' A floral perfume created by Jean-Paul Guerlain and launched by Guerlain in 1984. It is sold in a flacon designed by Robert Granai. A top note of violet, with a fruity tone from bergamot, lemon and calycanthus, leads into an intensely floral heart which includes rose, jasmine, narcissus, ylang-ylang, orris, orchid and lily of the valley, with a touch of cassis. The base contains vetivert, cedarwood, patchouli, benzoin, musk and civet. The perfume is named after the chateau and gardens built in 1777 for Queen Marie Antoinette.

Jasmine Also called Jasmin and Jessamine. The name derives from the Arabic/Persian *Yasmin*. The essential oils yielded by certain species of jasmine (plants of the genus *Jasminum*) are among the most important of all fragrances used in perfumery. Species used in perfumery are as follows.

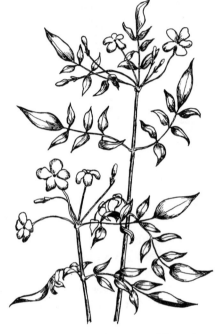

1. *Jasminum officinale*, the Common White Jasmine, a native of N. India and Iran, which was introduced into Europe in the 16th century.
2. *J. grandiflorum*, called Spanish or Catalonian Jasmine or Royal Jasmine. Native to southern Europe. This is the principal plant used in the perfumery trade, being first so used in Spain during the 16th century, and is cultivated in enormous quantity around Grasse and in Morocco, Spain, Algeria, Egypt and India.
3. *J. sambac*, called Zambac (Arabic *Zanbaq*) or Arabian Jasmine, sometimes also Tuscan Jasmine. Native to tropical Asia and introduced

Jasmine (*Jasminum grandiflorum*).

into Britain in the 17th century. In India this jasmine is known as Chameli and the oil as Motia, the oil being used in many Indian perfumes and also in hair oils, for which it is extracted by enfleurage using sesame seeds which are then pressed to extract the perfume.
4. *J. odoratissimum*, called Yellow or True Yellow Jasmine, a native of Madeira and the Canary Islands. The flowers remain fragrant when dried and have an odour of blended jasmine, jonquil and orange blossom.
5. *J. auriculatum*, sometimes called Julii, found in tropical Asia, especially Sri Lanka, Mauritius and Thailand.
6. *J. niloticum* of tropical Africa, the oil from which is used as a perfume in Sudan.

Arabian Jasmine was recorded in China, where it was called Mo Li, as early as the 3rd century AD, being cultivated then for the unopened buds, which were used by women to decorate their hair and were also used to give fragrance to tea. Oils of both Common Jasmine and Arabian Jasmine were being used by Arab perfume makers at least by the 9th century AD, the leaves being sometimes employed as well as the flowers.

An acre of land will yield about 500 lb of jasmine blossom (from *J. grandiflorum*), which is extracted by enfleurage, usually with olive oil. The yield of concrete is very small and of absolute considerably less, making the latter one of the most expensive perfume materials available. Since much of the production cost is a matter of labour charges, perfume makers now increasingly obtain their jasmine absolute from countries such as Egypt, where labour is cheaper. In the enfleurage process 3 lb of flowers are used to perfume about 1 lb of oil, an extract then being obtained by maceration in 1 pint of rectified spirit. Extraction is also undertaken by volatile solvents.

Jasmine has been the principal ingredient in a very large number of perfumes, including such classics as 'Arpège', 'Joy', and 'Chanel No. 5' and a whole range of high class modern perfumes from 'Amouage' through to 'Ysatis'. It appears among the principal ingredients in 83% of all quality perfumes and 33% of all men's fragrances. Its odour is unique and cannot be effectively imitated by synthetics.

For Red Jasmine see Frangipani.

Jatamansi *see* Spikenard

Java Almond *see* Elemi

Javo Oil *see* Citronella

'Jazz' A spicy–floral men's fragrance launched by Yves St Laurent in 1988. In the top notes, artemisia, coriander and juniper are given a spicy touch by nutmeg, cinnamon and cardamom, leading to a floral heart of jasmine, lily of the valley and geranium, with base notes containing sandalwood, patchouli, oak moss, sage, labdanum, frankincense and opoponax.

Jean Laporte *see* 'Métamorphose'

'Je Reviens' A classic, trend-setting perfume created by Maurice Blanchet for Worth in 1932. One of the earliest of the floral–aldehyde perfumes, it included spicy elements. Aldehydic top notes, mainly orange blossom, give way to a spicy floral heart founded on carnation, with hyacinth, jasmine, rose, tuberose and ylang-ylang. Vetiver, tonka and musk provide the principal base notes. The principal flacon, in the shape of a star-spangled blue orb, is by Lalique.

Jessamine *see* Jasmine

Jesuit's Tea *see* Ambroisia

Jewish Frankincense *see* Storax

'Jicky' A famous 19th century perfume created by Aimé Guerlain, introduced by Guerlain in 1889 and now regarded as one of the greatest of all perfume classics. It is sometimes described as the first modern perfume. Classified as a semi-oriental fougere-type fragrance, it contains citrus top notes, mostly lemon, but with hints of mandarin, bergamot and rosewood. In the middle notes, which are floral and woody, jasmine and patchouli predominate, with rose, orris and vetivert. The base notes are led by vanilla, with balsamic undertones. The perfume is marketed in a flacon by Baccarat.

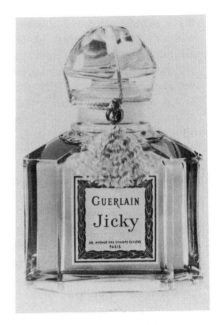

'Jicky'.

Jil Sander   A German perfume house forming part of the Benckiser group of fragrance companies. In 1980 it launched 'Jil Sander', a green–fresh perfume which includes galbanum, coriander and bergamot in the head, rose, jasmine, carnation and ylang-ylang in the heart and oak moss and vetivert among the base notes. Other Sander fragrances include 'Woman Two' (83), 'Woman III' (87) and 'Jil Sander No. 4' (91), together with four men's fragrances 'Man Pure' (81), 'Men Two' (83), 'Man III' (88) and 'Man IV' (91).

Jockey Club   A name given to many perfumes in the early part of the 20th century. The original perfume of this name is said to have attempted to imitate the fragrance wafted towards Epsom race course from nearby woods during the late spring meeting. (See Appendix B, recipe no. 66d.)

'Joie de Vivre'   A 'green' perfume (see Perfume Families) launched by Lenthéric in 1985. Created by Roure perfumers, its top notes include jasmine and rose, on a heart dominated by iris, with woody notes underlined by a base mainly of amber and sandalwood.

Jojoba Oil   An oil obtained from the seeds of a small bushy tree called the Pignut, or Goatnut, tree (*Simmondsia californica* = *S. chinensis* = *S. pabulosa*), native to Mexico and California. The oil, which is clear, waxy and scentless, is mostly used in aromatherapy and in cosmetic preparations, but provides a good base to which fragrant essential oils can be added when simple perfumes are being made at home (see Perfume Making at Home).

'Jolie Madame'   A classic chypre perfume introduced by Balmain in

1953. Created by Germaine Sellier of Roure, it has an unusual top note obtained from gardenia and artemisia with a touch of neroli, bergamot and coriander. The heart is floral, mainly jasmine, with underlying touches which include jonquil, tuberose, orris and rose. The base notes are mossy and leathery, dominated by patchouli and castoreum.

Jonquil   Also known as Rush Daffodil, Jonquille and Wild Jonquil, this plant (*Narcissus jonquilla*), native to S.W. Europe and N. Africa, is a species of Narcissus which has been cultivated in the south of France for its essential oil since the 18th century. The oil is the most strongly scented of the Narcissus oils (see Narcissus) and the most popular one used in perfumery, but the plant is difficult to cultivate successfully. High-quality perfumes using it include 'Parure' and 'Fleurs de Rocaille'. The dried flowers are used in pot pourri.

A closely related species, the Campernella Jonquil, or Campernella (*N. odorus*), produces a similar though less powerful oil. Although known since the 16th century, this plant appears to be a hybrid cultivated from early times and has not been found in the wild. It is grown widely and is cultivated in the south of France for its oil.

The fragrance of jonquil is often imitated synthetically.

Joss stick   *see* Incense

Jovan   *see* Yardley

'Joy'   A perfume classic of great distinction, introduced by Jean Patou in 1935 as an unusually luxurious scent which became the most costly

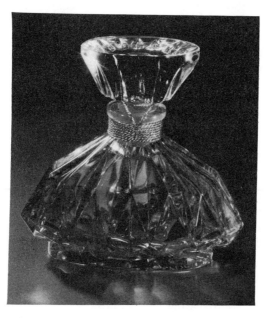

'Joy'.

perfume on the market. It was created for Patou by Henri Almeras. Its heart is in the main a blending of rose and jasmine. The top note includes rose, tuberose and ylang-ylang. The lower note is a restrained combination of sandalwood, musk and civet. The original 'Joy' flacon was designed by Louis Suë; it is also now sold in a crystal flacon by Baccarat and in flacons by Brosse.

Juglans regia   *see* Walnut Oil

Julii   *see* Jasmine

July Flower   *see* Clove-pink

Juniper   Also called Common Juniper, Genevrier, Ginepro and Enebro. A small, shrub-like tree (*Juniperus communis*) growing to about 6 feet high and found in Europe, N. America, N. Africa and northern parts of Asia. There are other species. The berries, which take three years to ripen, each contain three seeds. From the ripe berries a colourless or pale yellow–green oil, called Juniper Oil or Juniper Berry Oil, is steam-distilled; this oil which has a fresh terebinth or turpentine-like odour is mostly used in medicines, but it also appears in perfumery, usually

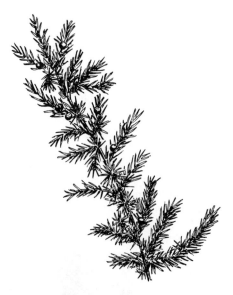

Juniper (*Juniperus communis*).

as a concrete or absolute (it is to be found, for example, in 'Mystere' and in the modern quality men's fragrances 'Polo' and 'Tsar'). The honey and pine-like aromatic scent of the plant once made it popular as a strewing herb to sweeten stale air. The leaves are still used in sachets and pot pourri.

An oil scented with juniper berries was used by the ancient Egyptians to anoint corpses during the mummification ceremony, and juniper also appears as an ingredient of the famous Kyphi incense. From early times juniper has been regarded as a magic plant, so featuring in ancient legends about evil spirits, probably because of its considerable medicinal and antiseptic properties. Juniper oil is still one of the most important oils used in aromatherapy.

Juniperus macropoda   *see* Cedar
              oxycedrus   *see* Cedar
              sabina   *see* Sassafras
              virginiana   *see* Cedar

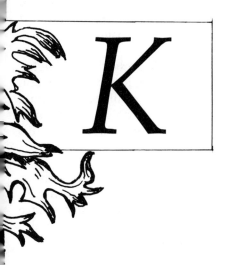

Kabushi Oil   An essential oil distilled in Japan from a small species of Magnolia tree (*Magnolia kobus*) native to Japan.

Kachi Grass Oil   A spicy, slightly lemon-scented essential oil obtained from the leaves and roots of Kachi Grass (*Cymbopogon caesius*), native to India, where it grows mostly in Mysore and Bangalore and is also known as Inchi Grass. Kachi Grass Oil is used in soaps, cosmetics and perfumes. See also Lemon Grass de Cochin.

Kalapa Tijoong   A tree also known as Kannarahan (*Horsfieldia irya* = *Myristica irya*) which is found from Sri Lanka to Indonesia. It has sweet-smelling flowers which are used locally in perfumery.

Kamynye Oil   A vanilla-like oil, used in perfumery as a fixative, which is extracted from a tropical African herb (*Hoslundia opposita*).

Kannarahan   *see* Kalapa Tijoong

Kapur Kachri   A fragrant perfume material obtained from the dried root of a species of Ginger-wort (*Hedychium spicatum*), which grows in northern India and Nepal and is used in Indian and other eastern perfumes. The roots are also burned in India as an incense. The word Hedychium comes from Greek meaning 'sweet snow' because of the pure white, sweetly scented flowers. The dried root has a violet-like scent. The roots are dried or powdered in India to place among clothes. See also Longosa Oil.

Karo-Karundi   A flowering shrub (*Leptactinia densiflora, L. senegambica* and *L. manii*) growing to about 6 feet high and found in tropical W. Africa. In Guinea an essential oil is distilled from the flowers and used in perfumery. The fragrance resembles jasmine with orange flower and acacia.

Karaya Gum   Also called Kateera Gum. A gum obtained by puncturing the bark of a tree *Sterculia urens* indigenous to tropical Asia. The gum appears in small irregular white or yellowish, semi-transparent tears. It provides a bonding agent useful in making incense pastes.

Kateera Gum   *see* Karaya Gum

Kazanluk   A town and area in the centre of the important rose-growing region of Bulgaria known as the Valley of the Roses. The region produces attar, mainly from the Damask rose, by distillation and on a large scale for the perfume industry, exporting much of it to France. Over a thousand varieties of Damask rose are now cultivated for this purpose. See also Grasse.

Keiri   *see* Wallflower

Kerleo, Jean   A distinguished French perfumer ('nose'). Commenced his career with Helena Rubinstein in 1955, becoming their head perfumer. Joined Jean Patou in 1967 and has created all the Patou fragrances since that date. Also created 'Lacoste'. President of the Société Technique des Parfumeurs de France 1976–79 and author of a book, *Le Parfum*.

Kesso Oil   *see* Valerian

Keura odorifera   *see* Pandanus

Khaluq   An unguent of the early Arabs made for women and forbidden to men. The ingredients varied. One recipe, which gives a good idea of the complexity of some of the Arab perfumes, was recorded by al-Kindi. It required dried safflower, which was mixed with rose-hips, cubeb oil and pounded cardamom and then kneaded with sesame oil. Peeled mahaleb fruit, ground rose flowers and honey were added. This preparation was fumigated 'twenty times a day for three days' with an incense made of Indian costus, sweet hoof, sandalwood and camphor. Next it was aromatized several more times with a perfume called Muthallathah, made chiefly of rosewater and dragon's blood. It was then mixed with saffron and camphor and kneaded with jasmine oil. Finally extra saffron was added. Exact measures for all these ingredients were prescribed by al-Kindi, who added: 'It is quite wonderful'.

Khasia Patchouli Oil   *see* Patchouli

Khazama   *see* Marjoram

al-Kindi, Yaqub   An Arab savant who lived mostly in Baghdad c. 800–870 AD and is known as 'the philosopher of the Arabs'. Wrote some 250 works on subjects as diverse as philosophy, mathematics, music and astronomy. His *Book of Perfume Chemistry and Distillations* contained some 107 perfume recipes and instructions, using 106 different ingredients derived from plants, 11 from animals and 9 from minerals; it is the principal source of our knowledge about early Arab perfumes (see Arab Perfumes).

King's Clover   *see* Melilot

Kiou-Nouk   A clear, semi-liquid resin obtained by a special process from frankincense to provide a more aromatic, less sickly odour than that of frankincense itself. It is an excellent fixative and blends well with almost any of the essential oils.

Klein, Calvin   *see* Calvin Klein

Knot Grass Oil   An oil obtained from the common weed Knot Grass (*Polyganum aviculare*), which grows all over the world and is also known as Red Robin, Hogweed and by very many other local names. It appears mixed with other oils in sone of the early Arab perfume recipes.

'Knowing'   A quality floral–chypre perfume launched by Estée Lauder in 1989. Created by the perfumers of Firmenich, it features an unusual floral ingredient, pittosporum, in an elaborate top note also containing rose, mimosa, tuberose, davana and fruity notes from plum and melon. The heart is mainly jasmine, lily of the valley, patchouli and orris,

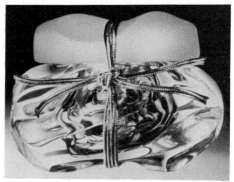

'Knowing'.

with a spicy touch from bay. The base notes come from oak moss, amber, sandalwood, vetivert and musk. It is sold in a lead crystal flacon, with a gold cord, which was designed by Ira Levy.

Koot   *see* Costus

Koriak   *see* Cyperus

Krizia   *see* Sanofi

Kuro-moji Oil   A Japanese perfume oil with a balsamic fragrance similar to myrtle which is distilled from the seeds, leaves and twigs of two related mountain shrubs, *Lindera umbellata* and *L. fericia*, native to Japan.

Kuchoora   A perfume material derived from a species of Curcuma (*Curcuma zerumbet*) which grows in India; it is used in Indian perfumery. The roots are dried and powdered, when they provide a camphor-like fragrance.

Kullum tree   *see* Macassar Oil

Kyphi   An oil and fat-free incense paste made by the ancient Egyptians. It was based on wine and raisins, with a number of aromatic herbs and resins added, including juniper berries, frankincense, myrrh and honey. Different recipes exist for Kyphi, including recipes inscribed on the walls of the temples at Edfu and Philae and one recorded by Dioscorides. Plutarch described it as a mixture of sixteen herbs and resins, including myrrh, henna, cardamom, juniper, saffron, honey and raisins, all steeped in wine. Democritus added spikenard among the ingredients and noted that the mixture was beaten into a paste and then allowed to solidify. Kyphi was a sacred perfume of great importance to the Egyptians, who burned it in their temples at sunset and in their homes during the night.

Kypros   An ancient Greek perfume mentioned by Theophrastus. It contained cardamom and a sweet-scented material called Aspalathus which had first been steeped in sweet wine. It was used by men and was believed to counter lassitude.

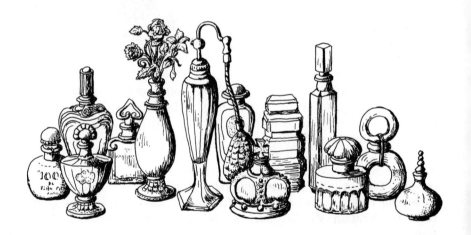

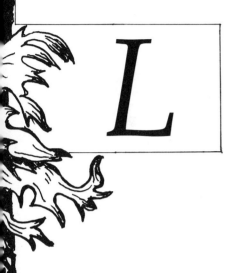

Labdanum   Also called Ladanon, Ledanon, Black Balsam, Storbon and Gum Cistus. A brownish, sweet-scented oleo-resin obtained from shrubs of the genus *Cistus*, known as the Rock Rose, found in the Mediterranean area, N. Africa and the Middle East. The resin exudes in sticky droplets on hairs on the underside of the leaves and on the stems. It is usually extracted by volatile solvents, or sometimes just by boiling the branches, and is then purified by maceration with an alcohol, yielding 1–2% of volatile oil. Labdanum is of great importance in modern perfumery: its fragrance closely resembles ambergris; it is economic in use and mixes well with other perfumes; it is a valuable fixative in many bouquet perfumes; and it provides the main material (Ambrein) used for manufacturing synthetic ambers. It is used not only in many quality perfumes (e.g. 'Amouage', 'Cuir de Russie' and 'Jazz'), but also in soaps, cosmetics, deodorants and even insecticides. Perfumers often call it Amber, and 'Amber' or 'Labdanum' appears among the main constituents of some 33% of all modern quality perfumes and 20% of all quality fragrances for men.

Of some seven species of *Cistus* used in perfumery, the two principal ones are as follows.

1. *Cistus ladanifer* (= *C. polymorphus*), a shrub growing up to 12 feet high, with white flowers, which is sometimes called Gum Cistus.

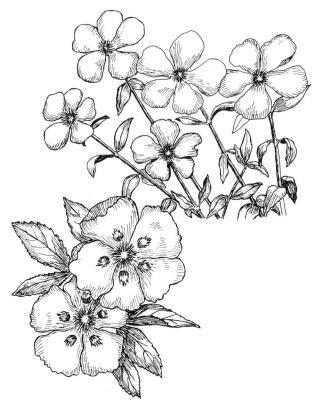

Labdanum (*Cistus incanus* (above), *Cistus ladaniferus*
(below)).

It grows wild in southern France, Spain and N. Africa and is cultivated in those countries and also in Greece and Corsica. This is the
main labdanum-producing species of the present time. The resin,
also called Guma Labdanum and Droga de Jara, has a fragrance
described as ambered, warm and leather-like.

2. *C. incanus* (= *C. incanus* ssp. *creticus* = *C. villosus* ssp. *creticus* =
   C. creticus). Growing up to 3 feet high, with pink flowers, this is the
   plant which for the most part provided the labdanum of ancient
   times; it is found in eastern Mediterranean areas, particularly Crete
   and Cyprus, and in the Middle East, including Arabia. (The botanical
   names of species of *Cistus* have been changed in recent years following taxonomic research.)

Labdanum does not appear to have been known to the Egyptians of
earliest times, but was listed by Herodotus in the 5th century BC as
an ingredient in many kinds of perfumes and one of the principal
aromatics brought from Arabia. It was possibly the 'myrrh' of the oldest
parts of the Old Testament (see Balm of Gilead). Herodotus observed

that the Arabs combed it off the beards of goats which had browsed among the bushes; it seems probable that at this time only the Arabs had learned how to collect this gum; Dioscorides later described its gathering by drawing leather thongs over the leaves, a system still employed in Crete. Labdanum was one of the main ingredients of the original chypre perfume and a constituent of the Royal Unguent of Parthia. The early Arab perfume makers used it in their recipes, and during the Middle Ages it was an important ingredient of pomanders.

'Lace'   A wide-selling floral–chypre perfume created for Yardley in 1964 by the perfumers of Roure. The top note, mostly provided by tangerine and ylang-ylang, gives way to a floral heart containing jasmine and rose, with musky, ambery and woody base notes.

Lacinaria   Also called Liatris, Deer's Tongue, Hound's Tongue and Vanilla Trilisia. A herb (*Trilisia odoratissima* = *Liatris odoratissima*) found in the eastern USA. The dried leaves, which have an odour of coumarin and vanilla, have been used for perfuming tobacco and were for a long time a major source of coumarin for use in perfumery.

Ladanon   *see* Labdanum

Lagerfeld   A perfume house established in 1975 by the Swedish–German fashion designer and photographer Karl Lagerfeld (b. 1939), who in his career has designed for Balmain, Patou, House of Chloé and Chanel as well as producing collections in his own name. In 1975 he produced 'Chloé', to be followed by 'K.L.' (82) and two men's fragrances, 'Lagerfeld' (78) and 'Photo' (90). The company now belongs to Unilever.

'L'Aimant'   A famous classic floral perfume introduced by Coty in 1927. Francois Coty, who was assisted by the perfumer Vincent Roubert, is said to have taken five years to perfect it. The top note contains bergamot and citrus notes, and the heart is a bouquet of jasmine, rose and geranium. The base note includes vanilla, vetivert, musk and civet.

'L'Air du Temps'   A celebrated classic floral perfume brought out by Nina Ricci in 1948.

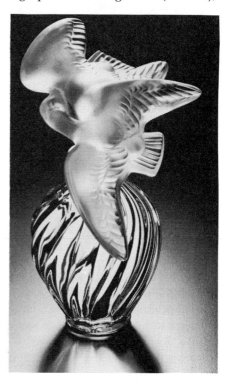

'L'Air du Temps'.

Created for Ricci by Francis Fabron of Roure, it was designed to be a perfume which would leave a memory as the wearer passed by. Under a top note of gardenia and bergamot, the heart is a spicy floral fragrance based on carnation, jasmine, rose, ylang-ylang and orris. The base note is mainly sandalwood and musk. The perfume comes in a well-known crystal flacon, featuring doves on the stopper, which is made by Lalique, and also in flacons by Brosse.

Lalique   Founded in 1905 by Rene Lalique (1860–1945), already at that time a leading jeweller, the firm of Lalique is now one of the world's foremost manufacturers of high-quality glass crystal ware, being particularly noted for its Art Deco designs of the 1920s and for its own distinctive decorative style of post-war years. Approached by Francois Coty in 1905 to design perfume bottles, Rene Lalique subsequently created flacons for a number of other famous perfume houses, such as Houbigant, Worth and Roger et Gallet. The firm has continued to make such flacons until the present day. The original flacon for 'Je Reviens' (Worth) was produced by Lalique, and Lalique currently provides the flacons for Nina Ricci's 'L'Air du Temps' and 'Nina' among others. See Perfume Containers.

Lancôme   A company founded in Paris in 1935 by Armand Petitjean, a perfumer (d. 1981), to produce fragrances and beauty products; it entered the UK market in 1946 and is now particularly noted for its skincare products. Lancôme's first perfume, 'Conquête', was launched in 1935. Subsequent fragrances have included 'Magie' (1950, with a flacon by Lalique), 'Balafré' (67), 'Climat' (68), 'Sikkim' (71), 'Magie Noire' (78) and 'Trésor' (52 and 91). The company's headquarters and main factory are at Chevilly Larue, near Paris, and since 1964 it has been owned by L'Oréal.

Languas galanga   see Galingale
      officinarum   see Galingale

Langwas   see Galingale

'La Nuit'   A chypre perfume introduced in 1985 by Paco Rabanne, for whom it was created by the perfumers of Roure. It has fruity top notes of tangerine and lemon mixed with, among other ingredients, myrtle, artemisia and cardamom. The heart includes peach, rose, jasmine and a spicy effect from pepper, while the base contains oak moss, patchouli and cedar. The bottle was designed by A. Ricard.

Lanvin   Parfums Lanvin was founded by the Paris couturier and costume designer Mme Jeanne Lanvin (1867–1946), who launched her first perfume 'My Sin' in 1925, following it in 1927 with the highly successful 'Arpège'. Subsequent Lanvin perfumes include 'Scandale' (31), 'Rumeur' (34), 'Prétexte'(37) and 'Clair du Jour' (83), together with men's fragrances which include 'Eau de Lanvin' (33), 'Monsieur Lanvin' (64), 'Vetyver' (64) and 'Lanvin for Men' (81). The early perfumes, including 'Arpège' were created by André Praysse. It was once said that the volume of flowers needed each year to make Lanvin perfumes equalled in bulk the size of the Arc de Triomphe. The company is now controlled by the Vuitton family.

Laretia acaulis   *see* Galbanum

Laroche   *see* Guy Laroche

L'Artisan Parfumeur   *see* 'Métamorphose'

Lathyrus odoratus   *see* Sweet Pea Oil

Lauder   *see* Estée Lauder

Laurel   *see* Bay

Laurel, Indian   *see* Ain

'Lauren'   A 'fruity–fresh' floral perfume devised by Parfums Ralph Lauren (now owned by L'Oréal) in 1978 with the creative perfumers of IFF. Fruity green fragrances in the top notes give way to a cool floral heart of ylang-ylang, mimosa, orange blossom and marigold, with base notes of cedar, sandalwood and oak moss. The flacon, in the form of a crystal cube, was designed by Bernard Kotyuk.

Laurus camphora   *see* Camphor

　　　cinnamonum   *see* Cinnamon

　　　nobilis   *see* Bay

　　　sassafras   *see* Sassafras

Lavandin   *see* Lavender

Lavandula   *see* Lavender

Lavender   There are several species of lavender, producing different types of lavender oil through steam-distillation of the freshly cut flowers and stalks, and they are grown on a considerable scale to meet the huge demands of the perfume industry. The main species are:

1. Old English Lavender (also called English Lavender) (*Lavandula vera* = *L. officinalis* = *L. augustifolia*), which has the finest aroma. A bush some 3–5 feet high, it grows best in Britain, where it was once cultivated intensively in Surrey (providing Mitcham Lavender Oil) and is still produced in large quantity elsewhere, including Norfolk, where Yardley still have large lavender estates. Other principal areas of cultivation are Tasmania and the south of France. Examples of quality fragrances which contain Old English Lavender are 'Blue Grass', 'Paco Rabanne' and 'Silvestre'.

2. Two sub-species of *L. vera*, named botanically *L. delphinensis* (Lavender of Dauphine) and *L. fragrans*, are cultivated in the south of France, providing what is called French Lavender.

3. Spike Lavender (*L. spica* = *L. latifolia*) a coarser variety native to mountainous areas in the Mediterranean region. Also called Lesser Lavender, Broad-leaved Lavender or Nardus Italica, this is grown in France, Spain and Yugoslavia and provides Oil of Spike (Essence

d'Aspice), sometimes called Spike Lavender Oil. The quality of this oil, which has a camphorous odour, is inferior but the yield from the plant is three times that of *L. vera*; it is used in men's fragrances, low-grade lavender perfumes and soaps. This lavender was mentioned by Theophrastus and some authorities believe that it was the Spikenard of the Old Testament;

4. French Lavender (*L. stoechas* = *Stoechas officinarum*), also called Stoechas, Arabian Stoechas, Stichados, Stickadore, Cassidony and Candy Rosemary. A small, attractive-looking plant plentiful in France, Spain and Portugal, it provides Stoechas Oil, distilled in Spain, which has a camphorous odour more like rosemary than lavender and is used medicinally as well as in perfumes and soaps;

5. Bastard Lavender, a hybrid lavender crossed between *L. spica* and *L. fragrans*. This is grown in France for an oil with a slightly camphorous fragrance known as Lavandin, mainly used in soaps but found also in some modern perfumes (e.g. 'You're the Fire').

The dried stems of flowers and leaves from all these lavenders are used in sachets and pot pourri and have for long been placed among linen and clothes to scent them.

Lavender has been a favourite perfume material since the time of the Greeks and Romans. The Romans made much use of it (particularly of Stoechas) in their bath water, and the name 'Lavender' may derive from the Latin *lavare* – to wash. From medieval times it was used not only in pot pourri and sachets and for scenting linen and clothes but also to strew on the floors of churches and houses. In Tudor times it was also used in Britain to stuff quilted jackets and caps.

Until 1906 lavender oil was extracted by water-distillation, but in that year a more efficient technique of dry steam-distillation was introduced. An acre of ground will grow about 3500 plants of English Lavender, yielding around 15 lb of oil. Total world production is enormous, with the south of France alone at one time processing nearly 5000 tons of lavender flowers every year. The oil has for long also been valued medicinally because of its antiseptic and antibiotic properties, and it is highly valued in aromatherapy.

Lavender Cotton Oil Also called Cotton Lavender and sometimes French Lavender, the leaves of the Lavender Cotton plant (*Santolina chamaecyparissus*), a shrub native to the western Mediterranean area, provide an essential oil with a camphor-like fragrance. The plant is not a true lavender. The oil is occasionally used in perfumery, and the dried leaves are used in sachets and pot pourri.

Lavender Water A toilet water popular in England since the 17th century, when it was prepared by distilling freshly picked lavender which had been immersed for a few days in alcohol. There are now many different recipes in use, one of the simplest being made by mixing 1 oz of Lavender Oil into $1\frac{1}{2}$ pints of spirits of wine, with an added drop of musk. (See Appendix B, recipes nos 49–52.)

Lavendula   *see* Lavender

Lawang Oil   An essential oil with a clove-like fragrance distilled from a species of cinnamon tree (possibly *Cinnamomum culilawan*) found in Indonesia.

Lawsonia alba   *see* Cyprinum
　　　inermis   *see* Cyprinum

Leather Notes   A term applied in perfumery to certain fragrances which are suggestive of leather. They are popular in the composition of many masculine perfumes and some feminine ones, especially chypre-type perfumes. See Perfume Notes.

'Le Dix'   A classic aldehyde perfume by Balenciaga, for whom it was created by Roure perfumers. It was introduced in 1947. The aldehydic top notes contain suggestions of bergamot, lemon, peach and coriander and give way to a heart based principally on rose, jasmine and orris. The lower notes are woody and balsamic, with vetivert, patchouli, sandalwood, rosewood, musk and civet.

Ledum palustre   *see* Marsh Rosemary

'L'Égoïste'   Sold outside the UK as 'Égoïste', this woody–spicy men's fragrance was created by Jacques Polge for Chanel, being a revised version of a fragrance they had previously marketed in Europe as 'Bois Noir'. It was launched in 1990 with notably lavish TV advertising. On a strong base built mainly on sandalwood and ambrette, it obtains spicy notes from cinnamon and coriander, with added touches which include rosewood, mandarin, tangerine and rose.

'Le Jardin d'Amour'   A wide-selling aldehydic floral–oriental scent launched by Max Factor in 1986. Composed of 192 ingredients, it contains rose, with orris, coriander and black pepper, in the top notes, leading into a heart which is primarily composed of neroli, tuberose, geranium and ylang-ylang, and base notes of sandalwood, vanilla, amber and musk. The flacons are made by Bermioli Luigi of Italy.

'Le Jardin de Max Factor'   A wide-selling light floral perfume introduced by Max Factor in 1982. It was created by the perfumers of Dragoco. The top note is fruity–floral, with neroli, honeysuckle, peach and bergamot. In the floral middle note jasmine, rose, lily of the valley and magnolia predominate, while the base contains amber, cedar, myrrh and a hint of musk.

'L'Élisir d'Amore'   A quality toilet water launched by Crabtree & Evelyn in 1989 as a fragrance in toiletries sold in conjunction with the Royal Opera House in London. It is based on a popular handkerchief perfume of the 19th century and contains a floral medley on a woody base.

Lelong, Lucien   A leading Parisian couturier who established the Lucien Lelong perfume house with the launching of his first perfume, 'Tout le

Long', in 1925. There followed 'A' and 'B', both in 1927 and both in Lalique bottles, and a series of other fragrances which included 'Indiscret' (35), 'Cachet' (48) and 'Édition Limitée' (50) (his last). Lelong bottles were noted for their startling modernity.

Lemon Balm   *see* Balm

Lemon Grass Oil   Also called Camel Grass Oil. An essential oil obtained by steam-distillation from Lemon Grass (*Cymbopogon citratus* = *C. schoenanthus* = *Andropogon schoenanthus* = *A. citratus*), native to the Middle East and India. The plant is also known as Camel Grass, Rush, Scented Rush and Camel Rush. In western perfumery it is principally used in soaps, but in India it is found in both perfumes and medicines. It is cultivated in India, Sri Lanka, the Seychelles, the Far East, central Africa, central America and the W. Indies as a major source of citral, one of the chief constituents of the oil. In dried form the plant is also used in pot pourri and sachets. The oil is sometimes called Oil of Verbena because of its similarity with Verbena Oil. The early Arab perfume makers used it in perfumes based on sesame and cotton seed oil, recognizing, as did Dioscorides, that the best quality came from N. Arabia (until recently it was used in Arabia for scenting a bath). It is believed to be the Calamus of the Greeks and Romans.

Lemon Grass de Cochin   Also called Oil of Inchy and Lemon Grass des Indes Orientales. An essential oil distilled from a grass, East Indian Lemon Grass (*Cymbopogon flexuosus* = *Andropogon flexuosus*), native to south India but cultivated elsewhere, including Vietnam, central America, the W. Indies and Madagascar. It has the scent of violets and lemons and is used in the perfume and soap industries. The oil from the wild plant, growing in India, is similar to Palma Rosa Oil. See also Kachi Grass Oil.

Lemon Nettle   *see* Balm

Lemon Oil   Also called Cedro Oil. An essential oil extracted by expression from the fruit peel of the Lemon tree (*Citrus medica* var. *limonum* = *C. limon*). The tree is believed to have originated in subtropical Asia, probably in northern India; it was introduced into Europe by the Arabs from about the 8th century AD, probably through Sicily and Spain, and is now found all round the Mediterranean, especially in Sicily and southern Italy, and in many other areas, notably California, where it was first grown in 1887. About 1000 lemons will yield 1 lb of oil. The oil is used in flavourings, liqueurs and medicines as well as in perfumery, soaps and cosmetics. Dried lemon peel is sometimes used in sachets and pot pourri. Lemon oil with an unusually delicate fragrance is obtained from the Yuzu Lemon tree of Japan. Lemon oil appears in a very large number of modern quality perfumes, giving top notes a fresh sparkle, and is particularly popular in men's fragrances. Some examples of perfumes containing it are 'Cristalle', 'Mon Parfum',

'Jicky', 'Shalimar' and 'Calandre'.

Lemon Scented Gum Tree *see* Eucalyptus

Lemon Scented Iron Bark Tree *see* Eucalyptus

Lemon Scented Tea Tree Oil *see* Ti-tree

Lenthéric Founded in 1875 in Paris by a hairdresser, Gillaume Lenthéric, who became a fashionable perfumer, the House of Lenthéric is now one of the leading perfume and cosmetics companies in the world. In 1990 it was sold by the Beecham Group to its management. Its fragrances, designed for the middle market, include 'Tweed' (1933), 'Just Musk' (73), 'Tramp' (75), 'Panache' (77), 'Mystique' (81), 'Joie de Vivre' (85), 'Style' (87), 'Fashion' (89), 'Panache Evening Edition' (89) and 'Fleur' (91), together with a fragrance for men 'Hallmark' (86).

Lentisk *see* Mastic

Léonard A French fashion house which formed its own perfume company, Parfums Léonard, in 1969. It produced 'Fashion' in 1970, followed by 'Eau Fraiche' (74), 'Tamango' (77), 'Léonard pour Homme' (80) and 'Balahé' (83).

Leptactinia densiflora *see* Karokarounde

       senegambia *see* Karokarounde

       manii *see* Karakarounde

Les Senteurs *see* 'Apogée'

Levisticum officinale *see* Lovage

'L'Heure Bleue' An innovative classic floral–oriental perfume by Guerlain dating from 1912 which was created by Jacques Guerlain. The effect is sweet and spicy. Bergamot, with hints of lemon, neroli, tarragon, coriander and sage, sets a fresh top note, giving way to a heart of carnation supported by jasmine, rose, orris, ylang-ylang and other fragrances on a base note principally comprising sandalwood and musk, but supported by, amongst others, St John's wort. It is sold in a flacon by Baccarat.

Liatris *see* Lacinaria

Liatris odoratissima *see* Lacinaria

Libanotris *see* Acerra

Lichen *see* Fragrant Moss/Oak Moss/Tree Moss/Hazelcrottle and Ash Tree Lichen

Light Notes The term light is used in perfumery to denote fragrances which have a fresh floral, citrus, fruity or green content without any sweet or balsamic elements. See Perfume Notes.

Lignum Aloes *see* Aloewood

Lignum Aspalathum *see* Rosewood Oil

Lignum Rhodium *see* Aloewood

Liiorin Gum *see* Balsam of Copaiba

Lilac A fragrant oil, also in perfumery called Syringa, which is obtained from the flowers of the Common Lilac (*Syringa vulgaris*) and related species, a shrub which originated in Iran and eastern Europe and is now grown widely in temperate regions. The oil is used in quality perfumes (e.g. 'Chamade', 'Soir de Paris', 'Florissa' and 'Tweed').

The plant was introduced into Europe through Spain by the Arabs in about the 16th century and originally the flowers were used in pomanders. The extraction of this fragrance by volatile solvents was not possible until the discovery of carbon dioxide as a solvent (see Volatile Solvents). However, many lilac perfumes are now made synthetically from chemical substances. The dried flowers are used in sachets and pot pourri. See also Mock Orange Blossom.

Lillie, Charles Sometimes regarded as the first professional British perfumer. He owned a shop in the Strand, London, in the early part of the 18th century and was the author of a book *The British Perfumer*.

Lily An essential oil used in perfumery is obtained from the flowers of two species of Lily: the Madonna Lily (*Lilium candidum*) (in the early days of Christianity it was dedicated to the Madonna as a symbol of purity), also called the Annunciation Lily and Bourbon Lily, a plant native to the Mediterranean area and S.W. Asia; and the Easter Lily (*L. longiflorum*), also of Mediterranean origin. Both these plants are cultivated widely, but the fragrance of lily in perfumery is nowadays mostly created synthetically, with the exception of some high-quality perfumes such as 'Zinnia'.

The lily has been used in perfumery since ancient times. It was popular in Egypt, where a perfumed ointment was based on 'the flowers of 2000 lilies' (probably here the blue water lily), and the ancient Greeks used Madonna lilies to make a perfume called Susinon.

Lily of the Valley Also called Muguet, a perfume obtained from the highly scented flowers of Lily of the Valley (*Convallaria majalis*), a small plant native to Europe but now grown all over N. America and northern areas of Asia. The plant is also called May Lily, Convallaria, Our Lady's Tears, Jacob's Ladder and Male Lily. Country lore held that the fragrance of these flowers drew the nightingale towards his mate. There is no evidence of its use in perfumery in ancient times; the 'Lily of the Valleys' quoted in the Bible is thought to have been Hyacinth.

In early days Lily of the Valley fragrance could only be obtained by infusing the flowers into olive oil or sweet almond oil. In modern perfumery the perfume is extracted by volatile solvents as a concrete or absolute and no essential oil is distilled. It is usually sold with a synthetic (Hydroxy citronellal), which almost duplicates the fragrance, added up to 50%, and it is the resulting product which is properly known as Muguet. Muguet provides the most exquisite lily fragrance available and is very highly regarded by perfumers. Some 14% of all modern quality perfumes contain it, for example 'Opium', 'Roma' and

'Florissa', and it appears in some 10% of men's fragrances. See also Farnesol.

Lime Oil   An oil obtained both by expression and by distillation from the rind of the fruits of the Lime tree (*Citrus medica* var. *acida*), which is grown for this purpose principally in the W. Indies. The tree is indigenous to India. The oil, which is among those now modified for safety or environmental reasons (see Perfume Creation), is mostly used in flavouring, but it is also found in high-class perfumes (e.g. 'Amouage') and eau de colognes, especially those containing coriander. It is also a source of citral.

Lime Tree   *see* Tilleul

Linaloe Oil   Also called Rosewood Oil (q.v.), Bois de Rose Oil and Essence de Bois Rose. An essential oil with a balsamic, floral, slightly rose-like odour; it is steam-distilled from wood chips from a tree called Rose Femelle (*Aniba rosaeodora* = *Aydendron rosaeodora*), native to the lower Amazon area. It is used extensively in lily and lilac-type perfumes and in colognes.

A similar oil with the same name is distilled in Mexico and the USA from the bark and fruits of the Linaloe Wood tree (*Bursera delpichiana*), also called the Mexican Linaloe Wood tree, native to Mexico. It is used in perfumes, soaps and cosmetics. The older trees of this species are preferred as they produce more oil.

Another form of Bois de Rose oil, also called Cayenne Linaloe Oil and Azelia Oil, is obtained from the Cayenne Linaloe tree (*Aniba panurense*) of Brazil. See also Sandalwood.

Linaloe Oil is an important source of linalol.

Linalol   An alcohol used in perfumery which is contained in Linaloe and some other essential oils, including linaloe wood, petitgrain, coriander and lavender. It has an attractive spicy–floral odour and is used in perfumes with honeysuckle, lilac or lily fragrances.

Linden Tree   *see* Tilleul

Lindera benzoin   *see* Spicewood

fericia   *see* Kuromoji

umbellata   *see* Kuromoji

Linear Fragrance   A term which has recently come into use in perfumery to describe a new style of perfume which started to become popular in the late 1980s. Instead of the classical perfume structure of top, middle and lower notes (see Perfume Notes), linear fragrances are designed to produce a strong and instant effect which remains constant. This is mostly achieved with a floral bouquet (e.g. 'Giorgio, Beverly Hills', 'Fendi', 'Carolina Herrera' and 'C'est la Vie'), but in some cases with other effects (e.g. a spicy–fruity effect in 'Poison'), in all cases supported by traditional woody, mossy or amber base notes.

Linseed Oil   Derived from the seed of Flax (*Linum usitatissimum*), a plant indigenous to temperate areas of Europe and Asia. In early times the oil was used as a lamp oil and in cooking. In ancient Egypt it provided a base oil for perfumes (see Egyptian Perfumes).

'L'Interdit' Givenchy's first perfume, launched in 1957 in tribute to Audrey Hepburn. A floral–aldehydic fragrance created by Roure perfumers. Top notes are pepper, clove and a touch of galbanum, amplified by aldehydes. The heart, containing mostly rose, jasmine and violet, is supported by base notes which include sandalwood, vetiver, patchouli, iris, amber and frankincense.

Linum usitatissimum   *see* Linseed Oil

Lippia   Oil obtained from the leaves of several species of *Lippia* is used in perfumery. From *Lippia citriodora* comes Verbena Oil (q.v.). Of the other species the principal is *Lippia dulcis*, a shrub which grows up to 18 feet high in tropical America and Mexico.

Liquid Storax   *see* Storax

Liquidamber orientalis   *see* Storax

        styraciflua   *see* Storax

Litsaea citrata   *see* May-chang

      cubeba   *see* May-chang

Litsea Cubeba Oil   An essential oil with a coriander-like odour obtained by steam-distillation from the ripe fruit of a species of Litsea tree (*Litsea cubeba* = *L. citrata* = *Tetranthera polyantha*), native to S.E. Asia and China, where it is known as May-chang. The oil has an importance in perfumery as a raw material from which citral is obtained.

Little Dragon   *see* Tarragon

Living Flower Technology   A technique recently developed by IFF which is designed to capture the exact fragrance of flowers. A single living flower is encapsulated in a vacuum for 6 to 12 hours and the fragrance emitted by it is then analysed on a gas liquid chromatograph, said to provide an exact chemical description of the aroma which can then be imitated synthetically. The technique has been used for some of the ingredients of quality perfumes (e.g. osmanthus, carnation and jasmine in 'Red' and others in 'Eternity'). It is now being extended to include herbs, spices and fruits.

Llorente, Jacques   A leading designer of perfume bottles. He has produced designs for, among others, Hermés, Louis Feraud, Van Cleef & Arpels and Worth.

Lobaria fraxinea   *see* Ash Twig Lichen

      prunastri   *see* Oak Moss

      pulmonaria   *see* Hazelcrottle

Longosa Oil   An oil extracted from the fragrant flowers of a species of Hedychium (*Hedychium flavum*), native to N. India and cultivated for this oil on the island of Nossé Bé, north of Madagascar. It has a peppery fragrance, with a background reminiscent of ylang-ylang, jasmine, orange blossom and tuberose. See also Kapur-kachri.

Lonicera caprifolium   *see* Honeysuckle
   fragrantissima   *see* Honeysuckle
   periclymenon   *see* Honeysuckle

Lorbeer   *see* Bay

L'Oréal   Based in Paris, L'Oréal is now the largest of all the conglomerates in the international toiletries, cosmetics and fragrances business. Its subsidiaries include Cacharel, Courrèges, Giorgio Armani, Guy Laroche, Lancôme, Ralph Lauren, Phas, Helena Rubinstein and Vichy.

'L'Origan'   A classic perfume introduced by Coty in 1905 which set a trend for floral perfumes of a sweet, spicy nature. The top note was chiefly bergamot, with underlying hints of mandarin, coriander, pepper and peach. The middle note contained a blend of clove and carnation, with ylang-ylang, orchid, rose, jasmine and orris. In the woody lower notes sandalwood was supported by, among others, cedarwood, labdanum and musk.

Loris Azzaro   An Italian designer of fashion, fashion accessories and theatre costumes who established his business in Paris in 1965. In 1970 he marketed the perfume 'Azzaro', followed by 'Azzaro 9' (84) and a men's fragrance 'Azzaro pour Homme' (78). All three are contained in bottles designed by Pierre Dinand.

'Lou-Lou'   An unusually strong oriental–floral perfume created by Jean Guichard of Roure for Cacharel, who launched it in 1987. Top notes of jasmine, orange blossom, cassie and ylang-ylang lead into a heart of heliotrope and musk, with base notes provided by tonka, vanilla, frankincense and sandalwood. The flacon, which is blue opaline, was designed by Annegret Beier.

Lotus   A name given to perfumes with a heavy oriental-type fragrance made by compounding natural perfume materials such as patchouli, benzoin or storax with various modifying artificial ones. No perfume oil is extracted from the Lotus plant.

Lovage   Also called Bladder Lovage, Cornish Lovage, Garden Lovage, Italian Lovage, Old English Lovage, Lovage Angelica and Sea Parsley. A perennial plant (*Levisticum officinale* = *Angelica levisticum*) growing up to 5 feet high, native to the Mediterranean area but now found widely and cultivated in England, France and elsewhere. An essential oil, known as Oil of Lovage, is distilled from the whole plant and has a limited use in perfumery as well as being used in flavouring. Its scent is spicy and persistent, reminiscent of a mixture of angelica or celery with oak moss. The dried roots and leaves, which have good fixative properties, are used in sachets and pot pourri

   Lovage was well known to the Greeks and Romans for its medicinal and flavouring properties and for its value in overcoming unpleasant odours.

Love-in-the-Mist   *see* Nigella Oil/Gith

Low Note   Also called Lower Note, Base Note, Back Note and Dry-off. A term used in perfumery to describe the third and last phase in the process of a perfume's evaporation on the skin, when the most lasting ingredients, such as woody or animalic scents, become most discernible. The term also covers the ingredients which provide that effect. See Perfume Notes.

Lucca Gum   *see* Olive Gum

'Lumière'   A fresh–floral quality perfume created by Nicolas Mamounas and perfumers of IFF for Rochas, who launched it in 1984. Green top notes, which include hawthorn, honeysuckle, coriander and orange flower, herald a middle note dominated by gardenia, jasmine and magnolia, with a base note built on sandalwood and ambergris. The bottle was designed by Carré Noir.

Lungwort   *see* Hazelcrottle

Lupinus arboreus   *see* Tree Lupin

'Lutèce'   A quality floral perfume launched by Houbigant in 1986 and named after the early Roman name for Paris. The aldehydic floral top note includes rose, jasmine and lily of the valley, developing into a powdery, floral heart of rose and peony with a touch of mandarin. Amber heads the base notes.

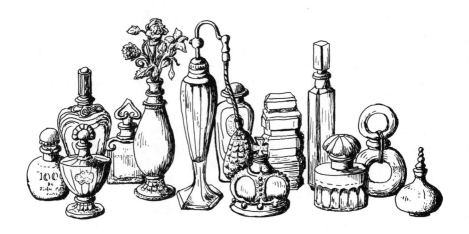

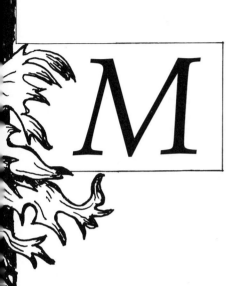

Macalep Oil   *see* Magalep

'Macassar'   The name of a trend-setting, spicy, leather-type fragrance for men introduced as an eau de toilette by Rochas in 1980. It was created by Nicolas Mamounas. Its main ingredients are bergamot and artemisia in the top note, jasmine, carnation, patchouli and vetivert in the middle note, and oak moss and leather-fragrance in the base.

Macassar Oil   An oil derived principally from the seeds of the Ceylon Oak (*Schleichera trijuga*), also called the Kussum tree and Malay Lacktree, of Malaysia and Indonesia, but in earlier times possibly from the seeds of safflower. It also contained ylang-ylang among its ingredients. It was widely used in Victorian times as a hair preparation, giving rise to the 'anti-macassar' used on chair backs, designed to protect upholstery against oily stains.

Mace (and Nutmeg)   Mace, also called Macis and Arillus Myristicae, and Nutmeg both come from the fruit of the Nutmeg tree (*Myristica fragrans = M. officinalis = M. aromatica*). In French, *muscadier* (a name also used in English) is the nutmeg tree, *muscade* meaning nutmeg and also musk-like; our word nutmeg derives from an earlier word *notemuge* – early English 'note' = nut and early French *mugue* = musky. The tree, which grows to about 35 feet high, is native to the Molucca islands and is now cultivated in Indonesia, Sri Lanka, Malaysia and Grenada, mainly for nutmeg used as a spice.

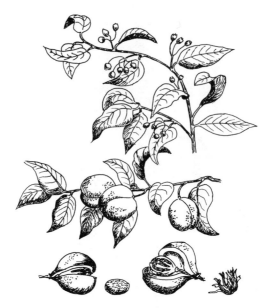

Mace and nutmeg (*Myristica fragrans*).

Nutmeg is the kernal of the fruit (or nut). Oil of Nutmeg is usually obtained from kernals unsuitable through damage etc. to be sold as a spice. The oil, expressed, steam-distilled or extracted, is used to give perfumes, colognes and lavender waters a spicy or masculine note, and it is found in many quality fragrances (e.g. 'Blue Grass', 'Panthère', 'Sybaris' and 'You're the Fire'). However, most distilled oil is used as a flavouring. The distilled oil is sometimes called Nutmeg Butter and, misleadingly, Oil of Mace. Mace is the wrapping ('arillus') round the kernal and provides a very similar, though less pungent, oil by distillation which is used occasionally in sandalwood-type soaps. Mace is also used dried in sachets and pot pourri. Nutmeg was known as early as Roman times, and the early Arab perfumers used both types of oil. Mace should not be confused with English Mace, a name sometimes given to costmary.

Macrotomia cephalotus   *see* Alkanet

Maceration   Also called digestion. An ancient method of obtaining aromatic substances from flowers and other plant parts by boiling them or heating them to a high temperature in water or oil, which absorbed their aroma. It has the disadvantage that with many materials the heat will damage the fragrance. But the technique is still sometimes practiced in modern perfumery with certain materials, using oils or fats heated to about 60°–70°C, into which the materials are immersed up to 15 times for periods of an hour or two at a time, the fat then being cleansed of residue and purified. The principal materials still sometimes so treated are cassie, hyacinth, jonquil, mimosa, orange flower, rose, narcissus and violet.

Madagascar Jasmine   *see* Stephanotis

'Madame Rochas' A classic aldehydic–floral perfume created by Guy Robert for Rochas, who first marketed it in 1960 and re-launched it in 1989. It has some 200 ingredients. The principal top notes are orange blossom, broom, honeysuckle and neroli, covering a floral heart dominated by ylang-ylang, tuberose, jasmine, orris and rose, with a woody base, chiefly sandalwood and cedar, backed by hints of musk and amber. The container is a replica of an 18th century scent bottle in crystal by Baccarat.

Magalep Also called Mahaleb, Macalep, St Lucia Cherry, Hurtleberry, Austrian Cherry and Perfumed Cherry. A deciduous tree (*Prunus mahaleb*) growing up to 40 feet high in Europe and W. Asia and cultivated in Britain since the 17th century. The fragrant wood (called St Lucia Wood) is used for walking sticks, tobacco pipes, etc. and an essential oil is occasionally distilled from it for use in perfumery. The seeds (cherry stones) are used in sachets and pot pourri. In early times the flesh of the seeds was used in their recipes by Arab and Persian perfume makers, who knew it as *mahlab*. During the 17th century the seeds were threaded on cords as aromatic beads. The flesh in the seeds was at one time expressed for its juice, or ground into a pulp called Milk of Magalep, which was strained, mixed with other fragrant substances such as rosewater, and used in washballs.

Magma From Greek, a thick unguent. The word was also applied to the dried dregs from old unguent bottles, which the Greeks and Romans collected and added to scented powders in order to improve their fragrance. (See Greek Perfumes.)

Magnolia This name is used for many synthetic perfumes, usually containing jasmine, neroli and rose.

Magnolia glauca   *see* Sassafras

       grandiflora   *see* Sassafras

       kobus   *see* Kabushi Oil

'Ma Griffe' A classic, trend-setting chypre perfume first produced by Carven in 1944. Created by Roure perfumers, the initial impact is green, with gardenia in the top notes modified by citrus, galbanum and clary sage. The floral middle notes, mostly jasmine and rose, are supplemented by, among others, sandalwood and vetivert. In the base notes, storax and oak moss predominate, with hints of cinnamon, benzoin, labdanum and musk. The cube-shaped bottle was designed by Jacques Bocquet.

Majorana hortensis   *see* Marjoram

Malabathrum A perfume material used in unguents by the Romans (see

Roman Perfumes) which was imported from N. India in considerable quantity and is referred to several times by Pliny. It is thought to have been a dried aromatic leaf from a species of cinnamon found in N. India and known as the Indian Cassia tree (*Cinnamomum tamala*). In Sanskrit it is called *Tamala pattra*, from which the word Malabathrum derives. The bark of this tree is still used as a substitute for cinnamon.

Malay Lacktree   *see* Macassar Oil

'Ma Liberté'   An unusual spicy–floral perfume created by Jean Kerleo and launched by Jean Patou in 1987. It has top notes which include lavender, clove, pepper and vanilla, leading to a heart of jasmine with cedar, vetivert and patchouli, on a powdery base note containing sandalwood, vanilla and musk.

Malus communis   *see* Apple

    pumila   *see* Apple

Mammea longifolia   *see* Nag Kesar

Mamounas, Nicolas   Chief perfumer for Rochas. His creations include 'Mystère', 'Macassar', 'Lumière' and 'Globe'. Founder of the School of Perfumery in Versailles.

Mandarin Oil   An oil expressed from the fruit peel of two species of the Mandarin Orange tree (*Citrus reticulata* = *C. nobilis* and *C. madurensis*), which are cultivated in Italy, Sicily, Spain, Florida, Argentina and Brazil for this purpose. The oil, which has a fragrance similar to Sweet Orange Oil, is used in colognes and in some floral perfumes, including quality perfumes (e.g. 'Diva', 'Jicky' and 'Mitsouko'). The dried peel is used in sachets and pot pourri. The tree is native to Cochin-China, being brought to Europe and America in the 18th century. The leaves and twigs provide a kind of Petitgrain Oil. See also Tangerine Oil.

Mang-tsao tree   *see* Japanese Star Anise

Maniguette   *see* Grains of Paradise

Mansau, Serge   A sculptor and prominent designer of contemporary scent bottles. He has designed, among others, for Cardin, Caron, Dior, Fath, Laroche, Léonard, Molyneux, Oscar de la Renta, Patou, Révillon and Rochas. See Perfume Containers.

Manzanilla   *see* Camomile

Marigold   The orange-flowered Common Marigold (*Calendula officinalis*), native to S. Europe and the Middle East but now cultivated widely, provides from the flowers a small amount of essential oil, also called Calendula, which is produced as a concrete or absolute for use in perfumery. The dried flowers also have medicinal uses.

Certain marigolds of the *Tagetes* genus also provide an essential oil, by steam-distillation from their seeds, called Taget or Tagetes Oil, which is used in perfumery. They include the French Marigold (*Tagetes patula* = *T. minuta*), also known as Indian Carnation, native to tropical America but now cultivated widely. Taget (or Tagette) Oil has an intense, cloying, fruity fragrance resembling apple, and is used in cosmetics and in many floral perfumes (e.g. 'Lauren', 'Boucheron' and 'Samba').

Marjoram Also called Sweet Marjoram and Knotted Marjoram. A bushy annual herb (*Origanum majorana = Majorana hortensis*) growing to about 1 foot high, probably native to Portugal but now found throughout Europe, N. Africa and the Middle East and cultivated widely. Oil of Marjoram is steam-distilled from the leaves and used for flavouring and in perfumery. Its scent resembles a cross between mint and thyme with a trace of nutmeg. Some 150–200 lb of the herb yield about 1 lb of oil. The dried leaves are used in sachets and pot pourri. Oil of Marjoram is also distilled from the Wild Marjoram (*Origanum vulgare*), a perennial herb growing in Asia, Europe and N. Africa with a strong, fragrant balsamic odour. In France this oil, which too is occasionally used in perfumery, is known as 'Marjolaine sauvage', the oil from *O.majorana* being known as 'Marjolaine douce'.

The name marjoram derives from Greek meaning 'joy of the mountains'. The ancient Greeks, who believed that if it grew on a grave it augured happiness for the departed, used it extensively in medicines, flavouring and perfumery. It was the sampsuchum of the ancient Egyptians, who gave its name to a long-lasting unguent and a scented oil popular in classical times. Both the seeds and the leaves of marjoram were used by the early Arab perfume makers.

An oil called Oil of Marjoram is also obtained from the leaves of a small species of thyme called Mastic Thyme (*Thymus mastichiana*). See also Origanum Oil.

Marsh Parsley *see* Peucedan Gum

Marsh Rosemary Oil An oil obtained from the leaves of the Marsh Rosemary (*Ledum palustre*), also known as Crystal Tea Ledum, one of the few plants which grows in Arctic as well as sub-Arctic regions. The leaves are also used by Eskimos as a tea. The oil has a bitter, coriander-like fragrance.

The name Marsh Rosemary is also sometimes used for American Sea Lavender (*Statice caroliana*), also called Ink Root, a sea-plant found on both sides of the Atlantic, from the roots of which a volatile oil is obtained for use in medicines.

Mary Chess A small high-quality perfume company founded in 1932 by Mrs Grace Mary Chess Robinson, an American living in London who was also known for her sculptured flowers. She created all her perfumes herself, using only natural ingredients. Her first perfume was 'White Lilac' (1933), followed by 'Tapestry' (34), 'Strategy' (35), 'Tuberose' (37) and 'Yram' (38). In 1978 the company also launched 'Chess d'Or'. The company produces a variety of other toiletries and holds royal warrants to supply the Queen Mother and other royalty. It is closely associated with the long-established fragrance firm Taylor of London, both being acquired in 1991 by The Fine Fragrances and Cosmetics Group (see also Caron).

Mastic   Also called Gum Mastic, Sweet Assa and Resina Lentisci. A gum obtained from the bark of the Lentisk tree (*Pistacia lentiscus*), a small shrub-like tree growing up to 12 feet high in the Mediterranean area and parts of Asia. It was introduced into Britain in the 17th century. The main sources of commercial supply of this gum are the islands of Cyprus, Scio and, for many centuries, Chios. The fragrance is very balsamic, with a penetrating, leafy odour recalling savin and turpentine. In early times the gum was used in pomanders and the oil was used to absorb other plant fragrances in the process of enfleurage. In modern perfumery the extracted oil is used as a fixative in various perfume compounds; it appears, for example, in 'Fahrenheit'.

Maté   An absolute used in perfumery which is developed from oil extracted from the leaves of the Yerba Maté tree (*Ilex paraguensis*), also called the Paraguay Tea tree, found in Argentina, Brazil, Paraguay and Uruguay. It has a rich, tea-like fragrance. The plant has been used in S. America since ancient times as a source of tea.

Matico   A climbing shrub (*Piper augustifolium*), also called Matico Pepper and Soldier's Herb, native to central America, Mexico and the W. Indies. The leaves provide an essential oil with an odour reminiscent of pepper, cubebs and mint. It is very powerful and hence used only in minute amounts, usually in carnation compounds. Matico was the name of a Spanish soldier who accidentally discovered the medical properties of the leaves when wounded in Peru.

Matricaria chamomilla   *see* Camomile
         discoidea   *see* Camomile
         parthenium   *see* Fever Chrysanthemum

Matthiola bicornis   *see* Night-scented Stock
         incana   *see* Stock

Mattipaul   A resin used for incense in Hindu temples. It is extracted from the trunk of the But tree (*Ailanthus malabarica*), also called the Thanh-that tree, found in India and Vietnam.

Maudlin   A perennial, sweet-scented yarrow (*Achillea ageratum*), also called Maudeline, Sweet Milfoil, Sweet Nancy, Camphor Plant, Balsamita Foemina and Sweet Yarrow. It grows up to 5 inches high and is native to Italy and Spain, being introduced into Britain from Italy in 1570 as a medicinal herb; during the 16th century it was a popular aromatic. The dried flowers and leaves are used in sachets and pot pourri to provide a balsamic note. It was at one time used with costmary to make washballs.

Mawah Oil   The name given to a variety of rose–geranium oil obtained from *Pelargonium graveolens*, which is produced in Kenya. See Geranium.

Max Factor   Max Factor, a theatre wig-master and make-up artist in Tsarist Russia, emigrated to the USA in 1904, forming his company, Max Factor & Co, in 1909 to provide make-up for the Hollywood film industry. By 1930 the company was selling 'Max Factor – the Make-up of the Stars' in 81 countries. It was purchased by Norman Simon Inc. in 1972, became part of the International Playtex Group in 1983, merged with the Revlon Group in 1987 and was bought by Proctor & Gamble in 1991. The UK branch of the company was opened in 1935 and has its main factory in Bournemouth. In 1980 it acquired the fashion house of Mary Quant.

The principal Max Factor perfumes currently marketed are 'Le Jardin de Max Factor' (82) and 'Le Jardin d'Amour' (86). Other fragrances, sold at Eau de Toilette strength, include 'Geminesse' (74), 'Blasé' (75), and 'Epris' (81), together with three fragrances, 'Intuition', 'Charade' and 'Desire', linked under the name 'Liaisons' and introduced in 1988.

May Blossom   *see* Hawthorn

May-chang   *see* Litsea Cubeba Oil

Meadowsweet Oil   An oil used in perfumery which is distilled from the flower buds of the Meadowsweet plant (*Filipendula ulmaria* = *Spiraea ulmaria*), also called Queen of the Meadows, Dolloff, Bridewort and Ulmaria. It is native to temperate Europe and Asia and is also now found in N. America. The flowers have an almond-like scent. Queen Elizabeth I was particularly fond of it as a strewing herb. Gerard, writing in about 1600, observed that the smell of the leaves 'makes the heart merry and delighteth the senses'. The dried leaves and flowers are used in sachets and pot pourri. See also Dropwort.

Mecca Myrrh   *see* Balsam of Makkah

Medici, Catherine de   1519–1589 The daughter of the Italian Duke of Urbino who in 1533 married the future King Henry II of France. She was the mother of three future kings and a powerful influence in the French court. She had a considerable interest in perfumery and brought an Italian with her who established a successful perfume-making business in Paris. She was instrumental in setting up a laboratory in Grasse for the study of perfume-making in order to rival the fashionable Arab perfumes of the time, for which she is regarded by some as the founder of the French perfume industry.

Megaleion Perfume   Also called Megalium. An ancient Greek perfume described by Theophrastus. It contained 'burnt resin' and oil of balanos (which was first boiled 'for ten days and nights'), into which were mixed cinnamon, cassia and myrrh. A colourant was added. Theophrastus noted that this perfume and Mendesian perfume were the most troublesome to make, since they contained many costly ingredients. It was believed to be good for wounds. Being fairly heady it was, Theophrastus observed, best suited for women, especially as it was very long-lasting.

The Romans also used Megalium, which in Pliny's time was composed of balanos oil, balsam, calamus, sweet-rush, xylobalsam, cassia and resin.

Mehndi *see* Cyprinum

Melanthion *see* Gith

Meleguata Pepper *see* Grains of Paradise

Meleleuca Oil *see* Ti-tree Oil

Meleleuca alternifolia *see* Ti-tree Oil

                    bracteata *see* Ti-tree Oil

                    leucadendron *see* Cajuput

                    viridiflora *see* Cajuput

Melia A species of Melia known as the Bead tree (*Melia azedarach*), native from N. India to Malaysia and W. China and now cultivated widely. The name derives from its pea-sized, musk-scented seeds, which are used to make rosary beads.

Melilot Also called Sweet Clover. A sweetly scented, clover-like plant, growing up to 4 feet high, of the genus *Melilotis*, found widely in Europe and Asia, which is sometimes used in perfumery. The Common Yellow Melilot (*Melilotis officinalis*), also called Sweet Lucerne, Kings Clover, Wild Laburnum and Hart's Tree, is found in Europe, temperate Asia and N. Africa and was once cultivated extensively in Britain for fodder. The White Melilot (*M. alba*) and Corn Melilot (*M. arvensis*) still grow wild in Britain but are less abundant. All three species have a sweet hay-like fragrance, remarkably attractive to bees (the name derives from 'Mel', meaning 'honey', and Lotus, hence signifying 'honey-lotus'), due to a high content of coumarin. The dried flowers and leaves are used in sachets and pot pourri and sometimes to scent tobacco (also for flavouring cheese). A fourth species (*M. bungiana* = *M. suavolens* = *M. graveolens*) is found in S.E. Asia and the dried flowers are used as a source of coumarin.

Melilot was known to the Romans (it is listed by Dioscorides) for its medicinal properties and was used by medieval Arab perfume makers.

Melinum A perfume oil made from quince flowers which, according to Pliny, was used in unguents in conjunction with omphacium, cyprinum, sesame oil, balsam, sweet rush, cassia and southernwood.

Melissa *see* Balm

Melissa officinalis see Balm

Melon A melon-like fragrance is occasionally used in modern quality perfumes (e.g. 'Knowing'). It is normally created with synthetics.

Memecyclon The leaves of the tree *Memecyclon tinctorium* (= *M. edule*), found in regions bordering the Indian Ocean including Yemen and Ethiopia, provide a yellow dye which was held in such high esteem as a colouring agent by the early Arab perfume makers that al-Kindi even provided a recipe for imitating it.

Mendesian Perfume   A perfume of the ancient Egyptians (see Egyptian Perfumes) originally made in the city of Mendes. It was popular also in Greece and Rome, the Greeks calling it 'the Egyptian'. Theophrastus recorded that it contained a number of expensive ingredients, including cinnamon and myrrh, was colourless, and was one of the most long-lasting of all perfumes. He also observed that it could cause headaches, to counter which it was sometimes mixed with fragrant wine to make it sweeter. Pliny noted that it was made of 'behen-oil, resin and myrrh'. See also Megaleion Perfume.

'Men's Club'   An eau de cologne introduced by Helena Rubinstein in 1966 for use by men. The fragrance is floral, with spicy aldehydes in the top note, rose and jasmine in the heart and musk and cedarwood in the base.

Mentha aquatica   *see* Bergamot Mint

  arvensis   *see* Peppermint

  citrata   *see* Bergamot Mint

  longifolia   *see* Mint

  odorata   *see* Bergamot Mint

  piperata   *see* Peppermint

  pulegium   *see* Mint/Pennyroyal

  rotundifolia   *see* Mint

  spicata   *see* Mint

  sylvestris   *see* Mint

  viridint (viridis)   *see* Mint

Mespilodaphne sassafras   *see* Safrole

'Métal'   A fresh–floral perfume launched by Paco Rabanne in 1979. It was created by Firmenich perfumers. Citrus fruits in the top note introduce a floral bouquet in the heart which includes jasmine, ylang-ylang, narcissus and an unusual rose ingredient. Sandalwood provides the main base note. The perfume comes in a bottle designed by Pierre Bellereaud.

Metallic Note   A term used in perfumery to denote a fragrance reminiscent of metal, providing a clean, cool effect. Metallic notes are used in perfumes to assist in promoting an effect, not as main fragrances. See Perfume Notes.

'Métamorphose'   A floral perfume created in 1979 by Jean Laporte, whose fragrances, which include a wide variety of quality toilet waters, soaps, burning oils, etc., are sold through his company L'Artisan Parfumeur in Paris and London. 'Métamorphose', a blend of 52 essences, contains top notes which include blackcurrant buds and tangerine, a heart mainly of rose, jasmine, iris and carnation, and a base dominated by sandalwood. It is sold in a flacon with an opalescent crystal stopper in the form of a butterfly.

Methyl Salicylate   The principal odorous constituent of Oil of Gaultheria

(Wintergreen) and found in many other volatile oils. It provides a pungent, minty odour. It is now manufactured synthetically from coal tar and is much used in modern perfumery.

Metopian Unguent   A perfumed unguent of the ancient Egyptians, Greeks and Romans. It was based on oil of bitter almond and contained honey, wine, myrrh and calamus or, according to another source (Dioscorides), oil of bitter almond and unripe olives perfumed with cardamom, sweet rush, sweet flag, honey, wine, myrrh, seed of balsamum, galbanum and turpentine resin. Pliny recorded that the Roman version was pressed out of bitter almonds, with the addition of omphacium, cardamom, rush, flag, honey, wine, myrrh, seed of balsam, galbanum and terebinth-resin.

Mexican Mock Orange   A shrub (*Philadelphus mexicanus*), also called Mock Orange Blossom, from the flowers and branches of which a scented water has been distilled since early times as a perfume. The fragrance resembles that of true orange blossom. See also Mock Orange Blossom.

Mexican Orange   *see* Orange Blossom

Mexican Tea   *see* Ambroisia

Michelia champaca   *see* Champaca
  fuscata   *see* Banana Shrub
  longifolia   *see* Champaca
  montana   *see* Champaca

Micro-fragrance   Also called micro-encapsulation and 'scratch-and-sniff'. A technique devised by the Minnesota Mining and Manufacturing Co. (3M) in 1970 by which large numbers of microscopic capsules containing a fragrance are coated on to paper, so that their odour is released when they are broken, e.g. by scratching with a fingernail. The system was first used to advertize a perfume by Coty. It has also been developed for use in a powdered form. See also Encapsulation.

Microtonia cymosa   *see* Patchouli

Middle Note   Also called the Heart or Body. In perfumery this relates to the main fragrance of a perfume, which becomes dominant after the top notes have faded away on the skin. It usually consists of floral, spicy or woody components. See also Low Note.

Mignonette   Also called Reseda Oil. One of the principal essential oils of perfumery obtained from flowers. The plant (*Reseda odorata*), native of N. Africa, is an annual growing to about 2 feet high and now cultivated widely; it is grown commercially in the south of France for its oil. The oil, obtained from the flowers mainly by extraction with volatile solvents but sometimes by maceration or enfleurage, has a violet-like fragrance. While some 1200 kilos of flowers are needed to provide 1 kilo of concrete, the scent is so powerful that it can be used only in minute quantity and then at a strength of about 1 part to 500 parts of alcohol.

The name Reseda may derive from Latin *resedo*, meaning to heal; in Roman times the plant was regarded as a charm against various ailments. The name 'mignonette' signifies 'little darling'. The plant was introduced into Britain in about 1750.

This plant should not be confused with the so-called Jamaica Mignonette, which is a variety of Henna.

Milfoil   Also called Yarrow, Common Yarrow, Soldier's Wound Wort, Blood Wort, Sanguinary, Devil's Nettle and by a number of other local names. A perennial herb (*Achillea millefolium*) found in temperate regions of the northern hemisphere. Milfoil Oil, distilled from the leaves, is used medicinally as well as in perfumes; it has a pungent, spicy, rather medicinal fragrance. The dried flowers are used in sachets and pot pourri. In ancient times Milfoil was regarded as a plant of the Devil and used for divination in spells.

'Mille' ('1000')   A quality floral–woody perfume created for Jean Patou in 1972 by Jean Kerleo. The brand name is in the numeral form '1000'. Top notes of osmanthus and damask rose cover a floral heart containing jasmine, violet and rose (Centifolia), with a base of patchouli and sandalwood. The perfume is sold both in a flacon by Brosse and also in a jade green flaconette after the style of a Chinese snuff box.

Milk Parsley   *see* Peucedan Gum

Mill Mountain   *see* Calamint

Mimosa Oil   The scent of the fragrant yellow flowers of the Mimosa tree (*Acacia dealbata* and *A. floribunda*), native to Australia but now cultivated widely, also called the Silver Wattle tree, is highly esteemed in perfumery. In the south of France, where the trees have been cultivated since about 1839, the perfume is extracted as a floral absolute by means of volatile solvents. Some 200 tons weight of mimosa flower heads were at one time being used in Grasse every year. Examples of modern quality perfumes containing mimosa are 'Lauren', 'Nina' and 'Vanderbilt'.

Mint   A perennial plant of many species of the genus *Mentha*, which grows widely. Mentha was a nymph in Greek mythology who was metamorphosed into the plant, and the name Mentha was originally used as a generic name by Theophrastus. Mints are frequently mentioned in Greek and Roman works for their value as strewing herbs and in medicines, flavourings and perfumes.

One of the most important species of mint for commercial uses at the present time is Spearmint (*Mentha spicata* = *M. viridis*), cultivated in China, Japan, Brazil and the USA for the essential oil (Spearmint Oil), obtained by steam-distillation from the flowering tops. Used mainly as a flavouring, this also helps to provide a 'green' note in perfumery (e.g. 'Turbulences')

Other mints used in perfumery are bergamot mint, pennyroyal and peppermint. The mint of the Bible was probably Horsemint (*M. longifolia* = *M. sylvestris*), found in Europe and N. Africa.

Mint Geranium   *see* Costmary

Minty Note   A term used in perfumery to describe a fragrance reminiscent of mint, e.g. peppermint or spearmint. Such fragances are usually used to provide a special, fresh effect in a Top Note. See Perfume Notes.

Mirabelle   *see* Plum

Mirbane Essence   Also called Oil of Mirbane. The first chemical perfume to be produced commercially, made from nitric acid and benzene (nitrobenzene). Devised in the 19th century, it had a fragrance crudely resembling sweet almonds, and was used for scenting soaps.

'Miss Dior'   A trend-setting chypre perfume brought out by Dior in 1947. The perfume was created for Dior by Paul Vacher. The top note is green and aldehydic, with suggestions of galbanum and bergamot. The heart is floral, with jasmine, rose and gardenia predominating. The base provides warm, woody and mossy touches, with patchouli, oak moss and ambergris the main constituents. The bottle was designed by Guéricolas.

'Mitsouko'   The earliest of the chypre family of modern perfumes (see Perfume Families) after Coty's original perfume named 'Chypre'. 'Mitsouko' (the name means 'mystery') was created by Jacques Guerlain and brought out by Guerlain in 1919. It has fresh, fruity top notes derived from bergamot, with touches of lemon, mandarin, neroli and peach (the first use of a synthetic peach fragrance in a perfume). The heart is floral, based on jasmine, rose and ylang-ylang, but with a spicy touch derived from clove. The base notes include oak moss and benzoin, with hints of sandalwood, labdanum, myrrh, cinnamon and musk. The flacons are by Baccarat and Brosse.

Mock Orange Blossom   Also called Mock Orange, German Jasmine, Seringa and occasionally Syringa. A shrub (*Philadelphus coronarius*) growing up to about 8 feet high and native to Italy and central Europe, but now grown widely (together with other related species of *Philadelphus*). The flowers have a strong fragrance reminiscent of the blossom of orange trees. An essential oil used in perfumery is obtained from the flowers and is used in modern quality perfumes (e.g. 'C'est la Vie'). The flowers are also dried for inclusion in pot pourri. But the fragrance is more usually made by synthesis. This plant should not be confused with the Orange Blossom plant. The stems of both Mock Orange and Lilac are easily hollowed out by removing the pith, and they were once used for making flute-like musical instruments (Greek *syrinx* = a flute), giving rise to the name Syringa for both plants. See also Neroli, Sweet Orange and Mexican Mock Orange.

Molinard   A perfume house which commenced in 1849 as a small shop in Grasse selling 'perfumed waters'; it set up its own distillery in 1894. Molinard's prestigious clientele included Queen Victoria. In 1920 the company moved its headquarters to Paris and began to expand, but its factory remains in Grasse, where it also maintains a Museum of Perfume. Its perfume 'Habanita', launched in 1924, was an immediate success. Perfumes which followed included 'Xmas Bells' (26), 'Calendal' (29), 'Le Baiser de Faune' (30), 'Les Iscles d'Or' (30). '1811' (30) and 'Madrigal' (35). Latterly it has produced 'Nirmala' (55), 'Rafale' (75), 'Molinard de Molinard' (80) and a men's fragrance 'Teck' (90). Most of these were sold in flacons by Baccarat or Lalique.

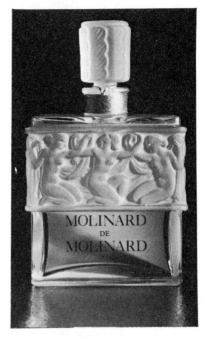

'Molinard de Molinard'.

'Molinard de Molinard' A fruity green floral perfume introduced by Molinard in 1980. The top notes are dominated by galbanum and blackcurrant buds. The heart contains jasmine, rose, narcissus, ylang-ylang and lily of the valley, and the base note includes labdanum, frankincense, amber, vetivert and musk. It was presented in a flacon much sought after by collectors, known as 'Beauty', which features a relief decoration of water nymphs and was made by Lalique; this flacon was first used for the Molinard perfume 'Les Iscles d'Or' and has subsequently also been used for 'Habanita'.

Molyneux A couture house founded in Paris in 1919 by a British fashion designer Edward Molyneux (1891–1974), who won the MC during the Great War. He reopened his House in Paris after the Second World War, retiring in 1967, when his nephew assumed control of the company. It is now a part of the Sanofi group. The company launched its first perfume, 'Vivre', in the 1930s and this was relaunched in 1971, to be followed by 'Quartz' (77), 'Gauloise' (81), 'Initiation' (90), and a fragrance for men, 'Captain' (75).

'Mon Parfum' A chypre perfume launched under the house name Paloma Picasso, in association with L'Oréal, in 1984. It was created by Créations Aromatiques perfumers. Top notes of ylang-ylang, lemon, bergamot, angelica and hyacinth lead into a heart mostly composed of jasmine and rose, with a woody base note obtained from oak moss, iris, sandalwood and patchouli supported by amber and musk. The flacon, an unusual design by Paloma Picasso and Bernard Kotyuk, consists of a bottle in a glass ring and is made by Brosse.

Monarda didyma   *see* Bergamot/Thyme

Monarda Oil   *see* Bergamot

'Montana'   A quality perfume launched in 1987 by Montana Parfums, perfume house of Claude Montana, the prominent Paris fashion designer. Created by Roure perfumers and described as 'avant garde chypre', it contains a green, fresh, fruity and spicy mixture of top notes, including marigold, ginger, pepper, blackcurrant buds and orange flower, which herald a floral and woody heart of jasmine, rose, narcissus, patchouli, sandalwood and oak moss. Base notes include ambrein, musk, frankincense and leather-fragrance. The flacon, a design in spiral layers of frosted glass, won a French Glass Industry prize in 1988. In 1990 the company launched a spicy–woody men's fragrance 'Montana pour Homme', containing tangerine, pepper and nutmeg in the top notes, geranium, nasturtium, patchouli and sandalwood in the middle notes and amber, frankincense and musk in the base, and also 'Parfum d'Elle'. Montana is now marketed in association with Charles of the Ritz, a part of the Revlon group.

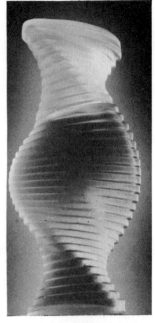

'Montana'.

Montpellier   A town in the S. of France near Marseilles which, in the 16th century, was prominent as a perfume-making centre and well known for its botanical gardens, where perfume plants were cultivated. Its importance faded as that of Grasse increased.

Moringa aptera   *see* Ben Oil

   oleifera   *see* Ben Oil

   peregrina   *see* Ben Oil

   pterygosperma   *see* Ben Oil

Moschus moschiferus   *see* Musk

Moss   *see* Fragrant Moss/ Oak Moss/ Tree Moss/ Ash Tree Lichen and Hazelcrottle

Mossy Note   A term used in perfumery to describe the general odour of oils obtained from mosses and lichens (see Moss above). Such oils are used in all types of perfumes. See also Perfume Notes.

Mouillette   *see* Fragrance Blotter

Mountain Balm   *see* Calamint

Mountain Mint   *see* Calamint

Mountain Pine   *see* Pine Needle Oil

Mousse de Chene   *see* Oak Moss

Mousseline   An Indian perfume based on vetivert. The name derives from 'muslin', as it was once used to give Indian muslin a distinctive scent before being exported to European markets.

Mpopwa   *see* Iguga

Mugo Pine Oil   *see* Pine Needle Oil

Muguet   *see* Lily of the Valley

Mugwort   *see* Tarragon

Mukul Myrrh tree   *see* Bdellium

Mumiya   *see* Pissasphalt

Mumuye   A gum which is used as a substitute for Gum Arabic and, in some parts of tropical Africa from which it originates, as a perfume. It comes from a tree *Combretum hartemannianum*.

Musa paradisiaca   *see* Banana

  sapientum   *see* Banana

Muscadier   *see* Mace

Muscatel Sage   *see* Clary

Muscone   A chemical obtained from musk and also made synthetically which has a significant value in perfumery because of its powerful properties as a fixative.

Muscovy   see Musk Geranium

Musk   Probably the most powerful of all perfume fragrances, and certainly one of the most expensive. Musk comes from a preputial follicle which is removed from the abdomen of the male musk deer (*Moschus moschiferus* and three other species of *Moschus*), found in the Himalayas from Afghanistan to China. The follicle, usually known as a

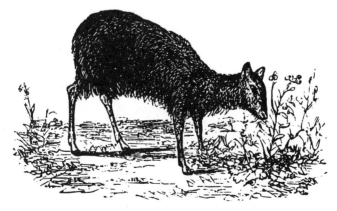

Musk Deer (*source* Rimmel, *Book of Perfumes*, 1895).

musk pod (or cod), is a sac about the size of a walnut and can be removed without harming the animal. The material extracted from the pod is in the form of solidified seeds (or grains). These contain the perfume in such concentrated form as to be most obnoxious unless diluted. Each pod holds less than 1 oz of grains. The odoriferous principal in the seeds is a substance called Muscone, which forms about 2% of the whole seed. The perfume is prepared in the form of a tincture by treatment with alcohol. The best-quality musk, known as Tonquin musk, comes from China and Tibet. Other varieties bear the names Cabardine, Yunnan and Assam (or Nepal) musk. The pods are called either Blue Skin or Grain Musk, according to their appearance.

Musk was unknown in classical times and reference to its use in perfumes does not appear until the 6th century, when Cosmas mentioned it as a product obtained from India. Soon afterwards both Arab and Byzantine perfume makers were employing it. There is a single and rather obscure reference to it in the Quran. Under the Abbasid Empire of the Arabs it was highly regarded, and the Caliphs of Baghdad (the 'emperors') used it lavishly; al-Kindi (early 9th century) included it in a large number of his perfume recipes and it became one of the more important luxury items (with silk, camphor and spices) brought back by Arab ships from China. It had a reputation as an aphrodisiac. Musk has been a key constituent in very many perfumes ever since its discovery, being held to give a perfume 'life', and musk or synthetic musk is now found among the principal ingredients of about 35% of all quality perfumes and quality fragrances for men.

So potent is musk that it can only be used in extremely diluted form. It is also exceptionally long-lasting and very important as a fixative. It is said that when musk is placed on a stored handkerchief the scent will last for 40 years. The early Arabs mixed musk in the mortar of some of their mosques and palaces, as they also did with rosewater, so that the buildings themselves would exude the fragrance.

There are many synthetic musks, early favourites such as Musk Ambrette, Musk Baur and Musk Ketone now being replaced by safer products, and with the increasing rarity and costliness of the original material they are being used more and more in modern perfumery. See also Sumbul.

Musk Ambrette   A synthetic musk perfume devised by Albert Baur in the 19th century. Its fragrance recalls ambrette as much as natural musk. It is one of the most powerful odorants known, but for safety reasons it is no longer used in quality perfumery (see Perfume Creation).

Musk Baur   A synthetic musk perfume, also called Tonquinol, patented by the German chemist Albert Baur in 1888. It was replaced by the chemical known as musk xylene, which for safety reasons is itself no longer used (see Perfume Creation). See also Musk Ketone.

Musk Geranium Also called Musk Storksbill, Musked Cranesbill, Ground Needle, Pick Needle, Muscovy and Geranium Moschatum. A seaside herb (*Erodium moschatum*) growing in Britain. The whole plant is aromatic when dried, having a fine musky odour. It was formerly used to scent washballs and is still used in sachets and pot pourri.

Musk Ketone A synthetic musk perfume devised by Albert Baur in the 19th century and said to be the sweetest of the artificial musks. It is a good fixative. Until recently it was regarded as one of the most acceptable of synthetic musk perfumes, but for safety reasons (see Perfume Creation) it is no longer used.

Musk Mallow *see* Ambrette

Musk Rat The fact that this animal, a rodent (*Ondatra zibethicus*) native to the USA, secreted a scent similar to musk has been observed since the 17th century. A chemical means of extracting it was discovered in the 1940s but has not proved commercially worth while.

Musk Root *see* Sumbul

Musk Seed *see* Ambrette

Musk Storksbill *see* Musk Geranium

Musk Xylene *see* Musk Baur

Musk Yarrow *see* Iva

Musked Cranesbill *see* Musk Geranium

Musky Sage *see* Clary Oil

'Must' A quality oriental perfume launched in 1981 by Cartier, for whom it was created by Givaudan perfumers. Mandarin, orange flower, rose and jasmine top notes introduce woody and musky middle and base notes, mostly of vetivert, sandalwood, musk and ambergris. The flask, made by Cartier, is decorated with gold. See also 'Panthère'.

Myoporum crassefolium *see* Anyme Oil

Myrica acris *see* Bois d'Inde
       cerifera *see* Candleberry Wax
       gale *see* Bog Myrtle

Myrica Oil *see* Bois d'Inde

Myristica fragrans *see* Mace
       ilya *see* Kalapa Tijoong

Myrobalan *see* Emblic

Myrocarpus fastigiatus *see* Cabreu Oil
       frondosus *see* Cabreu Oil

Myrospermum erythroxylon *see* Bois d'Olhio

Myroxylon balsamum *see* Balsam of Tolu
       balsamum **var.** *pareira* *see* Balsam of Peru
       balsamum **var.** *punctatum* *see* Quino-Quino
       pereira *see* Balsam of Peru
       toliuferum *see* Balsam of Tolu

Myrrh A gum-resin obtained from myrrh trees, of which the principal species is *Commiphora myrrha* (= *Balsamodendron myrrha*), also known as

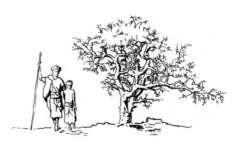

Myrrh (*Commiphora myrrha*).

True Myrrh or Herrabol Myrrh, native to Arabia, Somalia and Ethiopia; it is a very thorny, scraggy-looking tree which grows up to 15 feet high. Other species include: *C. habbessinica* (= *C. abyssinica* var. *simplicifolia*), also known as Qafal, which is native to the same region; *C. foliacia*, found in Dhofar (S. Arabia); and *C. kataf*, also known as Qataf, found in S.W. Arabia (see under Opoponax). Other species of *Commiphora* produce bdelliums, which are very similar to myrrh and often confused with it. Opoponax, for example, has also been called 'Sweet Myrrh'. Some authorities refer to True Myrrh as 'Male Myrrh' and Opoponax as 'Female Myrrh'. The Arabian Balsam tree, called Balsam of Makkah, is also a species of *Commiphora* and has been termed Makkah Myrrh, adding to the difficulties. The word 'myrrh' derives from Semitic (Arabic) meaning 'bitter', as it has a very bitter taste.

Myrrh obtained from *C. myrrha*, and possibly that from other species noted above, exudes in small 'tears' which darken in colour and often conglomerate as they harden. The odour is distinctive and pleasantly aromatic, though not pronounced. The resin is used in modern perfumery as a steam-distilled essential oil (the yield is 5% or more), its main function being to provide a balsamic tone and fixative. It is found among the principal ingredients of about 7% of all modern perfumes, especially oriental-type ones. It also has a particular use in making broom and honeysuckle compounds. Examples of modern quality perfumes using myrrh oil are 'Amouage', 'Opium', 'Roma' and 'Salvador Dali'. Myrrh is also used in pomander pastes and in some types of pot pourri.

Historically, myrrh is one of the most important of all perfume materials. Although the 'myrrh' collected by the ancient Egyptians during the 2nd millennium BC from the 'Land of Punt' was probably opoponax, as also may have been 'myrrh' referred to in some of the earliest parts of the Old Testament (see Bible Perfumes, Labdanum and Balm of Gilead), there is no doubt that True Myrrh from S. Arabia was a valuable item of commerce by the 5th century BC, when it was mentioned by Herodotus. By that time it was already an important material in Egypt for embalming. Both Theophrastus and Pliny noted its prime value as a perfume fixative, observing that it would last for 10 years, even improving with time. Greek and Roman perfume makers extracted myrrh-oil, generally referred to as stacte (q.v.), from the resin; this had the longest life of any perfume oils then known, and in consequence myrrh appears in a large number of their compound perfumes. Its use in perfumes and incenses continued into Byzantine times, but the early Arab perfume makers appear to have dropped it in favour of animal perfumes, such as ambergris and musk, which they had brought from the Far East and which were even better fixatives (see Arab Perfumes).

Myrrh, British   *see* Sweet Cicely

Myrrh, Garden   *see* Sweet Cicely

Myrrh, Sweet-scented   *see* Sweet Cicely

Myrrhis odorata   *see* Sweet Cicely

Myrtle   A tall, aromatic, evergreen, shrub-like tree (*Myrtus communis*) growing to about 20 feet high, found in southern Europe, the Middle East and India. Myrtle Oil, sometimes called Eau d'Anges, which has a spicy, nutmeg-like fragrance, is steam-distilled from the flowers, leaves and twigs. It is used in many modern fragrances (e.g. 'La Nuit', 'Antaeus' and 'Sybaris') and also in soaps. The dried flowers and leaves are used in sachets and pot pourri. An oil distilled from the fruits is used in the Levant and the Orient as an aromatic tonic.

   In classical times, myrtle was sacred to Venus and a bride would wear it on her wedding day. It was also worn by winners at the Olympic Games. In Greece it is still a symbol of love and immortality. The ancient Egyptians used it medicinally and for fumigation and made a hair ointment from it. Both Theophrastus and Pliny observed that the myrtle grown in Egypt had the most powerful scent, Theophrastus quoting it as an example of a perfume made from leaves. The early Arab perfume makers used both berries and young leaves, and also the dried leaves, in their recipes.

Myrtle Flower   *see* Iris, Yellow

Myrtle Grass   *see* Calamus/Iris, Yellow

Myrtle Sedge   *see* Calamus

Myrtle Wax   *see* Box Myrtle

Myrtus communis   *see* Myrtle

Myrurgia   A privately owned Spanish perfume house established early in this century. Its perfumes include 'Maderas de Oriente' (1981), 'Flor de Blason' (26), 'Embrujo de Sevilla' (33), 'Joya' (50), 'Nueva Maja' (60), 'Orgia' (73), 'Oasis' (80) and 'Only' (for Julio Inglesias) (89), together with men's fragrances including 'Hidalgo' (71), 'Vorago' (89), 'Massimi Dutti' (90), 'Aca Joe' (91) and 'Adolfo Dominguez' (91).

'Mystère'   A quality woody–chypre perfume brought out by Rochas in

1978. It was created by Nicolas Mamounas and contains nearly 200 ingredients. In the top note citrus and honeysuckle lead into a heart in which the main components are magnolia, gardenia, frangipani and jasmine. The base notes are dominated by cedar and juniper. The bottles were designed by Robert Granai and Serge Mansau.

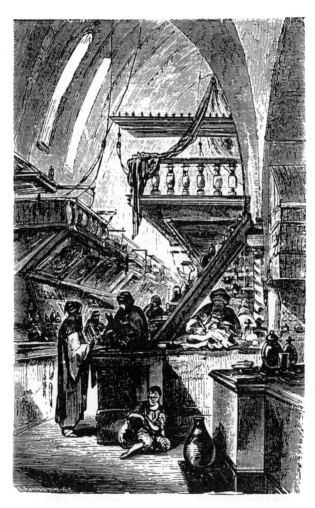

A perfume bazaar in the East (*Source* Rimmel, *Book of Perfumes*, 1895).

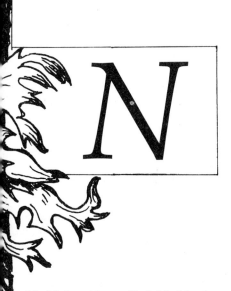

Naddah Also called Nadd. A very costly Arab incense which became popular among rich Arabs in medieval times. Its principal constituent was aloewood, to which was added ambergris, musk, frankincense and sometimes benzoin. *See also* Arab Perfumes.

Nag Kesar An Indian tree (*Mammea longifolia*), also called Surgi or Surunggi. The flowers yield an essential oil used in Indian perfumery.

Nagar Motha *see* Cyperus

'Nahema' A quality floral perfume with fruity, woody and amber notes. Created by Jean-Paul Guerlain, it was brought out by Guerlain in 1979 and is named after a princess in the *Arabian Nights Tales*. Peach, bergamot, calycanthus and passion fruit in the top notes lead to a heart dominated by rose, with traces of hyacinth, ylang-ylang, jasmine, lily of the valley and lilac. The base note includes balsams of Peru and Tolu, benzoin, vanilla, storax, vetivert and sandalwood. The perfume is sold in a bottle by Robert Granai.

Nair Oil Also called Ner Oil. An essential oil distilled from the leaves of a shrub called Nair or Ner (*Skimmia laurifolia*) found in the Himalaya region. The oil is used for scenting soaps. The leaves of this shrub are also used locally as an incense.

'Narcisse Noir' One of the earliest 'oriental' perfumes, created by Ernest Daltroff for Caron in 1911. Its top note is bergamot, with underlying fragrances which include mandarin, petitgrain and lemon. They yield to a dry floral effect in the middle notes, preponderantly from jasmine and narcissus, with low notes based on civet, musk and sandalwood.

Narcissus   Narcissus Oil, one of the most popular fragrances used in perfumery, is obtained from several species of Narcissus, most notably *Narcissus poeticus, N. tazetta, N. jonquilla* and *N. odorus* (see Jonquil). It is usually used in modern perfumery in the form of a floral concrete or absolute, and appears as one of the principal ingredients in about 11% of all modern quality perfumes (e.g. 'Fatale' and 'Samsara').

   Narcissus poeticus, called Poet's Narcissus or Pheasant's Eye Narcissus, is indigenous to Europe and cultivated for the essential oil in Holland and the south of France. The oil is extracted by enfleurage and volatile solvents and its scent resembles a blending of jasmine with hyacinth. Poet's Narcissus is generally believed to be the Narcissus of ancient times, although *N. tazetta* and *N. jonquilla* have also both been proposed.

   Narcissus tazetta, the Bunch-flowered Narcissus, or Polyanthus Narcissus, is a native of southern Europe and is now grown widely, including in the Levant, western Asia, N. Africa, N. India, China and Japan. The main area of cultivation for the essential oil is in the south of France. A species in which it is crossed with *N. poeticus,* known as Poetaz Narcissus, is also used in perfumery. See also Daffodil.

   In Greek legend, Narcissus was a youth who killed himself after falling in love with his reflection in a pool, his body then disappearing, to be replaced by the flower. Pliny states, however, that the plant was named from the Greek *narce* (= to be numb) on account of its narcotic properties, and not from 'the fabulous boy'. Theophrastus described the cultivation of narcissus in 300 BC. The Romans used the flower to make a perfume they called Narcissinum. Narcissus Oil was used in early Arab perfumes. The scent of the flowers at strength in a closed room is deleterious and the oil has to be used cautiously.

Narcotic   A term used in perfumery to describe exceptionally strong and heavy fragrances obtained from some flowers (e.g. jasmine and tuberose) and animalic ingredients, which need to be used with careful discretion in a perfume. See Perfume Notes.

Nard   *see* Spikenard

Nardostachys jatamansi   *see* Spikenard

Native Myrtle   *see* Backhousia

Nauli Gum   A gum yielding anethole collected from the Java Almond tree (*Canarium commune*), found in the Solomon Islands.

Neocallitropsis araucarioides   *see* Araucaria

Nepeta glechoma   *see* Ground Ivy
         lederacea   *see* Ground Ivy

Ner Oil   *see* Nair Oil

Nerol   A chemical substance obtained from natural sources such as oil of

Petitgrain or Helichrysum and manufactured synthetically from pinene since 1902. It is used in many perfumes, especially orange blossom, magnolia and rose compounds.

Neroli   The perfume oil known as Neroli is steam-distilled from the flowers of the Bitter Orange tree (*Citrus aurantium* var. *amara* = *C. bigaradia*), also called the Bigarade tree or Sour Orange tree. Native to S.E. Asia, this tree is believed to have been brought into Europe in the 12th century by the Arabs (who initiated the custom of wearing orange blossom at weddings as a sign of fecundity). The perfume probably obtained its name from a Prince of Neroli, an Italian, whose wife scented her bath and her gloves with it in the 16th century. Neroli Oil is produced today principally in the south of France, but also in Spain, Morocco, Tunisia, Algeria, Egypt, Sicily, Syria and the USA. It has a distinctive odour which combines spiciness with sweet and flowery notes. Only the steam-distilled oil is called Neroli Oil. It is used as a principal ingredient in about 12% of all modern quality perfumes and colognes and also in flavouring. The liquid remaining after distillation of the essential oil is subjected to extraction by an alcohol, producing Orange Flower Water, also called Oil of Neroli Water, which is used both in perfumes and in flavourings. At one time Orange Flower Water was more popular in perfumery than the essential oil itself.

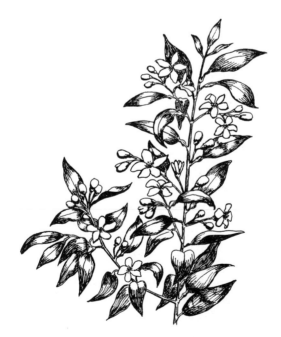

Neroli (*Citrus bigaradia*).

Essential oil is also obtained from the flowers of the same tree by extraction either with volatile solvents or with warm fats. This is called Orange Flower Oil and from it a concrete and absolute are prepared which are much used in high-grade floral perfumes and colognes (e.g. 'Beautiful' 'Ivoire' and 'Montana'). About 12% of all modern quality perfumes contain Orange Flower among their main ingredients.

The same tree also produces an oil used in perfumery called Oil of Bigarade, Oil of Oranges or Bitter Orange Oil (q.v.), which is obtained from the fruit peel by expression.

Additionally, an essential oil used in perfumery is obtained from the leaves of the same tree. This is Oil of Petitgrain (q.v.).

An inferior variety of Neroli Oil is produced from the Sweet Orange tree (q.v.).

Neroli Petolae   *see* Sweet Orange

Niaouli Oil   *see* Cajuput

Nicotiana   Also called the Tobacco Plant. An annual from several species of *Nicotiana*, including *Nicotianum alatum*, *N. tabacum*, *N. affinis* and *N. persica*, all native to America but now cultivated widely. The flowers, which have a very fragrant scent, provide a concrete and absolute by extraction which are used in making perfumes, particularly masculine ones. They are also dried for use in sachets and pot pourri. However, most perfumes of this fragrance are made synthetically.

Nigella Oil   An essential oil distilled from the seeds of Love-in-a-Mist (*Nigella damascena*), a hardy annual growing to about 2 feet high and native to southern Europe. It has a fragrance suggesting ambrette seeds.

Nigella Romana   *see* Gith

Nigella sativa   *see* Gith

Night-scented Stock   The flowers of this plant (*Matthiola bicornis*), native to Greece and growing up to 15 inches high, open up and give out a strong scent at night time. An essential oil containing this fragrance is obtained from the flowers for use in perfumery, but the fragrance is mostly manufactured synthetically. See also Stock.

Night Hyacinth   *see* Tuberose

Nikkel Oil   An essential oil distilled from the leaves and twigs of the Saigon Cinnamon tree (*Cinnamomum laureirii*), indigenous to Japan and also cultivated in China and Indonesia, mainly for its bark which is used as a spice. The oil has a fragrance reminiscent of lemon and cinnamon.

'Nina'   A quality floral perfume with woody undertones created for Nina Ricci in 1987 by Argeville perfumers. The top notes, which include orange blossom, bergamot and mimosa, lead to a floral heart containing rose, iris, jasmine, violet and ylang-ylang. The base comes from sandalwood and vetiver, with basil, marigold and cassis. It is sold in a distinctive flacon by Lalique.

Nina Ricci   A French fashion house founded in Paris by Nina Ricci (1883–1970) in 1932 with the support of her husband, a jeweller. After the war the house resumed its business under their son Robert, who introduced its first fragrance, 'Coeur-Joie', in 1946. This was followed by 'L'Air du Temps', one of the great classics of perfume, in 1948. Subsequent fragrances have included 'Capricci' (1960), 'Mademoiselle Ricci' (67), 'Farouche' (73), 'Fleurs de Fleurs' (82) and 'Nina' (87), together with three men's fragrances, 'Signoricci' (65 and 75), 'Phileas' (84) and 'Ricci Club' (89). The company is now established all over the world, and its factory at Ury, near Paris, opened in 1973, produces over 100 000 bottles of fragrances daily. Flacons for its principal perfumes are made by Lalique and are much sought after by collectors.

Nino Cerutti   Heir to a company founded in Italy in 1881 by three Cerutti brothers to produce woollen materials, Nino Cerutti (born 1930) is now head of a world-wide fashion house based in Paris. After producing a men's fragrance ('Nino Cerutti pour Homme') in 1979, the floral perfume 'Nino Cerutti pour Femme' was launched in 1987. Created by Jean-Claude Delville, it contains top notes of mandarin, galbanum, cardamom, peach and osmanthus, with a floral heart of tuberose, ylang-ylang, rose, jasmine, lily of the valley, orange blossom and hyacinth. The base notes include oak moss, sandalwood, patchouli, amber and vanilla. The bottle, designed by Serge Mansau, incorporates a tigella.

'Nocturnes'   An aldehydic floral perfume launched by Caron in 1981. It was created by Firmenich perfumers. The aldehyde top notes are fruity and green, with bergamot and mandarin. Stephanotis and other floral fragrances including lily of the valley, rose, jasmine and cyclamen, provide the heart, and the base is dominated by vanilla and sandalwood. The flask, black with a stylized flower, was designed by Pierre Dinand.

Norway Spruce Oil   An essential oil used in perfumery which is distilled from the needles of the Norway Spruce tree (*Picea abies* = *P. excelsa*). The tree is grown in Europe, N. Asia and the Balkans, primarily for lumber.

Nothopanax edgerleyi   *see* Raukawa

Nuanua Oil   An essential oil steam-distilled from the leaves of a species of *Nelitris* growing in Samoa. It has a fragrance reminiscent of ambergris.

Nut Grass   *see* Cyperus

Nutmeg   *see* Mace

Nutmeg Flower   *see* Gith

Nyctanthes A small tree (*Nyctanthes sambac*) found in Indonesia. The fragrant flowers, which have a scent similar to orange flowers, are used by Indonesian women as a hair decoration and in pot pourri. Another species, *N. arbor-tristis*, grows throughout India, where the fragrant flowers are used in pot pourri.

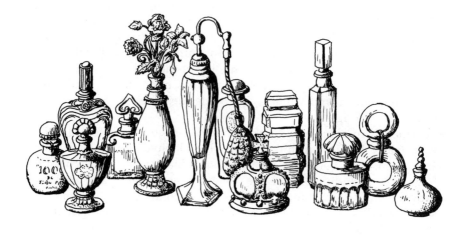

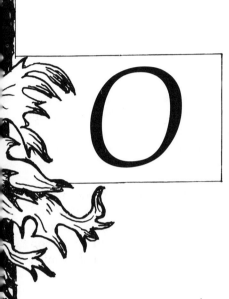

Oak Moss   In European perfumery the term Oak Moss (French *Mousse de Chêne*) relates to a lichen *Evernia prunastri* (= *Parmelia prunastri* = *Lobaria prunastri*), which is found growing on oak, spruce and fruit trees in mountainous districts throughout Europe and in N. Africa. In the USA the term also includes other lichens known in Europe as Tree Moss. The lichen is collected, mostly in France, Italy, Czechoslovakia, Yugoslavia and Morocco, and the fragrance, which is earthy and woody with a hint of musk and is sometimes classified as amber, develops over a period of storage; a resinoid and absolute are then extracted by volatile solvents. Oak moss is now a very important material for perfumers, making an excellent fixative. It is much used in chypre and fougere perfumes, or to provide a woody note, as well as in toilet waters, soaps and cosmetics, and appears as a principal ingredient in some 30% of all modern quality perfumes (e.g. 'Diva', 'Parure' and 'Red') and 37% of all men's quality fragrances (e.g. 'Ricci Club' and 'Polo'). The raw material is also used in sachets and pot pourri.

Oak moss was imported by the ancient Egyptians from the Greek islands to leaven and flavour bread, and is still so used in some Arab areas. In the Middle Ages, when Cyprus was the main source of supply, its fixative qualities were discovered and it began to be used in aromatic powders (see Cyprus Powder). See also Ash Tree Lichen.

'Obsession'   An unusually strong and spicy floriental perfume created by the perfumers of Roure for Calvin Klein in 1985. Mandarin, bergamot and vanilla in the top notes lead into a heart of jasmine, orange blossom, sandalwood, vetivert and other spicy notes, with a base which includes amber, oak moss, frankincense and musk. It is sold in a flacon by Brosse and bottles designed by Pierre Dinand.

Ocimum basilicum   *see* Basil

   minimum   *see* Basil

Ocotea caudata   *see* Safrole

   sassafras   *see* Safrole

Oenanthe   A perfume of ancient Greece made from vine leaves. It was mostly manufactured in Cyprus. Pliny listed it among the ingredients of the royal unguent of the Kings of Parthia.

Ogea Gum   *see* Balsam of Copaiba

Old Man   *see* Southernwood

Old Man's Beard   *see* Tree Moss

'Old Spice'   Sometimes regarded as the progenitor of the modern style of men's fragrances, 'Old Spice' was introduced by Shulton in 1937 and has been a top-selling mass-market men's fragrance ever since. A fresh, citrusy top note heads a spicy heart in which carnation and cinnamon predominate, underlined by a powdery base with traces of musk, vanilla and cedarwood.

Olea europaea   *see* Olive

   fragrans   *see* Osmanthus

Oleo Vermelho tree   *see* Bois d'Olhio

Oleum carvi   *see* Caraway

   dracunculi   *see* Tarragon

Olibanum   *see* Frankincense

Olive   The Olive or Common Olive tree (*Olea europaea*), also called Olivier, is native to the Mediterranean, Asia Minor and Syria, and is known to have been grown in Crete since at least 3500 BC. It is now also cultivated in Chile, Peru, S. Australia and elsewhere for its oil. Olive Gum, also called Lucca Gum, derived from this tree, is used in Italy in the manufacture of perfumes. Olive oil was produced by the ancient Egyptians mainly as a lamp oil, but they also prepared a perfumed oil by steeping fragrant flowers in it (see Balanos Oil). Theophrastus noted that oil freshly pressed from 'coarse olives' was the best for use as a perfume base. The early Arab perfume makers used it as a base in many of their compound perfumes, sometimes in conjunction with pitch. See also Omphacium.

Olivier   *see* Olive

Olla-podrida   A pot pourri made by perfume manufacturers out of their waste materials, such as spent plant and animal materials, to which are added inexpensive herbs such as thyme and rosemary, together with lavender and rose petals.

Oman Water *see* Ajowan

'Ombre Rose' A floral perfume produced in 1982 by the fashion designer and milliner Jean-Charles Brosseau in association with Jean Patou. It was created by Roure perfumers. Iris and vanilla in the top notes herald middle notes of ylang-ylang, lily of the valley and peach, with woody base notes. The perfume is sold in an unusual hexagonal flacon of black or frosted crystal with a floral pattern in bas relief, modelled after an antique flask.

Omphacium An oil or juice used in Roman perfumes which was squeezed out of unripe olives or dates. Pliny noted its use in Metopium unguent, 'oil of roses' and other compound perfumes.

'Only' A perfume launched in 1990 by Myrurgia in association with the singer Julio Iglesias. Top notes in a blend of ylang-ylang, marigold, bergamot and pineapple lead to a floral bouquet in the heart, chiefly rose, mimosa, jasmine, tuberose and violet, with woody and balsamic base notes containing vetiver, sandalwood, vanilla, musk and labdanum.

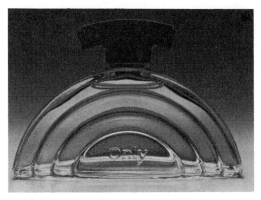

'Only'.

Onycha A word with the same derivation as 'onyx' (meaning in Greek a finger nail or claw) which is used as an alternative name for Sweet Hoof. In the Bible it appears as a perfume material, Exodus 30:34 quoting it as an ingredient in the holy incense of the Jews, and Ecclesiasticus 24:15 as 'a pleasant odour', but some authorities have suggested that in these contexts it may have been a plant material, possibly labdanum.

Ooka-ooka Tree *see* Tangloo Oil

'Opium' An oriental-type perfume created for Yves St Laurent by Jean Amic and Jean-Louis Sieuzac of Roure-Bertrand (now Roure) and first marketed in 1977. The top notes are a mixture of fruit and spices, with mandarin, plum, clove, pepper and coriander. In the floral middle notes lily of the valley, rose and jasmine predominate, underlined by a base note containing labdanum, benzoin, myrrh, opoponax, castoreum, cedarwood and sandalwood. The bottle was designed by Pierre Dinand and it also appears in flacons by Brosse.

Opobalsamum   *see* Balsam of Judaea and Balsam of Tolu.

Opoponax   Also known as Bissabol, Perfumed Bdellium, Female Frankincense and Coarse Myrrh of Aden. A gum-resin obtained from a bdellium tree, *Commiphora erythraea* var. *glabrescens*, found in Somalia and Ethiopia. The tree is closely related to myrrh. The gum has been known in the past variously as Sweet Bdellium, Sweet Myrrh and False Myrrh. Bissabol is the Indian name for it. It occurs in small yellowish-brown lumps flecked with white, and has a mild but persistent odour described by some as like crushed ivy leaves, by others as a blend of frankincense, celery, lovage and angelica. The oil is separated by distillation. Opoponax is being used increasingly in western perfumery, appearing in many high-class perfumes (e.g. 'Opium', 'Panthère' and 'Shalimar'). In India and China it is used in incenses. It is a good fixative, especially for pot pourri. It would appear that until the present century the substance known as Opoponax may have been an inferior gum derived from a closely related tree, *Commiphora kataf*, sometimes called the Opoponax Myrrh tree, which grows in S. Arabia and nearby regions of Africa. See also Cassie Ancienne.

Opoponax is also likely to have been the substance generally translated as myrrh which was imported into the Land of Punt by the ancient Egyptians (see Egyptian Perfumes), who regarded it very highly. It was probably also the substance known to the Romans as 'scented myrrh'.

A gum called Opoponax which is used in perfumery is also obtained from the lower stems of a perennial plant *Opoponax chironium*, found from the Mediterranean to Iran. Its fragrance has been described as like fenugreek with a background of lovage and costus.

Orange Blossom   Also called Mexican Orange. A flowering shrub (*Choysia ternata*) growing up to 6 feet high, which is native to Mexico but now grown widely. The flowers, with a sweet scent reminiscent of the flowers of orange trees, provide an essential oil used among the main ingredients in about 11% of all modern quality perfumes (e.g. 'Lou-Lou', 'C'est la Vie' and 'Madame Rochas'). See also under Mock Orange Blossom, Neroli and Sweet Orange.

Orange Flower Oil   An essential oil obtained from the flowers of the Bitter Orange tree by extraction (oil obtained from the same source by steam-distillation is called Neroli). See further details under Neroli.

Orange Flower Water   Also called Oil of Neroli Water. The distilled water left after distilling Neroli. It is a product of some commercial importance in itself and waters of several strengths are recognized.

Orange Oil   *see* Bitter Orange Oil/Bergamot Oil

Orchanette   *see* Alkanet

Orchid Oil   A fragrant essential oil extracted by volatile solvents from an orchid, *Orchis militaris* and related species. But the fragrance is also made synthetically. Examples of quality perfumes containing orchid are 'L'Origan', 'Rumba' and 'Red Door'.

Oregon Douglas Fir   *see* Douglas Fir

Oregano   *see* Douglas Fir

Organ   Also called Fragrance Organ and Perfumer's Organ. In perfumery, the work table and surrounding shelves with their bottles of perfume ingredients, at which the perfume creator sits to produce his perfumes. See also Mouillette.

Oriental Lignaloes   *see* Aloewood

Oriental Perfumes   Perfumes containing principal ingredients which are reminiscent of the East, giving them a strongly exotic, spicy or balsamic character. See Perfume Families.

Oriental Sweet Gum   *see* Storax

Origanum Oil   An essential oil with a thyme-like scent which is steam-distilled from the leaves and tops of Origanum (*Origanum heracleoticum* = *O. vulgare prisonaticum*), also called Rigani and Winter Marjoram, and related species. The plant is a perennial herb growing to about 2 feet high and native to the Mediterranean region. The oil varies considerably according to the species, which are mostly restricted to specific areas, including Crete, Cyprus and Algeria. It is similar to, though harsher than, Oil of Marjoram, which comes from other species of the same genus. Spanish Origanum Oil is distilled from Couched Thyme (*Thymus capitatus*), native to the Mediterranean region, and used in flavouring. See Marjoram and Thyme. Origanum Oil appears in many modern quality perfumes (e.g. 'Fatale').

Origanum dictamus   *see* Dittany

heracleoticum   *see* Origanum Oil

hortensis   *see* Marjoram

marjorana   *see* Marjoram

maru   *see* Hyssop

vulgare   *see* Marjoram

vulgare **var.** *prisonaticum*   *see* Origanum Oil

Orris   Also called Orrice, Arrace, Florentine Orris, Iris, Ireos of Florence, Illyrium Orrice and Illirick Orris. One of the most important of all perfume materials, orris derives from the dried rhizomes of certain species of Iris. Because Orris Oil, which is steam-distilled from the powdered rhizomes after some two years of storage, has an oily, yellow appearance, it is also called Orris Butter. It has a violet-like fragrance and is extensively used blended with ionone as a base for violet compositions and in other floral compounds. It has the property of strengthening other fragrances and is a good fixative. Orris (or Iris) appears as a principal ingredient in about 32% of all modern quality perfumes (e.g. 'Byzance', 'Fleur de Fleurs', 'Gucci No. 3' and 'Madame Rochas'). The dried roots are also used in sachets and pot pourri.

The best-quality orris is obtained from *Iris pallida*, native to the E. Mediterranean area and now mainly cultivated around Florence. The Florentine Orris (*I. florentina*) of southern Europe, also known as the White Flower de Luce (Fleur de Lys), is cultivated in Italy, France, Germany, Morocco and India. The German Iris, also called Flag Iris and Blue Flower de Luce (*I. germanica*), native to southern Europe, is less highly regarded as a perfume source.

The Iris, regarded from antiquity as a symbol of power and majesty, was named after the goddess of the rainbow because of the beauty and variety of its flowers. The ancient Egyptians held it as sacred and placed it on the sceptre of their kings. It was used in Greek and Roman perfumes from an early date. Theophrastus noted that the fragrance was at its best three years after the roots were gathered, and Pliny

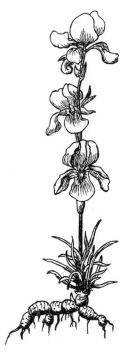

Orris (*Iris pallida*).

observed that the best came from Illyricum (modern Dalmatia). Macedonia, Elis and Corinth were famous for their Iris unguents. Although it had no part in Arab perfumes, it maintained its popularity in Europe. Orris powder once formed the basis of most sachets, tooth powders and hair powders, and pieces of orris root were made into beads for pomander bracelets and rosaries. A perfume was being made in the 15th century comprising orris root mixed with anise, and early in the 18th century orris was in wide demand, with orris powder being sold in silk or satin sachets for wearing on the body.

Oscar de la Renta   A perfume company formed by the prominent Spanish-born American–Dominican fashion designer Oscar de la Renta (b. 1932) with the launch of 'Oscar de la Renta' perfume in 1977; the company has subsequently issued two men's fragrances – 'Pour Lui' (81) and 'Ruffles' (87). It was acquired by Avon in 1988 but purchased from them by Sanofi in 1990.

'Oscar de la Renta' is a quality floral–oriental fragrance, created by Roure perfumers, favoured, among others, by Mrs Nancy Reagan, and winner of a Fragrance Foundation award. The top notes of orange flower, basil, coriander and cascarilla lead to a heart which includes ylang-ylang, broom, jasmine, rose and tuberose, and to base notes containing patchouli, sandalwood, vetivert, vanilla, myrrh and castoreum. It is contained in a crystal bottle with a stylized flower stopper designed by Serge Mansau.

Osmanthus   A floral concrete and absolute are obtained by extraction from the flowers of *Osmanthus fragrans* (= *Olea fragrans*), an evergreen tree growing to about 20 feet high in China and Japan. In China the flowers, known as Kwei Hwa or Mo Hsi, are used to scent tea and other foodstuffs. The fragrance is jasmine-like, with a suggestion of plums and raisins, and is found in high-class perfumes (e.g. 'Mille' ('1000'), 'Ciao', 'Nino Cerutti' and 'Red').

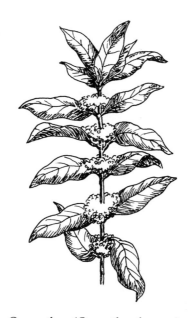

Osmanthus (*Osmanthus fragrans*).

Osmoxylon umbelliferum   *see* Ambon Sandalwood
Oswego Bee Balm   *see* Bergamot/Thyme
Oswego Tea   *see* Bergamot/Thyme
Osyris tenuifolia   *see* Sandalwood
Ouplate   *see* Costus
Our Lady's Tears   *see* Lily of the Valley
Oxystigma mannii   *see* Balsam of Copaiba
Oyster Oil   An essential oil with a typical pine fragrance distilled from the leaves of the Bay Pine tree (*Callitris rhomboides*) of Australia.

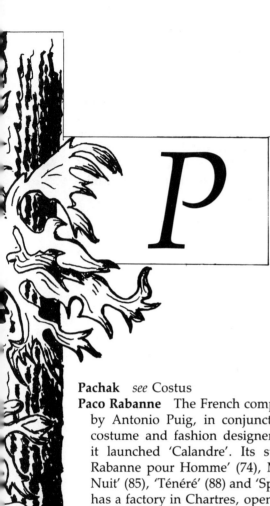

Pachak   *see* Costus

Paco Rabanne   The French company Parfums Paco Rabanne was formed by Antonio Puig, in conjunction with the Spanish-born avant-garde costume and fashion designer Paco Rabanne in Paris in 1969, when it launched 'Calandre'. Its subsequent fragrances have been 'Paco Rabanne pour Homme' (74), Métal (79), 'Soin pour Homme' (84), 'La Nuit' (85), 'Ténéré' (88) and 'Sport de Paco Rabanne' (90). The company has a factory in Chartres, opened in 1976.

'Paco Rabanne pour Homme'   A trend-setting fougere fragrance for men brought out by Paco Rabanne in 1973. Created by Givaudan perfumers, its main constituents are bergamot and lavender in the top notes, clary sage, carnation, rosemary and lavender in the middle notes, and tree moss and musk in the base. The bottle was designed by Pierre Dinand.

Paeonia foemina   *see* Peony
         officinale   *see* Peony

Pagoda tree   *see* Frangipani

Palma Christi   *see* Castor Oil

Palma Rosa Oil   Also called East Indian Geranium Oil. An essential oil with a rose–geranium-like scent steam-distilled from the leaves of a variety of Rosha (Rusa) Grass (*Cymbopogon martinii*) called Motia, which grows in drier areas of India, Pakistan, Afghanistan and Indonesia. It is used in quality perfumes (e.g. 'Vanderbilt' and 'Vol de Nuit') and soaps and as a source of geraniol, its principal constituent. Distillation of this oil, formerly known as 'Turkish Geranium Oil', commenced in the 18th century. See also Ginger Grass Oil.

Palo Balsama *see* Champaca Wood Oil

'Panache' A floral aldehyde perfume launched by Lenthéric in 1977. Green aldehydic top notes, with peach, thyme and pineneedle, lead into a floral green heart which includes jasmine, ylang-ylang, carnation and orris. Base notes are oak moss, cedar, musk, amber and myrrh. 'Panache Evening Edition', brought out in 1989, has chypre and amber notes.

Panaume *see* Sassafras

Panax edgerleyi *see* Raukawa

Pandanus Oil A honey-like essential oil extracted from the fresh male flowers of a water-loving tree resembling a date-palm, mostly found on or near beaches, called the Pandanus Tree or Thatch Screw Pine (*Pandanus odoratissimus = P. tectorus = Keura odorifera*). The tree is cultivated in India, the Seychelles, the Andaman Islands, Malaysia, Australia and certain Pacific islands, and also found in Arabia and Iran. The Indian name for the tree is Pandang and for the flowers and the perfume Keora (or Kewra). The odour is suggestive of lilac, honeysuckle and ylang-ylang blended with a prominent top note of hyacinth and tuberose. The oil was known to the early Arab perfume makers from at least the 8th century AD and was at one time an important export from Yemen.

'Panthère' A floral–woody quality perfume introduced by Cartier in 1987. Created by Firmenich perfumers, it has top notes of tuberose, orange flower, rose and jasmine, with a touch of mandarin and labdanum; these blend with woody middle notes which contain iris, sandalwood, vetiver, patchouli, nutmeg and oak moss. The base includes civet, musk, ambergris, vanilla

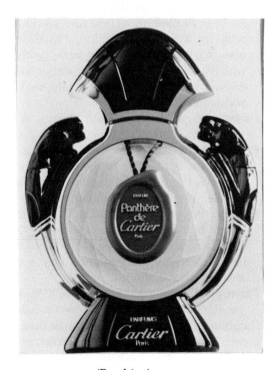

'Panthère'.

and opoponax. The flacon, made to a Cartier design, features stylized panthers.

Pao Rosa tree   *see* Rosewood Oil

Pao Santa   *see* Champaca Wood Oil

Para Beans   *see* Tonka Beans

'Paradoxe'   A leather–chypre perfume brought out by Cardin in 1983. It was created by Roure perfumers. Aldehydic top notes, with mandarin, lemon and bergamot, introduce a heart containing jasmine, hyacinth, ylang-ylang, iris and tuberose, with base notes which include pepper, frankincense, amber, musk and leather. The wheel-shaped bottle was designed by Serge Mansau.

Paraguay Lignum   *see* Champaca Wood Oil

Paraguay Tea Tree   *see* Maté

'Parfum d'Hermès'   A quality 'floriental' perfume created for Hermès in 1984 by Roure perfumers. Floral top notes, such as rose, jasmine and ylang-ylang, introduce a heart which contains iris, carnation and geranium, supported by a rich base of wide-ranging fragrances including myrrh, frankincense, labdanum, cedarwood, sandalwood, vetivert, vanilla and civet. The ring-shaped flacon, bound with silver metal and representing a stirrup link, was designed by Jacques Llorente.

'Paris'   An intensely floral perfume created by Sophia Grojsman of IFF for Yves St Laurent in 1983 and based principally on the rose. Floral top notes of mimosa, geranium, hawthorn and cassie lead to a heart of rose, backed by violet and orris, with woody and ambery base notes which include sandalwood, amber and musk. The flacon, faceted to give an impression of rose petals, was designed by Alain de Mourgues and is made by Brosse.

Parmelia furfuracea   *see* Tree Moss
            prunastri   *see* Oak Moss

Parquet, Paul   Chief perfumer for Houbigant in the late 19th century and one of the earliest perfumers to use synthetics in his creations, notably with 'Le Parfum Idéal', created in 1896. Parquet also created 'Fougère Royale', the first fougere fragrance.

Parsley   An oil steam-distilled from the seeds (Parsley Seed Oil) or leaves (Parsley Herb Oil) of the Parsley plant (*Petroselinum sativum = P. crispum*), native to Asia Minor but now found all over the world. It has a spicy, herbal fragrance and is used in herbal-type perfumes as well as in flavouring.

Parsnip Oil   An oil steam-distilled from the fruit, flowers and roots of the Parsnip (*Pastinaca sativa = Peucedanum sativum*), a vegetable plant cultivated in Europe since Roman times and introduced into America in the 17th century. It is now grown in temperate regions all over the world. The oil is aromatic, with a suggestion of vetiver, and is occasionally used in spicy, herbal-type perfumes.

'Parure'   An innovative chypre perfume, with a mossy, leathery, balsamic base note, created by Jean Paul Guerlain and introduced by Guerlain in 1975. The name means 'adornment'. Aldehydic top notes containing citrus, thyme, galbanum and clary sage introduce a floral bouquet of jasmine, rose, lilac, lily of the valley, narcissus, jonquil and orris, constructed on a base which includes balsam of Peru, ambergris, styrax and vetiver, together with moss and leather. The flacon has a distinctive petal-shaped stopper and was designed by Robert Granai.

Pastille Burners   Also called Perfume Burners (but see also under Burning Oil), these came into use in Britain in the 18th century as a means of burning an incense to clear the smell of food from a dining-room after a meal. They were made of silver, having a small urn with a pierced lid to hold a perfumed paste which was aromatized by a spirit burner underneath. Subsequently more simple pastille burners of china or earthenware were used widely to scent rooms, often in the style of a cottage with a smoking chimney in which the pastille was left to smoulder. The paste usually contained sandalwood, benzoin, cassia, cloves and balsam of Tolu. In France, more elaborate pastille burners of porcelain were used, sometimes in the shape of tree trunks. (See Appendix B, recipes nos 31 and 72.)

Pastinaca sativa   *see* Parsnip Oil

Patchouli   An essential oil steam-distilled from the dried and fermented leaves of a mint-like plant called Patchouli, Java Patchouli and Pucha-pat (*Pogostemon heyneansus* = *P. patchouli* = *P. cablin*) which grows up to 3 feet tall in Malaysia and Indonesia. It is also now cultivated in

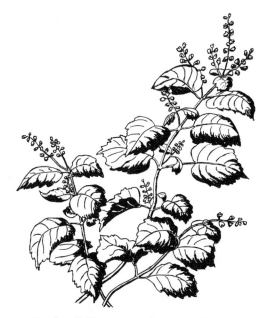

Patchouli (*Pogostemon heyneansus*).

India, China, Madagascar, the Seychelles, the West Indies, Brazil and Uruguay. The oil, which has a unique, cedar-like odour with spicy undertones which improves with age, is the most powerful of all the plant scents and one of the finest fixatives known. It is used particularly in 'heavy' and oriental-type perfumes, but only in very minute quantity because of its strength. It is usually diluted with attar of roses and dissolved in rectified spirit. One cwt of the leaves produces about 28 oz of essential oil. It appears among the main base note ingredients of some 33% of all modern quality perfumes and 50% of all men's quality fragrances. It is also used in soaps and the dried leaves are used in sachets and pot pourri.

Patchouli first became known in Europe early in the 19th century, when shawls scented with it were sent to Europe from India and became very fashionable. It is still used in the East to scent clothes and linen.

An inferior form of the oil called Khasia Patchouli Oil and Oil of Assam is distilled from the leaves of a woody plant (*Microtonea cymosa*), native to India and Assam. This oil is used in China and Vietnam as a perfume, particularly to scent soaps and fabrics.

Patou, Jean   A leading Paris fashion and perfume house formed in 1919 by Jean Patou (d. 1936) and still controlled by his family. Jean Patou commenced his perfumery business in 1925 with three famous perfumes, 'Amour-Amour', 'Que Sais-Je' and 'Adieu Sagesse'. In subsequent years the company issued 'Chaldée' (1927), 'Le Sien' and 'Moment Suprême (29), 'Cocktail Dry', 'Cocktail Sweet' and 'Cocktail Bitter Sweet' (30) and, in the same year, their most famous perfume 'Joy'; then 'Divine Folie' (33), 'Normandie' (35), 'Vacances' (36), 'Colony' (38), 'L'Heure Attendue' (46), 'Monsieur Net' (56) and 'Câline' (64); most of these, including 'Joy', were created by the company's perfumer Henri Almeras; several of them were relaunched in 1984 in flacons modelled after the originals by Louis Suë. 'L'Eau de Sport' followed in 1969, then '1000' (Mille) (72), 'Eau de Patou' (76), 'Patou pour Homme' (80) and 'Ma Liberté' (87). Patou's principal perfumer has, since 1967, been Jean Kerleo.

Peach   The peach tree (*Amygdalus persica* = *Prunus persica*) was probably introduced into Europe through Persia from China in Graeco–Roman times. Theophrastus knew of it as a Persian fruit. An oil obtained from the leaves, flowers and kernals has uses in herbal medicines. The early Arab perfumers used the flesh of the kernals. The fragrance of peach can be obtained by distillation of the fruit juice but is mostly produced synthetically. It is used to provide a fruity note in many modern perfumes (e.g. 'Habanita', 'Amouage', 'Femme', 'Climat' and 'Mitsouko').

Peau d'Espagne   A very expensive perfumed leather popular in Europe in the 16th century for making jerkins and other items of clothing for the wealthy. It was imported into Britain from Spain up to the time of the Armada. A preparation made of neroli, rose, sandalwood, lavender, civet, verbena, musk, clove and cinnamon was used to saturate the leather. See also Gloves, scented.

Pelargonium   *see* Geranium

Penhaligon's   Established as perfumers in 1870 by a Cornish barber, William Penhaligon, who had set up shop in London. The company fell apart after his death, until 1975, when it was revived and expanded by Sheila Pickles. In 1987 it became part of the Laura Ashley Group. Its customers have included Churchill and Rothschild, and it holds royal warrants to supply the Duke of Edinburgh and the Prince of Wales.

Penhaligon's make fragrances at Eau de Toilette and Cologne strength and sell a variety of high-quality toiletry articles, including antique silver-decorated scent bottles. Fragrances sold include 'Hammam Bouquet' (first introduced in 1872), 'Lords' (1911), 'Blenheim Bouquet' (1902) and 'English Fern' (1911), all for men; fragrances for women include 'Victorian Posy' (created for the Victorian and Albert Museum in 1979), 'Jubilee Bouquet' (77), 'Elizabethan Rose' (84), 'Bluebell' (78) and 'Cornubia' (91).

Pennyroyal   Also called European Pennyroyal, Pulegium, Pudding Grass and by a large number of local names. A species of Mint (*Mentha pulegium*) found in Europe, the Mediterranean area and the Middle East and cultivated in Japan, Spain, Morocco and Tunisia. Oil of Pennyroyal, also called Oil of Pulegium, is steam-distilled from the lightly dried herb, providing a minty, spicy and slightly bitter fragrance; it is used occasionally in perfumery in the reproduction of other fragrances and for scenting soaps, also in medicines and in the manufacture of menthol. The dried leaves are used (in moderation, as their odour is a strong one) in sachets and pot pourris.

Pennyroyal was a popular herb in classical times. The name Pulegium means 'flea plant', deriving from its use in rooms as a strewing plant to deter fleas. The Greeks associated it with Demeter, the goddess of Nature, and wore it behind their ears as a protection against sunstroke.

Peony   Also spelled Paeony. The Peony plant *Paeonia foemina* (= *P. officinalis*), also called the Apothecary's Peony (but there are several other species of peony) was believed in ancient times to shine during the night, so protecting shepherds and driving away evil spirits. The flowers, which are mildly fragrant, are used in sachets and pot pourri.

Pepper Oil   An oil obtained by steam-distillation from the unripe berries of the pepper vine (*Piper nigrum*), native to India and Malaysia but cultivated throughout the Far East for pepper. This oil has the distinctive odour of pepper. It is mainly used in fragrances for men, but appears in some modern quality perfumes (e.g. 'Le Jardin d'Amour' and

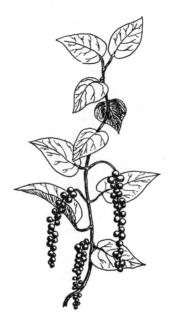

Pepper (*Piper nigrum*).

'L'Interdit'). Pepper was an important condiment in Roman times, but does not appear to have been used in early perfumery.

Peppermint   An essential oil steam-distilled from the fresh or partially dried flowering tops of several varieties of the Peppermint plant (*Mentha piperata*), a species of Mint cultivated widely in Europe, Japan and N. America. It is used in toilet waters and soaps, but mainly as a flavouring agent, especially in medicines and toothpastes. The dried leaves are used in sachets and pot pourri.

A form of Peppermint Oil known as Arvensis Peppermint Oil is distilled from varieties of Field Mint (*Mentha arvensis*) native to China and Japan and cultivated there and in Korea, Taiwan, Brazil and Paraguay. It has occasional uses in perfumery, but is mostly employed in pharmaceuticals and toothpastes.

Perfume

Perfume The word 'perfume' derives from Latin *per fume*, meaning 'through smoke', indicative of the importance of incense in the early use of fragrant materials. In its modern meaning, perfume is a concentrated essence of fragrant materials diluted in the minimum possible amount of a high-grade alcohol. The fragrancy content of a perfume sold over the counter (also known in this sense as an 'extrait') is about 15–30%, with the alcohol it is diluted in being 90–95% pure. Any mixture containing a lower proportion of fragrancy is an eau (water). The different types of eau (eau de parfum, eau de toilette, eau de cologne, for each of which see separate entries) contain progressively smaller amounts of the fragrancy essence and weaker solutions of alcohol. The word 'perfume' is also more loosely used in a sense synonymous with fragrance or aroma. Until a few years ago the British used the word 'scent' to describe the bottled liquid which in France and the USA has always been known as 'perfume', but this distinction is no longer made.

The liquid perfumes (including Waters) used in modern quality perfumery may be of three types. First, there are preparations based on what is generally termed the classical structure, introduced at the end of the 19th century, of top, middle and lower notes (see Perfume Notes); these are usually highly elaborate concoctions, containing anything from a few dozen ingredients to several hundred (e.g. 692 in 'Red'), both natural and synthetic, and are classified under a number of broad categories (see Perfume Families). Secondly, there are 'Single

Note' (or 'Single Fragrance') perfumes, which are made to provide the scent of a specific plant or flower or a simple posy of flowers or other fragrances, with few low notes; in some cases these will be composed of the essential oil of the flower in question, fortified with other ingredients to intensify the fragrance and to promote stability, smoothness and lasting power; in other cases (e.g. freesia) they may be made entirely of synthetic components, because the natural fragrance of the flower cannot be extracted, or can be reproduced more effectively and economically by such synthesis; in either case a 'single note' perfume will use a surprisingly large number of ingredients. Many 'single note' perfumes now marketed are fragrances first devised in the 19th century, or even earlier (e.g. 'Rose Geranium' and 'Lily of the Valley' by Floris) which are still sold by the perfume houses who originated them. Thirdly, there is a type of perfume which entered the market in the 1980s and to which the names linear fragrance, or sometimes horizontal fragrance, are applied; such perfumes are very strong and are designed to provide a powerful instant impression which does not change with time as do the classical three-note perfumes; in effect they may be seen as two-note perfumes, lacking top notes but with an unusually strong heart.

Perfume Burner   *see* Burning Oil

Perfume, Care of   Pliny wrote nearly 2000 years ago that unguents kept best in alabaster boxes (which were very cool), and that sunshine was detrimental to scents, which should be stored in the shade. This is broadly valid today. The enemies of delicate perfumes, as Guy Robert has written, are air, heat and light. A bottle of perfume should always be kept closed when not in use, preferably in a cool, dark place. Once the bottle is opened, some deterioration is inevitable because of the air let in, and this will become more apparent as the amount of liquid in the bottle reduces, because the bottle will then contain increasingly more air. The top notes, with their high evaporation rate, will suffer first, so that the character of the perfume will change. A quality perfume properly stored in an unopened bottle or in a bottle which is more or less full should last ten to twenty years, but in due course any air in the bottle will lead to oxidization, making the liquid dark and acidic, so it is unwise to try to retain a perfume for longer. Once the bottle has been opened and some of the perfume in it used, the best advice is to use all of it within a year or two, before the fragrance changes and starts to become unpleasantly oily and strong.

Perfume, Choice of   Different types of perfume suit different personalities and different occasions (see Perfume Families). The selection of what is the most suitable perfume for a particular person is very much a matter of personal preference and taste, depending on her life style and the circumstances in which she will be wearing it, but the trained consultants who serve behind most perfume counters will be able to give helpful assistance in making a choice. It should be remembered that perfumes can change with the body chemistry of an individual, so what is entirely satisfactory for one woman may not last so long on another and may even smell rather different.

It is advisable to try out a perfume by choosing one of the lighter concentrations, such as the eau de cologne, applying it to the pulse points on the wrist. It should not be rubbed into the skin, as that can impair the fragrance. It should be worn for at least an hour and preferably longer, so that the top, middle and lower notes in it will have time to unfold (see Perfume Notes). If it is still found to be pleasing after that time then it is suitable.

Body temperature affects the chemical balance of the skin and can change the character of a perfume, so a scent should not be chosen immediately after hard exercise or when a woman is feeling out of sorts and is possibly running a temperature.

If more than one perfume is being tested then the lighter one should be tried first and samples should be sprayed as far apart on the skin as possible (on the other wrist, and then, perhaps, on the top of the arm).

Perfume, Classification of Fragrances   The first comprehensive method of classifying the fragrances of perfume ingredients was proposed by Rimmel at the end of the 19th century. In his *Book of Perfumes* he set out a table identifying 18 different representative types of fragrance, grouping each into a class with other materials having a similar fragrance. His classification, slightly modified to accord with later terminology, was as follows.

Class	Type	Other fragrances
Almondy	Bitter almond	Laurels, peach kernals, mirbane
Amber	Ambergris	Oak moss
Anise	Aniseed	Badiane, caraway, dill, fennel, coriander
Balsamic	Vanilla	Balsam of Tolu, balsam of Peru, benzoin, styrax, tonka
Camphoraceous	Camphor	Rosemary, patchouli
Caryophyllaceous	Clove	Carnation, clove-pink
Citrine	Lemon	Bergamot, orange, cedrat, limes
Fruity	Pear	Apple, pineapple, quince
Jasmin	Jasmine	Lily of the Valley
Lavender	Lavender	Spike, thyme, serpolet, marjoram
Minty	Peppermint	Spearmint, balm, rue, sage
Musky	Musk	Civet, ambrette seed, musk plant

Class	Type	Other fragrances
Orange flower	Neroli	Acacia, syringa, orange leaves
Rosaceous	Rose	Geranium, sweet briar, rhodium
Sandal	Sandalwood	Vetivert, cedarwood
Spicy	Cinnamon	Cassia, nutmeg, mace, pimento
Tuberose	Tuberose	Lily, jonquil, narcissus, hyacinth
Violet	Violet	Cassie, orris-root, mignonette

Rimmel's system has remained a useful method of fragrance classification ever since, though increasingly limited in value as new fragrances, especially synthetic ones, have come into use. Piesse attempted to introduce an entirely different concept under which the odours were arranged on a basis of musical notes; by this he held that a perfumer could achieve an effective bouquet of fragrance by choosing odours which corresponded to a harmonious chord in music. The system no longer pertains, but the notion of fragrances as musical notes has remained (see Perfume Notes).

Various other attempts at more satisfactory methods of classification have been made since, ending with a table produced by W.A. Poucher setting out perfume materials against a scale of 100 according to measurements of their evaporation rates. This has the merit of being divisible into three sections, indicating fragrances suitable for the top, middle and lower notes of a perfume. Thus niaouli (1), the fastest evaporating of all perfume materials, appears with mandarin (2), coriander (3), lavender (4), bergamot (6), spike lavender (9), galbanum oil, kuromoji, lovage and nutmeg (11), and lemongrass, mimosa absolute and palma rosa (14) in the part of the scale listing fragrances suitable for 'top notes'. The 'middle note' fragrances are rated from 15 to 69, Poucher's list including rose otto, dill and storax oil (15), calamus, marjoram, orris absolute and violet leaves absolute (18), clove (22), geranium, jonquil absolute and ylang-ylang (24), orange flower absolute (31) and rose, tuberose and jasmine absolutes (43). 'Base note' fragrances rate from 70 to 100, with galbanum and opoponax resins at 90, angelica at 94 and, at 100, many of the important ingredients used as fixatives, such as ambergris, balsam of Peru, benzoin, costus, coumarin, labdanum, oak moss, olibanum (frankincense), patchouli, pimento, sandalwood, storax resin, tonka and vetiver. Space does not permit Poucher's table to be reproduced in full.

Perfume Containers The earliest perfume containers were made of terracotta, but the Ancient Egyptians began to develop the art of glass making from the 4th millennium BC and by about 1500 BC skilfully decorated glass perfume bottles were in use. Bottles, vases and pots of alabaster, onyx and porphyry were also used from early times, having the advantage of preserving the oils and unguents in them by keeping them cool. In Egyptian court circles perfume containers of silver were known. Some perfume materials and cosmetics were also kept in decorated boxes made of wood or ivory.

Greek perfume containers were made in a similar variety of substances, sometimes exquisitely carved. Greek ointment vials of pottery, called *Lekythen*, with a narrow neck, a single handle and decoration in black, are frequently found in tombs. The Greek *Aryballos*, a small unguent flask, was carried suspended from the owner's wrist by a leather cord. Some Greek scent bottles were made in the shape of human or animal heads.

In Roman times glass, onyx and alabaster remained the most normal materials for perfume containers (*Balsamaria* – and see also Alabastrum). They were produced in a wide variety of shapes and designs, often of the highest craftsmanship. Common perfumes for the less wealthy were sometimes sold in shell-shaped containers made of earthenware. Cosmetic creams were sold in glazed earthenware pots. Rich Romans sometimes used elaborate cases or boxes (*Narthecia*), often of precious metal, to hold their perfume and toilet requirements when they travelled or attended the public baths. Frankincense, burned as an incense on an altar or a turibulum both in temples and in the home, was kept in small boxes called *Acerra*.

As perfumery began to flourish in Europe, so skilfully wrought perfume containers of glass and metal were created by European craftsmen to hold their fragrant materials, though with little change in styles. Glass scent bottles were being made in France, England, Silesia, Bohemia and Italy from the 16th century. The pomander, carried in the hand or hanging round the waist, required a new type of container, which was originally ball-shaped and usually made of precious metal or ivory. The pouncet box held perfumed powders. Developing from the pomander came, in the 18th century, the vinaigrette, a tiny silver box holding a perfumed sponge. Novelty containers of this period included 'Oiselets de chypre' (see under Chypre), but most French 17th and early 18th century perfume was sold in white glazed earthenware pots.

The discovery of the Chinese porcelain-making secrets early in the 18th century made an important new material available for scent bottles, notably those produced at Meissen, Sevres and Chelsea. From the end of the 18th century the manufacture of small scent bottles of porcelain, glass, enamel and precious metal became a considerable art; enamelware scent bottles made at Battersea and Bilston at this period, for example, are now valuable collectors' pieces. A feature of the time was the decorated case containing two, three or four tiny bottles, so that the owner could vary the kind of perfume worn at different times of day. Perfume was usually sold in plain containers and transferred at home into these more decorative bottles.

By the middle of the 19th century, perfume and perfume containers were being manufactured on an industrial scale both in Europe and in the USA, the bottles being mostly made of glass. Popular glass styles included opaline (notably between 1825 and 1870), vaseline (between 1835 and 1900), cameo (from the 1870s), satin (notably in the 1880s), milk glass and cut glass (both from about 1890). Bottles, usually in coloured glass, decorated with overlaid patterns cut out of silver became fashionable from the 1870s. Double scent bottles were popular from the 1850s, Chatelaine Bottles and Tulip Bottles from c. 1880s. Atomizers were introduced early in this century. The principal glass makers of the period included the Cristalleries of Baccarat, Nancy, Saint-Louis, André Jolivet, and the Verreries of Argentueil and Viard et Viollet le Duc in France, Thomas Webb and Stevens & Williams in England, Val St Lambert in Belgium and Moser in Bohemia. In the 1890s the American firms of Tiffany and Carder brought out quality bottles of Art Nouveau style to compete with European products, while, from its foundation in 1903, the Steuben Glass Works of New York also produced scent bottles which are now highly valued by collectors. The Art Deco style was adopted by many perfume bottle makers from the 1920s. In the same period it became fashionable for women to carry their perfume with them, leading to a vogue for very small bottles which they could keep in their handbags. Bottles with fan stoppers were popular from the 1930s. From the end of the 19th century, growing competition had brought increasing demands from the perfumers for more appealing packaging not only in the shapes of the bottles but also in the designs of ribbons, labels and boxes, leading to an important new industry for supplying them.

Early in the 20th century the requirements of, in particular, Francois Coty (see Coty) on Baccarat and Lalique for new containers of very high quality for the commercial sale of perfume revolutionized ideas about the design of perfume flacons. In the 1920s the style of flacons chosen for the line of perfumes issued by Chanel also had a strong influence on flacon design. Notable designers of flacons at this time, in addition to René Lalique, included Maurice Martinot and Suë et Mare (see, for example, 'Joy' and 'Amour Amour'). Significant new manufacturing techniques were developed by Brosse.

Since the 1960s a large proportion of bottles used for brand-name perfumes, other than bottles prepared 'in house' by some perfume companies, has been designed by a comparatively small number of designers. Most prominent among these are Pierre Dinand, Serge Mansau, Jacques Helleu, Alain de Mourgues and Jacques Llorente, also the studios of Ira Levy, Annegret Beier, Joel Desgrippes, Robert Granai, Peter Schmidt and Bernard Kotyuk. Among many striking designs by these and other artists may be noted the 'in-house' flacons designed by

Boucheron and Cartier, the prize-winning designs for 'Chloé', 'Oscar de la Renta' and 'Montana', Paloma Picasso and Bernard Kotyuk's flacon for 'Mon Parfum', the Dali-inspired flacon for 'Salvador Dali', the opulent containers made by Aspreys for 'Amouage', the modernistic flacon for 'V'E' designed by Thierry Lecoule and Pierre Dinand's flacon for 'Vicky Tiel'. Flacons of the highest quality of design and workmanship continue to come from Baccarat and Lalique and distinguished glass and crystal flacons are also produced by Brosse.

Mention may also be made of the mass-production glassmakers who produce perfume bottles by the thousand to the drawings of the designers. Again most of this work is done by a comparatively small number of large firms, among whom the most prominent are Saint Gobain Desjonquères, B.S.N. Verreries de Manieres, Pochet et du Courval and Luigi Bormioli. Between them these four firms manufacture about 90% of all mass-produced perfume bottles. In the USA, the Wheaton Glassworks and Carr-Lowry Co. are notable among firms making bottles for leading perfume companies.

A notable development of recent times has been the popularity of 19th and 20th century scent bottles as collectors pieces. This hobby, already established for some years on the Continent and mainly confined to French perfume bottles, is now growing in Britain. In May 1990, Bonhams of London held the first auction sale in Britain devoted entirely to scent bottles, when Baccarat and Lalique pieces fetched up to £800. At a similar sale at the end of that year some rare pieces by these two makers obtained up to £3500 each. Highly prized and exceptionally rare Lalique flacons can now sell for around £10 000, and a record price of approximately £16 000 has been reached for one such item.

Perfume Creation   The decision to create and market a new perfume is necessarily a matter of hard commercial practicalities, usually based on market research. Whether the perfume is to be made for a perfume company or for a fashion house or other such concern which will sell it as a supplement to the main business, basic problems of type and cost must be settled at an early stage. A maximum price for the perfume must be determined, and a ceiling set on the cost of making and marketing it. The design of the bottle and packaging (see Perfume Containers) must reflect not only the type of fragrance and its brand name, but also the image which the company launching it wishes to convey about itself. It is within these considerations that the 'nose', or creative perfumer (also sometimes called a blender), will be engaged to start devising the new fragrance. In particular, it must be known from the very beginning how much money can be spent on materials. If the perfume is to sell to a mass market at a low retail price, rare and costly ingredients cannot be put into it.

The ingredients available to a perfumer come from the essential oils (and their concretes and absolutes) of about 400 different fragrant plant parts, together with a choice of some 4000 or more synthetic fragrances, which are chemicals either extracted from plant parts, and therefore intrinsically of natural origin, or manufactured from substances such as coal or crude oil. The yield of some essential oils, and especially of their concretes and absolutes, may be very low, and where this coincides with labour-intensive picking and collection the resultant perfume ingredient may be extremely expensive; tuberose absolute, for example, now costs more than its weight in gold. But the manufacturing process by which some of the synthetics are obtained can also be expensive, so that in perfumery 'synthetic' does not signify cheapness. Neither does 'synthetic' indicate something inferior to a natural product. Aldehydes, indeed, are used to sharpen and improve natural fragrances. While some of the very highest quality perfumes (e.g. 'Amouage' and 'Bal à Versailles') are created almost entirely out of costly natural oils and attars, or extracts from such oils and attars, the majority of high-quality modern perfumes use a liberal range of chemicals, together with natural materials, to obtain their effect. Without synthetics production of perfume on a mass scale to meet the demands of modern times would be impossible, because supplies of many ingredients would be insufficient and their cost prohibitive. In the case of some of the animal perfume materials, moreover, synthetics now enable perfumers to use substitutes which are not subject to criticism on ecological or 'animal rights' grounds. Similarly, several oils are now chemically modified, or even synthesized, to replace natural oils for safety or environmental reasons (e.g. because the original oil has been found to contain a trace of some toxic substance). The perfumer has to ensure that materials to be used meet internationally laid down standards in this respect. Oils now generally so replaced include balsam of Peru, bergamot, bitter orange, cassia, cinnamon, costus, lime, rue and styrax, together with some early chemically extracted or synthetic materials such as citral, musk ambrette, musk ketone and musk xylene.

Sitting at their organs, with shelves full of bottles of essential oils and synthetic preparations ranged around, perfumers will attempt by degrees to build up a composite fragrance which meets the specifications imposed. It requires years of experience to get to know and distinguish the hundreds of different fragrances which can be chosen from; the perfumers have had to learn what effect one fragrance may have on another when they are mixed together, how to smooth or sharpen a fragrance, how to bring odours to a common standard of strength so that one ingredient will not overwhelm another, how to achieve the effect of high, middle and low notes, and how to fix a perfume so that it will last. They must also know what ingredients will be available in the quantity required for manufacture of the perfume in bulk, for there is clearly no point in using something of which there is an inadequate supply. They must be skilled chemists.

Relying on a highly trained sense of smell, perfumers will test their compositions as they progress with fragrance blotters, small wands of blotting paper which are dipped into the mixture and allowed to dry before being sniffed. However, the olfactory nerve quickly tires, making the process a very slow one, and, with nuances of aroma to decide between, it may well be decided to wait for another day before going any further. As the composition develops, probably built up from the base notes, the perfumer will from time to time need to discuss it with the sponsor: an *haute couture* designer who has commissioned the fragrance may have very strong personal views about the nature of what is being prepared, and modifications may have to be made in the light of what such a sponsor says. Testing is also necessary over lengthy periods to ensure, for example, that the aroma will last the required amount of time when worn, that it will remain constant in different temperatures and climates, that it will remain consistent after being kept in a bottle for months. For these and other reasons a perfume may well take two or three years to develop. Francois Coty took five years to perfect 'L'Aimant'; the creation of Guerlain's 'Chant d'Arômes' lasted for seven years; Caron's 'Infini' was fifteen years in the making.

Most perfumes will contain 50 to 100 different ingredients, many of them considerably more (see Perfume). They must all harmonize perfectly with each other. Having finally achieved what is required by the perfumer and the sponsor, the perfumer will list the ingredients in a formula showing the exact strengths and quantities of everything the perfume contains, sometimes expressed in portions which add up to 1000. This formula, a valuable and highly confidential document, is the basis on which the perfume will then be manufactured (see Perfume Manufacture).

Perfume Families In today's perfume retail trade, perfumes are generally classified under one of seven family groups, called Perfume Families, or Fragrance Families, with names indicative of the type of perfume they comprise. These 'families' are the following.

1. Floral: the largest family, consisting of perfumes containing a preponderence of essential oils from flowers. Perfumes in this family are sometimes subdivided into four main sections – floral, floral–sweet, floral–fresh and floral–fruity–fresh. They are generally regarded as perfumes good for general daytime wear and for summer evenings.
2. Green: a fresher, sharper type of perfume than the florals, based on a blending of herbs, ferns, mosses and citrus fruits, designed to

create a general impression of meadows, green grass and leaves. Green perfumes are sometimes subdivided into sections called Fresh and Balsamic, the latter name indicating the softer, sweeter fragrance of resins and balsams. They are generally regarded as most suitable for outdoors and a sporty mood.

3. Aldehydic: also called Modern. These are perfumes with a rich, somewhat watery, tallowy fragrance derived from certain synthetic materials (see Aldehyde). They are sometimes subdivided into two sections – Aldehydic–floral and aldehydic–floral–woody–powdery. They are regarded as very sophisticated and modern (the first such perfume made was Chanel No. 5) and wearable all year round.

4. Chypre: named after the famous perfume from Cyprus of Roman times (see separate entry under Chypre). Perfumes in this family have a floral or green fragrance with deep Low Notes such as ambergris, making them very long-lasting. They are sometimes divided into three subsections with self-descriptive names: fresh–mossy–aldehydic, floral–mossy–animalic and mossy–fruity. They are mainly, but not entirely, designed for use by women, being regarded as appropriate for both day and evening wear, especially during winter.

5. Oriental: sometimes called Amber. A family of strong, spicy and exotic fragrances with a distinctive heavy sweetness obtained from lower notes such as musk, sandalwood and vanilla. They are regarded as most suitable for wear in the evening. A subsection with a lighter, floral feel, sometimes called semi-oriental–floral or floriental, is becoming increasingly popular; it is regarded as most appropriate for summer and daytime wear.

6. Tobacco/Leather: a family of fragrances reminiscent of tobacco and/or leather with a woody, spicy and sometimes animalic background. These fragrances are almost all designed for the growing trade in perfumed toiletries for men.

7. Fougere: fragrances in this family have a fresh, herbal, lavender character with mossy or hay-like backgrounds. Again, they are found mostly in toilet preparations for men.

In the never-ending pursuit for new types of fragrance many different effects are obtained by combining two or more of these basic Perfume Families together. Such combinations are sometimes referred to as Bouquets. A notable example is 'Red', categorized into a new perfume family called 'Fleuriffe Chypres'. *See also* Perfume Notes.

In male perfumery, which is for the most part a matter of fragrances contained in toilet preparations, including eau de toilettes, colognes and aftershave lotions, a different grouping of perfume descriptions is increasingly being adopted, under which fragrances are divided into ten basic families with self-descriptive names: floral, green, chypre, leather, fougere, citrus, lavender, spicy, woody and musky. There are, again, many permutations of these on the market.

Perfume Making at Home   In Elizabethan times most large households kept a part of the garden for cultivating fragrant plants to use in medical and toilet preparations, making perfumed pomanders, wash-balls, sachets, pot pourri, cassolettes and distilled waters from them in the 'still room' of the house. The home perfumer who wishes to revive this craft may be able to follow some of the recipes of earlier times, but many of them will prove impracticable, because many of the ingredients then used, such as ambergris and musk, are now pro-hibitively expensive, if not unobtainable. He, or she, does, however, have the advantage that many fragrant materials and essential oils are now readily available for purchase, and the laborious process of making them from the raw plants can be avoided.

Dry pot pourri is probably the easiest fragrant preparation to make, involving little more than the mixing of dried materials, of which a very wide range is nowadays available. The descriptions of plant materials in this book show whether they are suitable for pot pourri. Rose petals are the ingredient most commonly used. They should be collected on a dry morning free of dew and laid out to dry for about a week. Some-times coarse salt, or salt petre, is added as a preservative. A material with fixative properties should be included. (See Appendix B, recipes nos 1–5.)

Moist pot pourri is a little more complicated. The rose petals or other flowers and herbs should be spread out to dry for about two days, so that they are not completely dried. Layers of this material, mixed up with spices and gums which have been ground into a coarse powder, are then rammed down hard into a jar or basin with alternate layers of salt; a pinch of brown sugar and a few drops of brandy can be added; the container is then sealed tight and the mixture left to cure for at least 2 months, when it will emerge as a congealed mass which can be broken up into cakes. (See Appendix B, recipes nos 6–8.)

Pomanders are best made by mixing aromatic materials with gum arabic or tragacanth mucilage as a bonding agent. The selected in-gredients of the pomander, in the proporton of about 2 parts of gums and resins to 1 part of other dry ingredients, are finely powdered and mixed with a little of the mucilage until a paste is formed. A few drops of essential oil can be added and everything should then be well mixed by kneading. The paste is then shaped as required and left to dry. (See Appendix B, recipes nos 14–23.)

Incense is best made using powdered charcoal as a burning base in the proportion of about 14 parts to 6 parts of aromatic material. The latter should consist of 2 parts of powdered resins, such as labdanum, storax, terebinth or frankincense, mixed with 4 parts of other fragrant plant materials (e.g. dried bay leaves, calamus root, cloves, cubebs, lavender flowers, marjoram, rosemary leaves or thyme leaves). These are all mixed into a paste with a mucilage of gum arabic or tragacanth. A drop or two of essential oil can be kneaded in. The mixture is then shaped into small cones or rolled round sticks to make joss sticks, and these are allowed to dry. (See Appendix B, recipes nos 24–29.)

Sachets require very dry ingredients which can be ground into a coarse powder. Lavender has always been a favourite as a base, but orris, calamus, cedarwood, marjoram, sandalwood, oak moss, rose petals, verbena leaves, or patchouli leaves are good alternatives. A wide range of other materials, mostly similar to those that can be used in pot pourri, can be blended into this base. At least one ingredient with fixative properties should be included. (See Appendix B, recipes nos 9–13 and 73–74.)

Liquid perfumes provide the would-be home perfume markers with rather more problems, as will be apparent from the entry above on Perfume Creation. They cannot hope to simulate the quality fragrances produced by commercial perfumeries, which may contain several hundred ingredients, including many chemicals, and they can realistically aim only at very simple constructions. They will have to be prepared to purchase all their essential oils, some of which may be quite expensive. For a start a base will be needed on which the perfume can be built. This can either be an alcohol (vodka is sometimes used) or an oil; jojoba oil is regarded as a good, neutral, stable base oil, or, following the perfume makers of ancient Egypt and Greece, sesame oil could be used. The base should be prepared by the addition of such base notes (see Perfume Notes) as may be required, including fixatives, adding them drop by drop. The main body of the fragrance is then inserted, the chosen oils once again being added drop by drop. Ten drops of essential oils added to about half a pint of alcohol will produce a weak cologne-strength fragrance; for a stronger perfume a smaller amount of alcohol or base oil should be used (or, conversely, more essential oils). The mixture should be kept in a sealed container for at least a week in order to blend properly before it can be used. Home perfumers can experiment with the introduction of top notes as well (which should be added last); the evaporation rates mentioned in Poucher's table, referred to under Perfume, Classification of Fragrances, may assist in this, as will a study of which ingredients are used for which notes in the descriptions of perfumes contained in the body of this book. They might even experiment by using all the main ingredients shown for one of the celebrated perfumes and seeing what sort of a fragrance results. They will be a long way from producing 'Amouage', 'Joy' or 'Bal à Versailles', but they should get pleasing results and they will certainly find the experiment fascinating. (See Appendix B, recipes nos 38 onwards.)

Perfume Manufacture   There are two types of manufacturing operation in perfumery. The first is the manufacture, by distillation, expression, enfleurage, maceration, extraction, etc., of the essential oils and attars, concretes and absolutes, pomades and tinctures, together with the manufacture of all the many synthetic preparations, which provide the primary fragrances used by a 'nose' in creating a perfume (see Perfume Creation). Many of the factories where this work is done will be adjacent to the fields or plantations where the plant materials are grown, because such materials may need to be treated as soon as they have been collected if their full fragrances are to be preserved. It follows that these factories will be found all over the world where fragrant materials are harvested. The second operation is the comparatively simple process of assembling and blending together all the oils and essences of which a perfume is composed in accordance with the formula for that perfume devised by the 'nose' who has created it. These ingredients will be mixed to form a concentrate which is left

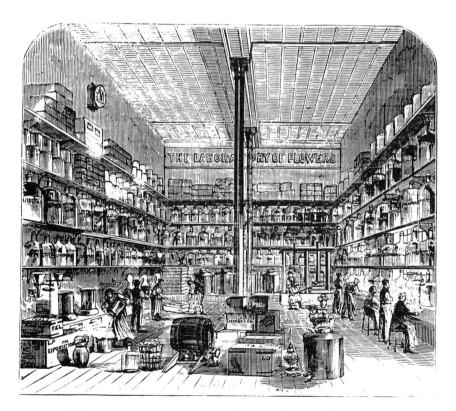

The 19th century perfume factory of Messrs Piesse and Lubin in London.

for several weeks until everything in it has blended completely and matured. The concentrate is then diluted in alcohol to its required strength as an extrait, eau de parfum, eau de toilette or eau de cologne (see Perfume) and left in copper containers to blend for a further few weeks. It is then ready to be bottled.

The design and manufacture of fragrance is now a very large-scale international business. A wide range of toiletries and other household items, from cosmetics, shampoos and soaps to aerosols, deodorants, furniture polishes and lavatory cleaners, now have fragrances added to make them more acceptable and hence to improve their sales. Equally important are flavourings, often derived from the same ingredients, for today's food manufacturers rely a great deal on artificial means to give their mass products an improved or simulated taste. The manufacture of perfume may be but a small part of the business of many of the score or so of large fragrance and flavouring manufacturers now operating. Among the bigger of such firms may be mentioned International Flavours and Fragrances (IFF), the largest company of all, and Quest International, the second largest, a British company based in Kent. The fragrance manufacturers have their own perfumers and can create a

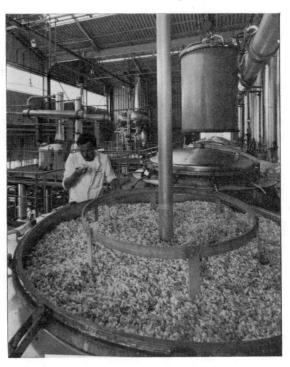

Jasmine being processed in a modern factory. (Photograph from Quest International.)

fragrance and produce it through all its processes of manufacture to the ready-for-sale product. The main companies specializing in the creation and manufacture of high-quality perfumes are IFF (see above), Roure (formerly Roure-Bertrand-Dupont) and the Swiss-based companies Givaudan and Firminich. Between them these four firms make around 60% of all the quality perfumes now marketed.

The large perfume houses have their own 'noses' and manufacturing facilities and may even own acres of land, perhaps around Grasse, from which to produce their own ingredients such as rose and jasmine. Some, like Chanel, have exclusive contracts with growers. But many distinguished perfume houses now obtain their perfumes under contract arrangements from a fragrance manufacturer, and when a fashion house or similar such business decides to add a perfume to its products it will almost invariably obtain it either from a fragrance manufacturer or from a perfume house with its own manufacturing facilities. Thus, Dior, Yves St Laurent, Paco Rabanne, Nina Ricci, Calvin Klein and Givenchy, among many others, have all had perfumes made for them by Roure, and companies such as Grès, Puig, Balenciaga, Révillon, Léonard, Caron and Coty have used IFF. In the world of perfumery the importance of these fragrance manufacturers, anonymous and almost unknown to the general perfume-using public, is thus considerable.

Perfume Notes   Perfumery takes some of its language from music, and the composition of a perfume is seen as a combination of notes. The broad structure of most modern perfumes is based on three layers of notes, referred to respectively as top notes, middle notes and lower notes.

The top note, sometimes called the head note, head or outgoing note, is the part of the perfume which is most apparent immediately it is applied to the skin. It consists of light, volatile fragrances, designed by the perfumer to give a good, and sometimes striking, initial impression. It may last only for a few minutes.

The middle note, also called the medium note or heart, is the main section of the perfume, which becomes dominant after the top note has faded away. It usually consists of floral, spicy or woody components which determine the basic character of the perfume. It is composed of ingredients made to last longer than the top notes (it is part of the skill of the perfumer to prepare his ingredients with an appropriate lasting power) and in a quality perfume it should be apparent for 4 hours or more.

The lower note, also called low note, base note, back note, depth note, body, body note and dry away, consists of underlying, long-lasting fragrances which provide the perfume with its fixatives and give it depth. It becomes most discernible as the middle note begins to fade, and in a quality perfume it should last for a few more hours or even for a day or two. It usually consists of animalic, woody, resinous or crystalline components.

In describing a perfume, the term note is also used for individual fragrances which influence the total effect (e.g. 'a sweet note provided by tuberose'). Many words are conventionally used in perfumery to describe individual fragrance notes. They include: amber, balsamic, camphoraceous, citrus, coniferous, dry, earthy, floral, fougere, fruity, green, hayfield (hay-like), herbaceous, heavy, leather, light, metallic, minty, mossy, narcotic, powdery, smoky, spicy, sweet, tobacco and woody. For the conventional meaning of these words see separate entries. New notes are still devised, e.g. the oceanic note in 'Dune', introduced in 1991.

See also under Perfume, Classification of Fragrances.

Perfumed Bdellium   *see* Myrrh and Opoponax

Perfumers Workshop   A New York fragrance firm producing quality perfumes which include 'Tea Rose' (75), 'Freesia', 'Gardenia', 'Muguet' and 'Samba' (87).

Perilla Oil   An essential oil obtained by steam-distillation from the leaves and flowers of Perilla (*Perilla frutescens* = *P. ocimoides*) a herb found from India to China, Japan and Korea. It has a powerful spicy, slightly cumin-like fragrance and is occasionally used in perfumery. (An oil with the same name is distilled from the seeds of this plant and used in paints and varnishes.)

Perkin, William   A British 19th century chemist who found how to synthesize coumarin, the first major discovery in the making of synthetic perfumes.

Petitgrain Oil   An essential oil with a sweet, flowery, Neroli-like fragrance distilled from the leaves, twigs and small unripe fruits of the Bitter Orange tree (*Citrus aurantium* var. *amara*), which also provides Neroli and Bitter Orange Oil. It is cultivated for Petitgrain Oil in Sicily, Spain, Italy, Paraguay, Brazil, Morocco, Tunisia, Algeria, Egypt and France. The oil is an important component in many perfume creations, especially in colognes and toilet preparations. Modern quality fragrances containing it include 'Narcisse Noir', 'That Man' and 'Special No. 127'. Eau de Brout is obtained from the distillation waters. The oil contains linalol.

A form of Petitgrain Oil known as Citronnier is distilled from the leaves and twigs of the Lemon tree (*Citrus limon*) in Mediterranean areas (see Lemon Oil). This has a softer, more lemony fragrance.

Another form of Petitgrain Oil is distilled in Sicily from the leaves and twigs of the Mandarin tree (*Citrus reticulata*) and known as Mandarin Petitgrain (or Petitgrain Mandarin) Oil. This has a more thyme-like fragrance.

Petroselinum crispum   *see* Parsley
                 sativum   *see* Parsley
Peucedan Gum   A resin said to resemble ammoniacum obtained from the roots of the herb Peucedan (*Peucedanum officinale* = *P. altissima* = *Selinum officinale*), also called Sulphurwort, Milk Parsley, Marsh Parsley, Sulphur Rod, Hog's Fennel, Hoar Strong and, in the USA, Chucklusa. This plant, growing to about 3 feet high, is related to dill and is found in Europe, Asia and N. America. The roots have a strong odour of sulphur and the resin was once used in herbal remedies. Another species of Peucedan (*P. galbaniflora*) is believed to have been the source of a fragrant gum called 'green incense' in ancient Egyptian inscriptions, and also to have produced the gum referred to as galbanum (q.v.) both in the Old Testament and by Pliny.
Peucedanum graveolens   *see* Dill
                 sativum   *see* Parsnip Oil
                 sowa   *see* Dill
Peumos boldus   *see* Boldea
Philadelphus coronarius   *see* Mock Orange Blossom
                 mexicanus   *see* Mexican Mock Orange
Phoenix dactilifera   *see* Date Palm
Phyllanthus emblica   *see* Emblic
Physocalymna floribundum   *see* Rosewood Oil
                 floridum   *see* Rosewood Oil
                 scaberrimum   *see* Rosewood Oil
Picasso, Paloma   *see* 'Mon Parfum'
Picea abies   *see* Norway Spruce Oil
       excelsa   *see* Norway Spruce Oil
Pick Needle   *see* Musk Geranium
Picked Turkey   *see* Gum Arabic
Picotee   *see* Clove-Pink
Piesse, Charles   A celebrated 19th century perfumer living in Nice. His book *The Art of Perfumery* was published in 1880. He is particularly remembered for his attempt to classify fragrances on a scale corresponding to musical notes (see Perfume, Classification of Fragrances).
Pignut tree   *see* Jojoba Oil
Pimenta acris   *see* Bois d'Inde
       officinalis   *see* Pimento Oil
Pimento Oil   Also called Pimenta Oil and Oil of Allspice. An essential oil, having a scent resembling cloves with a touch of nutmeg and cubebs (hence the name Allspice), which is steam-distilled from the leaves of the Pimento tree (*Pimenta officinalis* = *Eugenia pimenta*), also known as the Allspice tree or Jamaican Pepper tree. The tree, which grows to about 30 feet high, is indigenous to the W. Indies and

S. America and is also cultivated in Mexico, India and Réunion. The oil is used in quality perfumes (e.g. 'White Linen') and soaps to give a spicy touch, and is sometimes used to strengthen ylang-ylang and to modify the odour of carnation oils. It is an ingredient of Bay Rum. The dried leaves are used in sachets and pot pourri. The natural oil mainly consists of eugenol; when mixed in the proportion of 3 oz to 1 gallon of rectified spirit it becomes 'Extract of Allspice'.

An oil known as Wild Pimento Oil is also distilled in Jamaica from the leaves of *Amonis jamarcensis*. It has a fragrance resembling spike lavender.

Pimpinella anisum   *see* Anise

Pinaud   A prominent Parisian perfume house from the 18th to the early 20th century. In the late 19th century Pinaud produced a range of floral perfumes under the name 'A la Corbeille Fleurie' (The Flower Basket), followed by other famous perfumes including 'Brise Embaumée', 'Violette' and 'Bouquet Marie-Louise', all of which were sold in flacons by Baccarat.

Pineapple   The aroma of the pineapple fruit, from the pineapple plant (*Ananus comosus = A. sativus*), first found under cultivation in the West Indies in the 16th century (it has never been found growing wild), can be obtained by distillation of the fruit juice. However, as with most fruit fragrances, perfumers usually produce it more satisfactorily with synthetics. It is found in modern quality perfumes (e.g. 'Only').

Pinene   A chemical component in the essential oil of a large number of aromatic plants, including basil, bay leaves, bergamot, carrot seed, clary, coriander, cubebs, eucalyptus, frankincense, myrrh, myrtle, parsley, petitgrain, rosemary, sassafras, star anise and turpentine. It is mostly obtained by distillation from turpentine oil. It has a harsh, spicy, fir-like odour and is used in the manufacture of synthetic camphor, citronellal, geraniol and nerol.

Pine Needle Oil   An oil steam-distilled from the needles, young shoots and cones of many different coniferous trees of the genus *Pinus*, found in Europe, the USSR (CIS) and N. America. It is valued for its refreshing pine odour, and is used in pharmacy and toilet preparations as well as in soaps and perfumes. In the latter it is mainly employed in masculine and green or conifer-type perfumes (e.g. 'Alliage' and 'Panache').

The principal Pine Needle Oil used in perfumery comes from the Scotch pine (*Pinus sylvestris*) of north and central Europe. From the Dwarf Pine (*P. pumilio*) of central Europe is obtained Dwarf Pine Oil, also called Dwarf Pine Needle Oil. From the Mountain Pine (*P. mughus = P. mungo = P. montana*), another dwarf species found in Alpine regions of Europe, comes Mugo Pine Oil, which is also sometimes called Dwarf Pine Oil. The dried needles and cones of pines are also sometimes used in sachets and pot pourri.

Pine Needle Oil was known to the early Arab perfume makers, who obtained it from *P. orientalis*, *P. pinaea* and other species; one of al-Kindi's perfume recipes used it mixed with frankincense.

Pine Oil   An oil obtained by steam-distillation of wood chips from the heartwood and roots of various species of Pine tree (*Pinus palustris*, *P. ponderosa* and others). It is mainly produced in the USA, Finland, France, Portugal and the USSR (CIS). It has a harsh pine-like odour and is used in some low-cost perfumes and soaps.

P'Ing-She Fei-Tsao   A perfumed toilet soap made in central China by mixing the crushed pods of the Fei-Tsao tree (*Gymnocladus chinensis*) with camphor, musk, cloves, sandalwood and putchuk.

'Pink Lace'   A floral–chypre perfume by Yardley which was launched in 1988. Top notes, designed to give a sparkling, fruity effect, include lemon, coriander and camomile. The heart contains jasmine, rose and ylang-ylang together with a spicy touch from carnation. Base notes include sandalwood, frankincense, patchouli and vetivert.

Pinus montana   *see* Pine Needle Oil

    mughus   *see* Pine Needle Oil

    mungo   *see* Pine Needle Oil

    orientalis   *see* Pine Needle Oil

    palustris   *see* Pine Oil

    pinaea   *see* Pine Needle Oil

    ponderosa   *see* Pine Oil

    pumilio   *see* Pine Needle Oil

    sylvestris   *see* Pine Needle Oil

Piper augustifolium   *see* Matico

    clusii   *see* Cubeb

    cubeba   *see* Cubeb

    nigrum   *see* Pepper Oil

Pissasphalt   Perhaps the most extraordinary of all ancient perfume materials. A resin was used by the ancient Egyptians (see Egyptian perfumes) in their embalming processes, in conjunction with various aromatics, particularly cassia and myrrh. The Greeks and early Arabs recovered this substance from mummies in Egyptian tombs, by which time it had absorbed all the aromatics used with it and become a form of fragrant bitumen. This was re-used in perfumes. The Arabs called this material *Mumiya*.

Pistacia lentiscus   *see* Mastic/Terebinth Oil

Pittosporum   The fragrance of the flowers of a small tree, *Pittosporum dallii*, native to New Zealand but cultivated in Europe, is used as a special feature in the floral bouquet of Estée Lauder's 'Knowing'.

Plantain   *see* Banana

Pliny   Pliny the Elder (23–79 AD) was a lawyer and admiral who died in the Vesuvius eruption. His greatest work, *Natural History*, a vast compendium covering many subjects, contains much information about the perfumes and perfume materials of his time. See Roman perfumes.

Plum The fragrance of the plum (also called Mirabelle) found in modern perfumes is invariably created synthetically. It is often used to provide a fruity effect, appearing, for example, in such quality perfumes as 'Femme', 'Chant d'Aromes' and 'Xia-Xiang'.

Plumiera acutifolia see Frangipani

      alba see Frangipani

      bicolor see Frangipani

      rubra see Frangipani

Pogostemon cablin see Patchouli

        heyneanus see Patchouli

        patchouli see Patchouli

Poiret, Paul (1879–1928) The first French couturier to market perfumes designed to harmonize with his clothes. His perfume company, Parfums Rosine, was set up in 1910, using well-known artists, including Erté and Raoul Duffy, in the design of bottles and packaging.

'Poison' An innovative linear fragrance type of perfume created by Roure perfumers for Dior, who launched it in 1985. Designed to be audacious, it provides a spicy, fruity fragrance from wild berries in a combination of blackcurrant, red currant, raspberry and blackberry, given a spicy backing by coriander, pepper and cinnamon and a sweet note from orange blossom. The base contains ambergris, labdanum and opoponax.

Polar Plant see Rosemary

Polge, Jacques (b. 1943) The principal perfumer ('nose') of Chanel. His creations include 'Bois Noir', 'Coco' 'Antaeus' and 'L'Égoïste' for Chanel, 'Senso' and 'Diva' for Ungaro and 'Stephanie' for Bourjois.

Polianthus tuberosa see Tuberose Flower Oil

'Polo' A trend-setting chypre-type men's fragrance first produced in 1978 by Warner Cosm. and now marketed by Ralph Lauren in association with L'Oréal. Its main ingredients are juniper and artemisia in the top note, pine with spicy elements in the middle note, and patchouli, moss and leather-fragrance in the lower note. It comes in a flask designed by Bernard Kotyuk.

Polyganum aviculare see Knot Grass

Pomade Also called Pomatum. A perfumed ointment used on the hair and on the skin of the head. The word is also used by perfumers to describe fat saturated with the scent from flowers during a stage of the enfleurage process of preparing essential oils for perfumes. (See Appendix B, recipe no. 37.)

Pomander A solid ball of scented materials carried on the person. In ancient Greece women wore a necklace of small scented pastilles or beads, usually based on crushed-up rose petals, with other fragrant materials and a gum to bind them. From these derived the prayer beads, or rosary, first used by Byzantine Christians. In Renaissance times a large scented ball (*Oldano*) was attached to the end of a rosary, and after a time this came to be worn without beads, either on a chain round the neck or at the waist. These were carried both for pleasure and to ward off contagion, more particularly the plague. The Arabs then introduced into Europe the more practical alternative to ward off contagion of an orange stuck with cloves or stuffed with medicinal herbs, the latter sometimes soaked in vinegar. During the 16th century this aromatic orange was replaced in court circles by a very small (walnut-sized), oldano-like, ball-shaped receptacle made of filigreed gold, silver or ivory held by a chain to wear round the neck or from the wrist, and containing either solid perfume or aromatic vinegar soaked in a sponge (the predecessor of the vinaigrette). The solid perfume usually contained ambergris, giving rise to the name 'pomme ambre' (amber apple), from which the word 'pomander' derives. Some pomanders had segments for different perfumes. Pomanders went out of fashion in the 17th century, but have had some revival in home perfumery in recent years. See also under Cassolette, Pouncet Box and Perfume Making at Home. (See also Appendix B, recipes nos 14–23.)

Pomatum   *see* Pomade

Popinac   *see* Cassie

Popoie   *see* Iguga

Populus balsamifera   *see* Balm of Gilead/Tacamahac

Portugal, Oil of   *see* Sweet Orange

Pot Pourri   A mixture of fragrant materials placed in a bowl or jar and used for perfuming the rooms of a house. Pot pourri has been used since medieval times. The term 'pot pourri' is French, derived from Spanish for a stock-pot or mixed stew. Originally many pot pourri mixes sold by perfumers were simply the residues of their working material (now known as Olla-podrida (q.v.)). Early pot pourri was usually made of fresh, moist ingredients, with rose petals and orange flowers predominating, which were left to infuse for a month or two with salt added as a preservative, after which other powdered perfumes or essential oils were added before the composition was brought into use. Dry pot pourri, which is the type manufactured commercially at the present time, also traditionally has a preponderance of rose petals, but lavender and many other dried flowers are used in it as well. Salt is sometimes still added as a preservative, as also are small amounts of essential oils. Despite the name, most 'dry' pot pourri are not normally sufficiently dry to be used in sachets. Unscented flowers which keep their colour after drying are sometimes added to both moist and dry pot pourri to improve their appearance. Modern commercial pot-pourri production in the UK relies almost completely on imported materials, such as rose petals from Morocco and Turkey and jasmine from Italy. Blends of perfume oils (called 'revivers') are now made to freshen up pot pourri when their scent begins to fade.

Poucher, W.A. Author of *Perfumes, Cosmetics and Soaps*, a three-volume work which is regarded as a standard guide among perfumers. First published in 1923, it has since been reissued in several revised editions, the last in 1991.

Pounce *see* Sanderac

Pouncet Box A box originally used to contain pumice stone, needed in preparing parchment for writing, and later, when it was usually made of scented wood, to hold perfumed powder for use as a snuff or inhalant. Subsequently, in the Elizabethan period, the name came to be used for any type of box which held perfumed powders for placing between linen or blowing about a room or over the hair with bellows.

'Pour l'Homme' An innovative, trend-setting leather-type fragrance brought out by Van Cleef & Arpels in 1978 for men's toiletries. Its principal constituents are bergamot and thyme in the top note, carnation, artemisia and patchouli, giving a spicy, woody feel, in the middle note, and moss and leather-fragrance in the lower note.

Prasium majus *see* Balm

'Prestige Dry Herb' The first of the masculine scents with a fresh green fragrance. Issued by Wolff and Sohn as an eau de cologne in 1960. Principal ingredients are mandarin and galbanum in the top note, clove-pink in the middle note, and tree moss in the lower note.

Prickly Ash tree *see* Tomar Seed Oil

Prickly Juniper *see* Cedar

Priest's Pintle *see* Rose Rod

Printanier *see* Cassolette

'Private Collection' A 'green' perfume brought out by Estée Lauder in 1972. Green top notes containing citrus and hyacinth lead to a floral heart, with jasmine, narcissus and rose, over a mossy base of oak moss, cedar and musk. The flacon, of frosted glass with a gold cord, was designed by Ira Levy.

Proctor & Gamble A major manufacturer of toiletries and household goods, based in Ohio. It owns the Old Spice, Shulton and Santa Fe mens's toiletry companies, and in 1991 it acquired Max Factor and the German company Elena Betrix from Revlon.

Profumego An ornamental ball of copper or bronze containing incense paste which was used in Italy, and subsequently elsewhere in Europe, at the time of the Renaissance to perfume a room. It was either hung up by a chain or, sometimes, rolled along the floor.

Propolis Sometimes called Virgin Wax or Bee-glue. A sweet-smelling, sticky brown substance gathered from trees by bees for use as a cement in their hives. The aroma resembles storax. Propolis was used by

Persian and Arab perfume makers from as early as the 9th century AD, and in later times was used in preparing pomander beads. It is still used occasionally in pot pourri. See also Beeswax.

Protium attenatum   *see* Elemi
        chapeliesi   *see* Elemi
        guianese   *see* Elemi
        heptaphyllum   *see* Elemi

Prunus armeniacus   *see* Apricot
        mahaleb   *see* Magalep
        persica   *see* Peach

Pseudostuga douglasii   *see* Douglas Fir
        menziesii   *see* Douglas Fir
        mucronata   *see* Douglas Fir
        taxifolia   *see* Douglas Fir

Pterocarpus   A species of Pterocarpus (*Pterocarpus santalinus*), a small tree native to islands of the Indian Archipelago, provides a highly scented wood which is used in India and China for burning as incense and, when powdered, for scenting clothes.

Ptychotis ajowan   *see* Ajowan

Pucci   *see* Emilio Pucci

Puchapat   *see* Patchouli

Pudding Grass   *see* Pennyroyal

Puig   Pronounced 'Pooch'. The leading Spanish perfume and cosmetics company, formed in Barcelona in 1914 by Don Antonio Puig, initially to import French perfumes into Spain. It is still run by his sons. In 1969 Antonio Puig also founded the French firm Paco Rabanne, which is part of the Puig organization. He began to market his own perfume brands in 1925, and the success of 'Aqua Lavanda' in 1940 enabled the company to expand. Its headquarters and factory are in Barcelona. Puig fragrances have included 'Agua Brava' (68), 'Estivalia' (75) and 'Vetiver de Puig' (78). In the UK it currently markets two fragrances for men: 'Quorum' (82) and 'Sybaris' (88), both created by Sebastian Gomez, together with 'Carolina Herrera'.

Pulegium   *see* Pennyroyal

'Pure Silk'   A floral–chypre perfume created by Roure perfumers for Yardley, who launched it in 1982. Ylang-ylang and orange blossom blend with aldehydes in the top note, leading to a floral heart of rose, jasmine and woody tones, with vetivert, patchouli and oak moss the main components of the base note.

Pyrethrum balsamita   *see* Costmary

Pyrus coronaria   *see* Crab Apple
        malus   *see* Apple

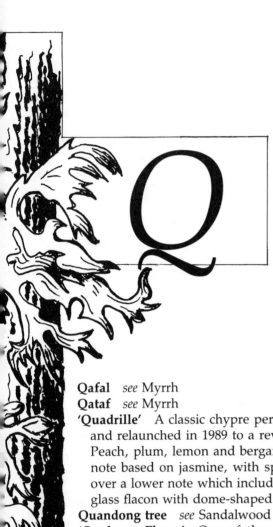

Qafal *see* Myrrh

Qataf *see* Myrrh

'Quadrille' A classic chypre perfume brought out by Balenciaga in 1955 and relaunched in 1989 to a revised formula created by IFF perfumers. Peach, plum, lemon and bergamot in the top notes introduce a middle note based on jasmine, with spicy touches from clove and cardamom, over a lower note which includes amber and musk. It is sold in an oval glass flacon with dome-shaped cap similar to the flacon of 'Le Dix'.

Quandong tree *see* Sandalwood

'Quelques Fleurs' One of the great classics of perfumery, created by Robert Bienaimé for Houbigant and first marketed in 1912. 'Quelques Fleurs' started a fashion for light floral perfumes and is regarded as the first true multifloral bouquet, for prior to it flower fragrances had mostly been single notes or mixed with many other ingredients. With fresh, leafy top notes, lilac, rose, jasmine, violet and orchid are among its main ingredients and the floral nuance penetrates into the base, but the details of its composition are safeguarded by the company's perfumers to preserve its mystique. The flacon now used, engraved with stylized flower petals, was designed in 1985 by Alain de Mourgues.

Queen of the Meadows *see* Meadowsweet Oil

Quercus infectoria *see* Gallnut

Quest International The largest fragrance and flavouring manufacturers in the world after IFF (see Perfume Manufacture). Quest was formed in 1986 by an amalgamation of the Dutch company Naarden with a number of other companies and is a subsidiary of Unilever. Quest's headquarters for its fragrance division are at Ashford, in Kent, and it has operational centres in 27 countries in Europe, Asia, Africa and America. The scale of its activities can be measured by the fact that in 1986 it handled 22 000 metric tons of fragrance compounds and ingredients. Its factory at Grasse produces high-quality essential oils, notably rose de mai, jasmine, orris, neroli and orange flower absolute. The company undertakes research and development work in the field of perfumery, including the creation of new fragrant materials ('ethyl safronate' and 'dewberry' being recent successful examples). At its 'fine fragrance centres' at Ashford and Neuilly, in Paris, and also in Brazil, the Netherlands, Japan and the USA, it has teams of creative perfumers to devise and test fragrances, which it then manufactures to the requirements of its customers. These may come not only from perfume firms but also from the much wider general field of companies making household products such as air fresheners, deodorants, fabric conditioners, shampoos and soaps, where the company's main fragrance business lies.

Quince The fruit of the Quince tree (*Cydonia oblonga* = *Pyrus cydonia*), native to Persia and the Caucasus but cultivated widely. Quince was used in perfumes by the ancient Greeks and Romans, the Romans calling the perfume they made from its flowers Melinum. Theophrastus, *c.* 300 BC, referred to the manufacture of 'quince-perfume', in which quince flowers were steeped in oil. It also appears in the recipes of al-Kindi (*c.* 850 AD) as an ingredient used in early Arab perfumes.

Quino-Quino A balsam resembling balsam of Peru and balsam of Tolu which is obtained from a tree *Myroxylon balsamum* var. *punctatum*, growing in Florida, Bolivia and Peru. It is used in incenses.

'Quorum' A men's fragrance created for Puig by Sebastian Gomez and launched in 1982. Top notes, including thyme, artemisia, rosemary, marjoram, bergamot and tangerine, head a spicy–floral heart with geranium, nutmeg, coriander, jasmine and clove among its contents. The base combines leather and tobacco notes with hints of sandalwood and oak moss. The flask was designed by André Ricard.

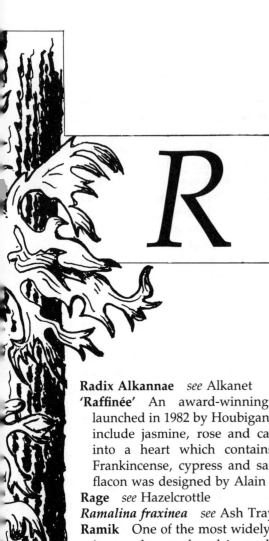

R

Radix Alkannae *see* Alkanet

'Raffinée' An award-winning high-quality floral–oriental perfume launched in 1982 by Houbigant. With over 200 ingredients, its top notes include jasmine, rose and carnation, with a touch of citrus, leading into a heart which contains hyacinth, mimosa, orris and tonka. Frankincense, cypress and sandalwood are included in the base. The flacon was designed by Alain de Mourgues.

Rage *see* Hazelcrottle

Ramalina fraxinea *see* Ash Tray Lichen

Ramik One of the most widely used of early Arab compound perfumes; it was also employed in medical preparations. Prepared on a base of mashed-up green gallnuts, its other ingredients varied – in one recipe recorded by al-Kindi it also contained date syrup and jasmine oil. The preparation was dried into small cakes which were hung up on a string. They appear to have been a form of pomander beads which would give off their aroma when warmed by being handled.

Ramin Oil An oil used in perfumery which is obtained from the wood of the Ramin tree (*Gonystylus bancanus* = *G. miquelianus* = *Aquilaria bancana*) of Malaysia. The wood of this tree is also burned as incense.

Ramy *see* Elemi

Raukawa A New Zealand herb (*Panax edgerleyi* = *Nothopanax edgerleyi*), from the leaves of which the Maoris extract a fragrant oil.

'Red' An innovative, wide-selling perfume launched in 1989 by Giorgio Beverly Hills under its Avon ownership. It is one of the first major perfumes to make use of living flower technology (q.v.) in the manufacture of some of its ingredients. A combination of floral, fruity, oriental and chypre notes, it has been classified as the first of a new perfume family called Fleuriffe Chypre and is claimed to contain a total of 692 ingredients. The top note, formed around osmanthus, includes orange flower, ylang-ylang, bergamot, peach and spicy notes. In the heart jasmine and carnation lead a bouquet which also includes rose and marigold. The base notes are led by amber, tonka, patchouli, sandalwood, musk, oak moss and vetiver.

Red Bee Balm *see* Bergamot

'Red Door' A floral perfume introduced by Elizabeth Arden in 1989. Strong, flowery top notes contain rose and ylang-ylang, and lead to flowery middle notes headed by jasmine, lily of the valley and orchid, with orange flower, lily, freesia and violet. In the woody base vetiver predominates.

Red Fir *see* Douglas Fir

Red Gum Oil *see* Storax

Red Jasmine *see* Frangipani

Red Robin *see* Knot Grass

'Red Rose' One of the best known in the range of floral perfumes brought out by Floris, 'Red Rose' was first marketed in 1868 and has been sold by them ever since. A favourite fragrance of the Grand Duchess Xenia of Russia, it became extremely popular in high society and was much praised by King Edward VII. Clary sage and rosewood in the top notes herald a heart which is predominantly rose, but with a touch of geranium, the whole being underlined by a lower note mostly of musk.

Reseda odorata *see* Mignonette

Reseda Oil *see* Mignonette

Resina Laretae *see* Galbanum

Resina Lentisce *see* Mastic

Resinoid A term used in perfumery to denote a resin which has been washed with benzene or alcohol to remove sticky soluble materials. See Infusion and Tincture.

Reuniol A mixture of geraniol and citronellol which is used as a base in making rose fragrances.

Réunion Island Situated in the Indian Ocean north of Madagascar, the French island of Réunion has been developed as one of the most important areas in the world for growing plants for the perfume industry. In particular, it produces geranium, ylang-ylang and vetivert.

Révillon A company established in 1839 by Louis-Victor Révillon, the son of a Count turned commoner, when he purchased a furrier's shop in Paris, developing it into a high-class business making coats and jackets of fur. In 1937 the company launched its first perfume, the very successful 'Carnet du Bal', following this up with 'Cantilène' (48), 'Detchema' (53), 'Révillon 4' (73) and 'Turbulences' (81), together with three men's fragrances – 'Partner' (60), 'Révillon pour Homme' (77) and 'French Line' (84). See also Caron.

Revlon   Founded in 1932 (to market a nail enamel) by Charles and Joseph Revson and a chemist Charles Lachmann (the L in Revlon), the Revlon Group, based in New York, is now the largest retail cosmetics house in the world. Its associated perfume companies have included Max Factor (sold to Proctor & Gamble in 1991 together with Elena Betrix), Halston, Almay, Boss and Charles of the Ritz. Principal perfumes still marketed under the Revlon label are 'Charlie' (1972), 'Xia-Xiang' (88) and 'Roma' (90). Other Revlon fragrances include 'Intimate' (55), 'That Man' (61), 'Braggi' (66), 'Ultima 2' (67), 'Norell' (69), 'Moon Drops' (70), 'Cerissa' (74), 'Chaz' (75), 'Scoundrel' (80) and 'Norell 2' (80), together with 'Unforgettable', launched in the US in 1990.

Rhinacanthus osmospermus   *see* Voanalakoly

Rhodiola integrifolia   *see* Rose Root

Rhodium Oil   Also called Rosewood Oil and Guadel Oil. An oil distilled from underground parts of the wood of two shrub-like species of *Convolvulus* (*Convolvulus floridus* and *C. scoparius*), known as Rhodium, Rosewood and Aspalathus and native to the Canary Islands. One cwt of wood yields about 3 oz of essential oil. The oil is clear and has a persistent fragrance reminiscent of a blend of rose, cedarwood and sandalwood. It was once much used for scenting soap balls and pomanders, but is not employed much in modern perfumery as it is easily imitated synthetically. The dried wood is still used in sachets and pot pourri. *C. scoparius* is also found in S. America, where the wood is used locally to make scented beads.

Although sometimes called Aspalathus (q.v.), rhodium has no connection with the Aspalathus of ancient times. Some species of the genus *Aspalathus*, which provide a fragrant wood, are sometimes called Rhodium; they are native to S. Africa and are not connected with the Rhodium of perfumery.

Rhododendron ferrugineum   *see* Alpine Rose

Ribes nigrum   *see* Blackcurrant Bud Oil

Ricci   *see* Nina Ricci

'Ricci Club'   A quality woody–citrus fragrance for men's toiletries brought out by Nina Ricci in 1989. Described as a 'sweet and sour' fragrance, it contains around 180 components. Fresh top notes containing citrus fruit oils, mostly grapefruit, together with spicy notes, cover a woody heart of guaiac wood, vetivert, rosewood and sandalwood, with 'sea-chypre' base notes which include oak moss, patchouli, myrrh, tonka and seaweed extracts.

Ricinus communis   *see* Castor Oil

Rigani   *see* Origanum

Rimmel, Eugene   (d. 1887).´A 19th century London perfume maker of French origin whose perfumery, the House of Rimmel, with a factory in Nice, was founded in 1834. In 1865 Rimmel published *The Book of Perfumes*, the foremost popular work on the subject written during that century. His company has now become Rimmel International, owned by Unilever, and mostly produces cosmetics.

'Rive Gauche'   A classic aldehyde perfume launched by Yves St Laurent in 1971. It was created by the perfumers of Roure. An aldehyde accord in the top note introduces a floral heart containing gardenia, honeysuckle, jasmine, ylang-ylang, orris, geranium and magnolia, with woody notes, mainly sandalwood and vetivert, preponderating in the base. The bottle designer was Pierre Dinand.

Robert, Guy   A prominent French perfume creator ('nose') from Grasse, where his family has owned a fragrance firm for over a century. His creations include 'Madame Rochas', 'Calèche', 'Équipage', 'Gucci No. 1', 'Havoc' and 'Amouage'. His uncle Henri Robert created 'Chanel No. 19', and 'Cristalle' and his son Francois Robert created 'Apogée'.

Robert Piguet   A fashion firm formed in Paris in 1928 by Robert Piguet (1901–53), a Swiss-born dress designer. He employed, among others, Dior, de Givenchy and Balmain before they set up their own businesses. Before he closed his House in 1951 he had marketed four successful perfumes: 'Bandit' (1944) (one of the first modern perfumes to use a leathery base note), 'Fracas' (48), 'Visa' (45) and 'Baghari' (50).

Robinia pseudoacacia   *see* False Acacia

Rochas   The Rochas company was formed in Paris in 1925 by the couturier Marcel Rochas (1902–55), who designed clothes and accessories, including costumes for many films. In 1944 his perfume division, Parfums Rochas, launched 'Femme'. Subsequent Rochas fragrances include 'Moustache' (49), 'Madame Rochas' (60) 'Monsieur Rochas' (69) and then, created by the company's chief perfumer, Nicholas Mamounas, 'Mystère' (78), 'Macassar' (80), 'Lumière' (84), 'Byzance' (87) and 'Globe' (90). The company is now owned by the German hair products group Wella.

Rocket (Garden, Dame's, White, Purple)   *see* Honesty Oil

Roger & Gallet   A firm tracing its past back to 1806, when Jean-Marie Farina, a perfumer, set up shop in Paris to market eau de cologne (q.v.). In 1840 he sold his business to Leonce Collas, who transferred it in 1862 to his two cousins Messrs Roger and Gallet. The company is now a very large business specializing in high-class toiletries and soaps, with a factory at Bernay, in Normandy, and forms a part of the Sanofi group. The original 'Jean-Marie Farina' eau de cologne is still sold, and its other fragrances have included 'Shendy' (1970), 'Vetyver' (74) and 'L'Homme', all for men, together with 'Open' (87).

'Roma'   An 'oriental–sweet–fruity' perfume launched by Revlon in 1990 in association with the designer Laura Biagiotti. It was created by perfumers of IFF. Fresh top notes obtained from cassis, bergamot and a touch of mint blend into a floral heart of jasmine, rose, lily of the valley and carnation. The balsamic base notes contain myrrh, ambergris, vanilla, patchouli and oak moss. The flacon was designed by Laura Biagiotti in association with Peter Schmidt.

Roman Coriander   *see* Gith

Roman Fennel   *see* Anise

Roman Perfumes   The earliest use of perfumes in Italy was among the Etruscans (in Tuscany) in the 8th to 3rd centuries BC, who used unguents and perfumes on the body and fashioned elegant incense burners, and among Greeks who settled in S. Italy and Sicily from early in the 1st millennium BC. Among the early Romans there was at first little interest in perfumes; an edict of 188 BC even forbade their sale. But by the 1st century BC Roman men and women were beginning to use perfume materials lavishly. The perfumes of the Greeks, together with the perfumes from Egypt used by the Greeks, were popular, and, as the Empire grew and trade expanded, previously rare or unknown materials began to be imported in quantity. Of local materials, the Romans were particularly fond of the rose (used considerably in the form of fresh rose petals), orris, violet and lily. Balsam of Judaea from Palestine was, as Pliny noted, foremost of all the scents. Saffron, mostly obtained from Asia Minor, was used widely. But it was the oriental perfume materials brought from Arabia and India which were most widely favoured. Pliny, who has provided a detailed account of the trade in aromatics and spices (see, for example, Frankincense), commented on the huge drain on the Empire's financial resources occasioned by it. Most important were frankincense, required for burning in the temples and on public occasions as well as in the home, and myrrh, a key ingredient in many perfume preparations, together with the materials then known as cassia and cinnamon and various other gums from Arabia and India. From Syria came storax and galbanum. Perfume materials brought from India included cardamom, clove, costus, malabathrum and spikenard, together with the flavouring spices such as ginger and, most important of all for use in food preparation, pepper. Many of these materials were sorted and processed in Alexandria, the Empire's industrial capital, before being shipped to Rome.

In addition to incenses, the Roman perfume makers produced three principal types of perfume: solid unguents (*Hedysmata*), usually a single scent based on a fat such as hog's lard; liquid unguents (*Stymmata*), usually a mixture of spices and flowers fixed with a resin, on a base oil such as balanos, sesame or olive, and perhaps with an added colourant such as cinnabar or alkanet; and scented powders (*Diapasmata*), made from dried materials like orris, marjoram, costus storax, labdanum and spikenard, which were used for sprinkling in garments. Scented oils were obtained from several plants in addition to those mentioned above, including calamus, balsam, melilot and narcissus. Pliny noted the ingredients of a number of compound perfumes used by the Romans, including mendesian (imported from Egypt), melinum, susinum and the imposing royal unguent, originally prepared for the kings of Parthia. Other unguents described by Pliny were based on fenugreek, iris, marjoram and cinnamon ('which fetches enormous prices'). Chypre was brought in from Cyprus. The town of Capua, south of Rome and noted for its roses, became the perfume centre of the Romans; here perfume makers (*Unguentarii*) produced floral unguents from several factories, particularly 'oil of roses', which, according to Pliny, was made with rose and crocus flowers, omphacium, cinnabar, calamus, camel grass, honey, salt or alkanet, and wine. Imported aromatics needed by the perfume makers of Capua could be obtained from the huge spice market set up by Vespasian in about 75 AD in Rome, where apothecaries bought many of the same ingredients for their medicines.

In the first two centuries AD the lavish Roman consumption of perfumes reached a peak. The perfume shops of Rome became social meeting places. Perfumes were used not only for the body (where they were even applied by some to the soles of the feet) and for clothing, but also for spraying on the walls and sprinkling on the floors. Horses and dogs were sometimes rubbed with scent. Fountains played perfumed water. At one imperial reception, Nero had the entire surface of a lake in the palace grounds covered with rose petals. At triumphs, the returning armies, bearing perfumed flags and standards, were showered with perfumed materials, while frankincense was burned along the processional route – all very different from earlier days, when Julius Caesar had liked his soldiers to smell of garlic!

The perfume bottles (*Unguentaria*) used by the Romans were made of alabaster, onyx or glass, or, for the cheaper unguents, of clay. The glass bottles were in a wide variety of shapes, many of them identical to the scent bottles of the present day (see Perfume Containers).

Rondeletia   A synthetic perfume made by combining various flower fragrances to represent the fragrance of the flowers of the Rondeletia shrub of Mexico and Cuba.

Ronima Gum   *see* Elemi

Ropion, Dominique   Formerly a leading 'nose' with Roure and now with Florasynth-Lautier. His creations include 'Ysatis', 'Amarige', 'Maxim's de Paris' and 'Safari'.

Roquette   *see* Honesty Oil

Rose Oil   Also called Rosewater, Attar of Roses and Otto of Roses. The rose is perhaps the most important of all the plants used in perfumery and has been so since the dawn of history. Rose oil is mentioned in a number of the medical inscriptions of the ancient Egyptians. Homer referred to the rose in about 600 BC and Theophrastus described how it was cultivated in 300 BC. The Greek poetess Sappho called it 'the Queen of the Flowers'. Both Horace and Pliny gave accounts of its cultivation in Roman times. The rose oil of these early days was probably obtained by a simple form of enfleurage, steeping the petals in another oil (Theophrastus noted that salt was added), but the Romans made lavish use of the fragrance by strewing fresh petals, stuffing cushions with them and wearing rose garlands. The early Arabs used roses in many of their perfumes and, by the 9th century, had discovered how to distil the petals with water to produce rosewater on a commercial scale. Large areas in Iraq, Syria and Iran were then devoted to rose-growing and distilling factories were established. The Caliphs of Baghdad received 30 000 bottles of rosewater as an annual tribute from Persia and Arab rosewater was traded as far as China. The popularity of this scent among the Arabs is demonstrated in the statement of one of the Caliphs: 'I am king of sultans and the rose is king of sweet-scented flowers; each of us is therefore worthy of the other'. (See also Arab Perfumes.)

The essential oil (attar or otto) of roses is obtained by redistilling rosewater. The oil sometimes occurs in the leaves as well as in the flowers. Production of attar of roses was developed on a substantial scale in Persia in the 16th century and introduced from there into Europe by the Turks. About 10 000 lbs of roses are needed to distil 1 lb of oil. The major rose-growing areas are now in Bulgaria (see Kazanluk) and the south of France (see Grasse), with further large-scale production in Turkey, Morocco, Tunis and India.

The species of rose known to the classical world was the red *Rosa gallica* (Turkish Rose), which originated in Iran and was cultivated in Asia Minor, the Balkans and Europe. The Damask Rose, or Rose of Damascus (*R. damascena*) is now the principal species cultivated for rose attar not only in Bulgaria but also in Iran and India. This was the rose most used by the early Arab perfume makers, who introduced it to Europe. In the south of France the principal species cultivated around Grasse was for centuries the Cabbage Rose (*R. centifolia*), also called the Painter's Rose because it features in many works of the Old Masters; this is also cultivated in Turkey and N. Africa. In France it is known as *Rose de Mai*, because it blooms during May. In recent years, however,

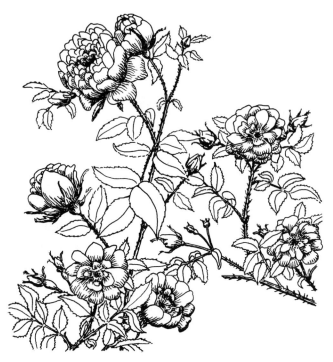

Rose (*Rosa centifolia* (top); *R. damascena* (right); *R. gallica* (bottom)).

a range of related new varieties has been developed at Grasse for the perfume industry. The fragrance of different species and varieties of rose varies; one expert has enumerated 17 different rose scents, some with a similarity to musk, myrrh, violet or clove. Rose oil appears as a main ingredient in 75% of all modern quality perfumes and in some 10% of all men's fragrances.

Dried rose petals continue to be an important ingredient of many sachets and pot pourri.

Rose de Grasse   A name used by perfumers to denote rose absolute and a high-class rose oil collected from rosewater.

Rose de Mai   See Rose Oil. A name used by perfumers in the south of France not only for the Cabbage Rose, which is the rose most cultivated there, but also for rose absolute obtained from this species of rose.

Rose Femelle   *see* Linaloe

Rose Geranium Oil   *see* Geranium

Rose Malloes   *see* Storax

Rosemary   Also called Compass Plant, Compass Weed, Polar Plant and Incensier. An evergreen shrub (*Rosmarinus officinalis*) growing to about 6 feet high, native to southern Europe and Asia Minor, but now found widely. The name signifies Dew of the Sea, because it thrives in the salt spray of Mediterranean coastal areas. It was introduced into Britain by the Romans. Rosemary is now cultivated in France, Spain, Yugoslavia, Tunisia and Britian for its essential oil, distilled from the leaves and flowering tops. Known as Oil of Rosemary, it has a pungently sweet, camphoraceous, lavender-like fragrance and is used in perfumes, colognes and soaps, and also medicinally and in making Vermouth. It appears, for example, in 'Tsar'. The dried leaves are used in sachets and pot pourri.

Rosemary has a considerable history. As it remained fresh and fragrant for longer than any other herb, it became, from ancient times, an emblem of friendship and fidelity and was included in the bride's wreath at weddings. Applied to the outside of the head, it was held to strengthen the memory, and thus became a symbol of remembrance, so that it was placed on corpses. In legend it was supposed to grow only in the garden of the righteous. The ancient Greeks burned rosemary as an incense and it has since been so used in religious ceremonies and exorcisms and as a fumigant. Although not known to the early Arab perfumers, there is record of it as a distilled oil in the 15th century. It was once much used as a hair wash and for scenting washballs. It was a major ingredient in Hungary Water. See also Marsh Rosemary.

Rose Perfume   The ancient Greeks, according to Theophrastus, used a perfume of this name which, in addition to rose petals, contained ginger grass and calamus steeped in sweet wine, with a portion of salt and alkanet added to give it a red colour. Theophrastus observed that it was held to be a cure for ear troubles, was 'good against lassitude', and that, being light, it was best suited to men. A similar 'oil of rose' was made by the Romans.

Rose Root   Also called Snowdon Rose and Priest's Pintle. A small herb (*Sedum roseum* = *Rhodiola integrifolia*) found in Europe and N. America (where the leaves are eaten by Alaskan eskimos). Rose Root was once much cultivated in English cottage gardens for its rose-scented roots, and is occasionally still used for scenting infused oils or broken into small pieces to add to pot pourri.

Rosetto, Giovanni   An Italian, the author of *Secreti Nobilissimi dell'Arte Profumatoria*, published in 1678, one of the first books devoted exclusively to perfumery.

Rosewood Oil   Also known as Brazilian Rosewood Oil and Tulip Wood Oil. An oil used in perfumery which is distilled from the wood of the Brazilian Rosewood tree (also called the Tulip Wood or Maschado tree) (*Physicalymna scaberrimum* = *P. floribundum* = *P. floridum*), found in tropical S. America. Another Rosewood Oil occasionally used in perfumery is extracted from the wood of the Pao Rosa tree (*Aniba terminalis*), native to the lower Amazon area of Brazil. Modern quality perfumes containing Rosewood include 'Jicky', 'Le Dix' and 'Vol de Nuit'. See also Linaloe and Rhodium.

Rosewood   *see* Rhodium/Sandalwood

Rosha Grass   *see* Ginger Grass Oil/Palma Rosa Oil

Rosine   *see* Poiret

Rotreps Oil   *see* Honesty Oil

Roudnitska, Edmond   Born 1905 and now the 'doyen' of French 'noses'. The creator of several of the Dior fragrances, including 'Diorissimo', 'Diorella' and 'Eau Sauvage'. His other creations include 'Eau d'Hermès' for Hermès and 'Femme' for Rochas. He has published a book *Une Vie au Service de Parfum*.

Roure   The oldest of the great fragrance manufacturing companies (see Perfume Manufacture), the firm of Roure was founded in Grasse in 1820 by Claude Roure, whose descendant Jean Amic still runs it as President. It was for long called Roure-Bertrand, after the Bertrand family became part owners through marriage, and in the 1920s became Roure–Bertrand–Dupont after joining up with an aromatic chemist named Dupont. In 1963 it was acquired by Hoffmann-LaRoche (as was Givaudan). Roure headquarters are at Argenteuil, near Paris, in a complex which also includes laboratories and plant for producing synthetic raw materials and compounds. In Grasse it maintains a factory for extracting and distilling natural products, together with a research centre (the hydrocarbon extraction process was a Roure development) and a perfumery school. The company established factories in New Jersey, USA, in 1930 and has since set up affiliates in ten other countries in all parts of the world. Its UK company is based at Harefield, in Middlesex.

Roure, one of the pioneers of modern aromatic chemistry, were the first fragrance producer to offer the couture houses facilities for creating and manufacturing perfumes on their behalf, Schiaparelli being one of their first such clients. While 30% of the company's business now lies in marketing fragrances for toiletries, cosmetics and various household products, its main output is still predominantly in the field of perfumes, of which it is the world's leading producer; one in five of all present-day quality fragrances, including many of the best-known top-selling perfumes, are created by Roure perfumers.

'Royal Copenhagen'   An unusual, trend-setting chypre fragrance produced by Swank in 1970 as an eau de cologne for men. Created by perfumers of IFF, the main ingredients are bergamot and lemon in the top note, rose, jasmine and patchouli in the middle note, and tonka, with other elements including honey, to provide a sweet lower note.

Royal Unguent   A perfume used in Roman times which was devised for the kings of Parthia and was described by Pliny as 'the very climax of luxury'. Pliny noted the contents as: balanos oil, costus, amomum,

Syrian cinnamon, cardamom, spikenard, cat-thyme, myrrh, cassia, storax, labdanum, opobalsamum, Syrian calamus and sweetrush, cinnamon leaf (malobathrum), serichatum, cyprus (see cyprinum), camel's thorn, all-heal, saffron, gladiolus, marjoram, lotus, honey and wine.

Ruchette   *see* Honesty Oil

Rue Oil   An oil distilled from the leaves and young shoots of Common Rue (*Ruta graveolens = R. officinale*), also called Garden Rue, Herby-grass and Herb-of-Grace, a herb growing to about 3 feet high, native to the Mediterranean area but now cultivated widely. Introduced into Britain by the Romans for its medicinal uses, it has for long been used in flavouring as well as in perfumes, having a special value in com-pounds with a sweet-pea fragrance, but is now among those oils syn-thesized or modified for safety reasons (see Perfume Creation). A similar oil, sometimes called Algerian Oil, is also produced from two other species of rue (*R. montana* and *R. bracteosa*) found in Algeria. In the Middle Ages rue was regarded as a powerful defence against witches.

'Rumba'   A wide-selling fruity–floral perfume launched by Balenciaga (following their acquisition by Bogart) in 1988. Fruity top notes come from peach, plum and bergamot, spiced with basil, and the floral heart includes jasmine, rose, carnation, orchid, magnolia and gardenia. The base contains patchouli, labdanum, cypress, oak moss and vanilla. The bottle is modelled after a Roman vase.

Rusa Grass   *see* Palmarosa Oil

Rush   *see* Lemon Grass Oil

Rush Daffodil   *see* Jonquil

Ruta bracteosa   *see* Rue Oil

     graveolens   *see* Rue Oil

     montana   *see* Rue Oil

     officinale   *see* Rue Oil

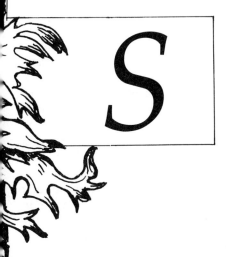

Sabina cacumina   *see* Savin

Sachets   Small bags containing fragrant materials either carried on the person or laid among clothes and linen to perfume them. In ancient times women in the East wore sachets containing powdered perfume materials hung round their necks and concealed under their clothes (see Bible Perfumes). This custom found its way into Europe in the Middle Ages at the same time that sachets began to be used to perfume linen and clothes and drive away moths and other insects. Body sachets of satin or silk filled with powdered orris were very popular early in the 18th century. More generally sachets contained a mixture of dried or powdered herbs, roots or fragrant wood, such as calamus, lavender, marjoram, orris, rose petals and rhodium; sometimes drops of essential oil were added, especially to provide a fixative. Sachets are still made on the same basis, a large variety of dried materials being suitable for them, and, like pot pourri, they can be produced at home. (See Perfume Making at Home and Appendix B, recipes nos 9–13 and 73–74.)

Safflower   Also called Carthamus and Dyer's Saffron. Species of safflower, notably *Carthamus tinctorius* (native to India, Iran and Asia Minor) and *C. lanatus*, or Bastard Saffron (native to Arabia and India) have been cultivated widely, notably in India and China, since ancient times for the yellow or red dye from their flowers and the oil from their seeds (used in cooking). The ancient Egyptians used the oil as a base and colourant for their perfumes (see Balanos). Early Arab perfume makers used it to colour their perfumes and to thicken saffron. See also Macassar Oil.

Safranol   The principal odorous constituent of Saffron; it is now made synthetically, the synthetic version being widely available.

Saffron   One of the most expensive of all perfume materials, and also one of the most ancient, saffron is derived from the dried stigmas and styles tops of the Saffron Crocus (*Crocus sativus* = *C. officinalis*), originating in Asia Minor and the Mediterranean area. The finest saffron now comes from S.E. Spain, and it is also cultivated in Iran and India. It is grown for its use in foodstuffs as much as for perfumery. Some 60 to 70 thousand flowers are required to produce 1 lb of saffron powder. Saffron Oil is obtained by extraction with volatile solvents and is used in minute quantity in perfumes, particularly oriental-type perfumes, providing a very rich, distinctive and slightly earthy note. The main odorous constituent is Safranol.

Saffron was cultivated in Crete in Minoan times and was popular in ancient Egypt, Greece and Rome, appearing as an ingredient in many famous perfumes of the day; the Romans also strewed it over the floors of public places to scent the air on special occasions (see Roman Perfumes). In classical times it was mostly cultivated in Cilicia, in Asia Minor. The Arabs, to whom it was one of the most important of all perfume materials, introduced its cultivation into Europe in the 7th century after the conquest of Spain. By the 16th century English saffron was considered the finest in the world, being grown in large quantity around Saffron Walden.

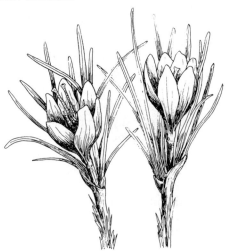

Saffron (*Crocus sativus*).

Safrole A form of Sassafras Oil, also called Brazilian Sassafras Oil, which is distilled from the wood of a tropical tree (*Ocotea sassafras* = *Mespilodaphne sassafras*) found in Brazil. It is used in perfumery, soaps, deodorants and for flavouring. A similar oil comes from two related species of this tree – *Ocotea cymbarum* (= *O. amara*) and *O. caudata*, also found in tropical S. America, the oil from the former also being called Acéite de Sassafras. Safrole also occurs naturally in the oils of sassafras, star anise, nutmeg, ylang-ylang, cinnamon leaf and camphor and is obtained commercially from camphor oil. It is used as a starting point in the synthesis of heliotropin.

Sagapenum An aromatic oil obtained from a gum taken from the stem of a herb, *Ferula persica*, native to Iran and the Caucasus. It was known to the early Arab perfume makers and was used in early medicines. A 16th century German treatise on essential oils listed it as one of the 'precious oils'.

Sage Oil An essential oil steam-distilled from the dried leaves of the Sage plant (*Salvia officinalis*), also called Garden Sage and Common Sage, a shrub growing to about 12 inches high, native to the Mediterranean area and Asia Minor and now cultivated widely. The oil is mainly manufactured in Spain and Yugoslavia. A similar oil, called Spanish Sage Oil, is distilled in Spain from the wild Sage (*S. lavendulaefolia* = *S. triloba*). Sage Oil provides a eucalyptus-like, spicy and herbaceous fragrance for perfumery, the Spanish Sage Oil fragrance being slightly more like that of Spike Lavender. Sage Oil appears in modern quality perfumes (e.g. 'Gem') and is used in soap fragrances. See also Clary Oil.

Saigon Cinnamon tree *see* Nikkel Oil

Sain *see* Ain

Saint Laurent *see* Yves St Laurent

Saj *see* Ain

Sal *see* Chua Oil

Salwa *see* Chua Oil

'Salvador Dali' A 'floriental' perfume, introduced by COFCI of Paris in 1983, comprising jasmine, rose and orange flower in the top notes and cypress and sandalwood in the heart, with a base of frankincense and myrrh. It was launched in a limited edition of large crystal flacons designed by Dali and based on the lips of Aphrodite in a famous Greek statue by Praxitales. The range now includes a men's fragrance 'Dali pour Homme'.

Salvia lavendulaefolia *see* Sage

    officinalis *see* Sage

    sclaria *see* Sage

    triloba *see* Sage

'Samba' A floral–chypre perfume launched by the American perfume company Perfumers Workshop in 1987. Head notes of peach, cassis, tagetes, citrus and galbanum lead to a heart which includes rose, jasmine, hyacinth, magnolia, violet, lily of the valley and clove, on a base of myrrh, oak moss, sandalwood and patchouli, with hints of violet and musk.

Sambucus nigra *see* Elder Flower Oil

Sampsuchinon Also called Sampsuchum. An ancient Egyptian unguent and scented oil mentioned by several classical authors. Recipes were recorded by Dioscorides. Sampsuchum was the Egyptian word for Marjoram. The unguent (sampsuchum) was made of fat mixed with marjoram and was said to be very long-lasting. The scented oil (sampsuchinon) contained marjoram, thyme, southernwood, myrtle leaves and other ingredients, on a base of olive oil.

'Samsara' A high-quality 'amber' perfume created by Jean-Paul Guerlain and brought out by Guerlain in 1989. In 1990 it won an Italian Academy of Perfume award. The name, from Sanskrit, means 'eternal return' and symbolizes serenity. The top notes contain sandalwood and jasmine, leading into a floral heart, mainly rose, narcissus, violet and orris. The base, dominated by amber, also includes vanilla and tonka, sweetened with a touch of ylang-ylang. The flacon is by Robert Granai.

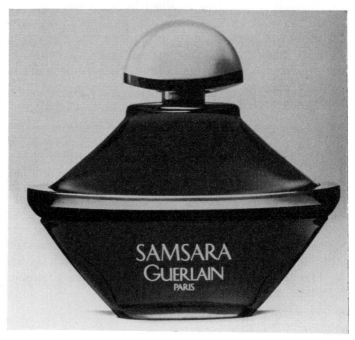

'Samsara'.

Sandal Oil   An aromatic oil used in perfumery which is extracted from the roots of a tree (*Aptandra spruceana*) found in Brazil. This perfume is also known as Castanha de Cotia and Sando de Maranhão Oil.

Another form of Sandal Oil (also called Sandalo Inglez) is extracted from the bark of another Brazilian tree, *Calophyllum brasiliense*.

Sandalo Inglez   *see* Sandal Oil

Sandalwood   The most renowned sandalwood oil, and the sandalwood oil of history, is distilled from the Sandalwood tree of India and Indonesia (*Santalum album* = *Sirium myrtifolium*), the best coming from Mysore. This tree, also called White Sandalwood, is a parasitic plant, attaching suckers to the roots of other trees, and grows up to 30 feet high. The oil is also called Sanders, White Sanders, Yellow Sanders, Citron Sanders and Santal. The oil is contained in the heartwood and is obtained only from very mature trees after they have been felled. The harvesting of sandalwood is now tightly controlled by the Indian Government. White Sandalwood is sometimes confused with Red Sandalwood (*Adenanthera pavonina*), which provides a useful red hardwood but is not aromatic.

Sandalwood oil, which is clear, viscid and strongly aromatic, is steam-distilled from the wood chippings, 1 cwt of wood providing about 30 oz of oil. It is often called Sandal. It retains its odour for a long time and is an excellent fixative. It has for long been one of the principal materials of Indian perfumery, being used both as a fragrance and, when

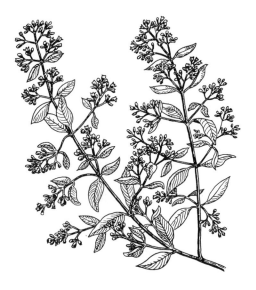

Sandalwood (*Santalum album*).

dissolved in spirit, as a base for other fragrances. It is much used in incenses. As it assimilates very well with rose, it is sometimes used in India mixed with Attar of Roses. In western perfumery it is one of the most valuable (and expensive) of raw materials available, being found in the base notes of many types of perfume and used to give classic notes to chypre, fougere and oriental-type perfumes. It appears as a principal ingredient in over 50% of all women's quality perfumes, and some 30% of men's fragrances.

Although some sandalwood seems to have reached the ancient Egyptians, there is no indication of its use in classical Greece and Rome until about the 2nd century AD. The early Arab perfume makers used sandalwood mainly in pulverized or sawdust form as a base for solid perfumes and incenses.

Other forms of Sandalwood Oil, with a slightly different and usually milder fragrance, are obtained from a number of other Sandalwood trees, including:

1. the Australian Santal tree, also called the Lanceleaf Sandalwood tree (*Santalum lanceolatum* = *S. cygnorum*), which yields Australian Sandalwood Oil;
2. the Quandong, or South Australian Sandalwood tree (*Eucarya acuminata* = *Santalum acuminatum* = *S. preissianum*), from which is obtained South Australian Sandalwood Oil;
3. the West Australian Sandalwood tree (*Eucarya spicata* = *Santalum spicatum* = *Fusanus spicatus*), yielding West Australian Sandalwood Oil;
4. the Fiji Sandalwood tree (*Santalum yasi*) of Fiji, from which Fiji Sandalwood Oil is made (but few of these trees now remain);
5. the East African Sandalwood tree (*Osyris tenuifolia*), which yields East African Sandalwood Oil;
6. the Polynesian Sandalwood tree (*Santalum marchionense*) of Polynesia, yielding Scented Sandalwood Oil, used locally as a body oil and for embalming;
7. the West Indian Sandalwood tree (also called Candlewood and Rosewood) (*Amyris balsamifera*), native to central America and the southern USA, which provides West Indian Sandalwood Oil, also called Cayenne Linaloe Oil (see Linaloe). It has a sweet, cedar-like odour and is used in low-cost perfumes.

'Sandalwood'   The brand name of a trend-setting woody fragrance for men brought out as an eau de cologne by Arden for Men (see Elizabeth Arden) in 1957. Its main ingredients are lavender in the top note, sandalwood and geranium in the middle note and tree moss and amber in the lower note.

Sandarac   Also called Pounce. A resin obtained from the Sandarac tree

(*Tetraclinis articulata* = *Callitris quadrivalvis*), also called the Arar tree, of S. Spain and N. Africa. In these regions it is burnt as an incense, as it formerly was by the Greeks and Romans. The essential oil is used in perfumery as a fixative. The Romans called the wood of this tree Citronwood, because of its lemon scent, and valued it highly for making furniture.

Sanders   *see* Sandalwood

Sando de Maranhão   *see* Sandal Oil

Sanguinary   *see* Milfoil

Sanofi   A French, state-owned group of companies, associated with Elf Aquitaine Oil, which has major interests in the cosmetics, toiletries and fragrance industries. It owns Nina Ricci, Yves Rocher (whose fragrances include 'Diamella', 'Samarcande', 'Trimaran' and 'Vie Privée') and Sanofi Beauté. The latter company comprises Van Cleef & Arpels, Roger & Gallet, Oscar de la Renta, Molyneux, Krizia (fragrances include 'K de Krizia', 'Moods' and 'Krizia Uomo'), Geoffrey Beene ('Grey Flannel' and 'Bowling Green'), Fendi, Perry Ellis, Stendhal and the US company Parfums Stern (acquired from Avon in 1990).

Santal   *see* Sandalwood

Santalol   An alcohol extracted from Sandalwood Oil and used in perfumery

Santalum acuminatum   *see* Sandalwood

album   *see* Sandalwood

cygnorum   *see* Sandalwood

lanceolatum   *see* Sandalwood

marchionense   *see* Sandalwood

preissianum   *see* Sandalwood

spicatum   *see* Sandalwood

yasi   *see* Sandalwood

Santolina chamaecyparissus   *see* Lavender Cotton Oil

Sasooroo   *see* Ambon Sandalwood

Sassafras   Also called Ague tree, Sassafrax, Cinnamon Wood and Panaume. A tall tree (*Sassafras officinale* = *S. alibidinum* = *S. variifolium*) growing up to 40 feet high in N. America from Canada to Florida. A fragrant oil called Sassafras Oil, with a spicy antiseptic odour midway between cinnamon and fennel, is distilled from the rootbark and wood; it is used in mainly lower-grade perfumes and soaps as well as medicinally and in flavourings. The oil contains a high proportion of safrole. Bark chips and powdered bark are used in pomanders, sachets and pot pourri.

A form of Sassafras Oil is also distilled from the bark and leaves of an Australian tree *Doryphora sassafras* and is used in perfumery. An oil called Oil of Sassafras is distilled from the root bark of two species of Swamp Laurel tree (*Magnolia grandiflora* and *M. glauca*) native to southern

USA. An oil called Australian Sassafras Oil is distilled from the bark of the Southern Sassafras tree (*Atherosperma moschatum*) of S. Australia and Tasmania. An oil similar in colour and odour to Sassafras Oil is also obtained from the leaves of a shrub *Amyris punctata*, which grows to about 12 feet tall and is native to the Middle East and N. India. See also Safrole.

Saturega calamintha   *see* Calamint
Satureia hortensis   *see* Savory
          montana   *see* Savory
Saussurea lappa   *see* Costus

Savin   Oil of Savin, used medicinally as well as in perfumery, comes from the twigs of the Savin (also called Savan and Savine) tree (*Juniperus sabina = Sabina cacumina*), a species of Juniper which grows from S. Europe to the Caucasus, in central and N. Asia and in N. America.

Savory Oil   An essential oil which is steam-distilled from the twigs and leaves of Summer Savory (*Satureia hortensis*), an annual herb growing up to 12 inches high, native to the Mediterranean region but now grown widely and cultivated for use in perfumes in France, Yugoslavia and the USA. It imparts a medicinal odour reminiscent of thyme and origanum, and is used extensively in herb-type perfumes. The dried leaves and flowers are used in sachets and pot pourri. A similar oil, valued more in flavouring than in perfumery, is distilled from Winter Savory (*S. montana*), a perennial shrub with sweet-scented flowers native to southern Europe.

Savory has been used in food flavouring since Roman times, and Winter Savory has been grown in Britain since the 16th century. Virgil described both Savorys as among the most fragrant of herbs (noting that on this account they were grown near beehives).

Scabwort   *see* Elecampane
Scarlet Monarda   *see* Bergamot
Scented Gum tree   *see* Eucalyptus
Scented Hairhoof   *see* Woodruff
Scented Maiden Hair   A fern (*Adiantum amabile*) found in Brazil. The young fronds have a scent which is imitated by chemical synthesis in commercial perfumery for Fougere-type perfumes. See also Fern.
Scented Mayweed   *see* Camomile
Scented Poplar   *see* Balm of Gilead
Scented Rush   *see* Lemon Grass Oil
Schiaparelli   A company formed in Paris in the 1920s by Elsa Schiaparelli (1890–1973) to make fashionable knitware, for which purpose she employed, by 1930, a staff of some 2000. With a very avant-garde approach, Schiaparelli, a close friend of Dali, was soon designing a wide range of clothes and accessories. In 1937 she presented her startling 'shocking pink' collection and produced the perfume 'Shocking' to go

with it. After her death the perfume house bearing her name also produced 'Shocking You' (76) and a men's fragrance 'Snuff' (77).

Schleichera trijuga *see* Macassar Oil

Scotch Pine *see* Pine Needle Oil

'Scratch-and-Sniff' *see* Micro-Fragrance

Screw Pine *see* Pandanus

Scrub Myrtle *see* Backhausia

Sea Holly Oil An essential oil distilled from the roots of a species of Erynga (*Eryngium campestre*), also called Sea Hulver and Sea Holme, a thistle-like plant growing up to 12 inches high on the Mediterranean and Atlantic coasts of Europe. It has a musk-like fragrance. In ancient times this plant was credited with many medicinal properties, and Plutarch related that goats became spell-bound when taking it in their mouths.

Sea Holme *see* Sea Holly Oil

Sea Hulver *see* Sea Holly Oil

Sea Parsley *see* Lovage

Sedum roseum *see* Rose Root

See-bright *see* Clary

Sellier, Germaine One of Roure's leading 'noses', whose creations include 'Jolie Madame' and 'Vent Vert' for Balmain and 'Fracas' for Piguet.

Serichatum A perfume material mentioned by Pliny which was grown in Arabia in Roman times and was sometimes used in Roman unguents. It has not been identified botanically.

Seringa *see* Mock Orange Blossom

Serpolet *see* Thyme

Sesame Oil Also called Bene Oil, Teel Oil and Gingle Oil. An oil obtained by expression from the seeds of the Sesame plant (*Sesamum indicum* = *S. orientale*), also called Oriental Sesame, Bene and Simsim. The oil was used in ancient Egypt as a lamp oil and in unguents and foodstuffs and it is still so used there to this day. It was also a base oil for perfumes of the ancient Egyptians (see Balanos and Egyptian Perfumes), the ancient Greeks and the early Arabs (see Arab Perfumes); the latter recognized two sorts of the oil from two different varieties of the plant. Theophrastus observed that sesame oil absorbed the scent of roses better than any other oil.

Seseli carvi *see* Caraway

Setawale *see* Valerian

Setwall *see* Valerian

Seville Orange *see* Bitter Orange Oil

'Shalimar' A famous classic oriental-type perfume created by Jacques Guerlain and brought out by Guerlain in 1925. It is named after the garden of Shalimar (Sanskrit – 'the abode of love') built in Lahore by the emperor Shah Jehan for his favourite wife Mumtaz. The top notes provide a citrus effect from lemon, supported by bergamot, mandarin and rosewood. The heart is floral, with rose, jasmine and orris, but given a woody effect by patchouli and vetiver. The base notes, which include traces of vanilla, benzoin and balsam of Peru, are dominated by opoponax. It is marketed in a flacon designed by Raymond Guerlain and made by Baccarat, and in flacons by Brosse.

'Sheherazade' A quality chypre perfume launched by Desprez in 1983. Named after the famous story teller of the *Arabian Nights Tales*, it was created for Desprez by IFF perfumers. Aldehydic top notes, which include bergamot and rosewood, head middle notes based on rose and carnation, with other constituents which include jasmine, ylang-ylang, orris and cassia. The base, which is sweet, ambery and powdery, includes vanilla, sandalwood, benzoin and opoponax. The perfume is sold in an elegant glass crystal flacon in oriental style designed by Pierre Dinand.

Shikimi *see* Japanese Star Anise

Shiseido A major Japanese cosmetics and perfume firm, founded as a pharmacy in 1872 in Tokyo by Yushin Fukuhara, which has marketed perfume in Japan and the USA since the early 1960s. It now sells 'Tactics' (1979), 'Murasaki' (80) and 'Nombre Noir' (82) in France but has not yet launched its perfumes in Britain. See also Aromachology.

'Shocking' A classic, trend-setting oriental-type perfume introduced in 1937 by Schiaparelli, for whom it was created by Jean Carles. Aldehydes with touches of bergamot and estragon provide the top notes, leading to a honey-like floral bouquet in the heart, and animalic base notes dominated by civet. The flacon, originally made in Czechoslovakia, represents a tailor's dummy and is draped with velvet in the signature 'shocking pink' colour.

Shorea robusta *see* Chua Oil

Shulton A major American toiletries company marketing some wide-selling fragrances for men, which include 'Old Spice', 'Blue Stratos', 'Insignia' and 'Mandate'. In 1990 it was acquired by Proctor & Gamble.

Siberian Pine Oil Also called Oil of Siberian Fir. An oil distilled from the fresh leaves of the Siberian Fir (*Abies siberica* = *A. pichta*) growing in northern USSR and central Asia. It has a typical pine fragrance.

Silphium *see* Asafoetida

Silver Pine Needle Oil Also called Silver Fir Needle Oil. An oil steam-distilled from the leaves of the Silver Fir (also called Silver Spruce and White Spruce) (*Abies pectinata* = *A. alba*), native to Europe and Asia Minor, the tree most popularly used as a Christmas Tree. The oil is used in perfumery and toilet preparations either on its own or blended with other fragrances. *See also* Pine Needle Oil.

Silver Spruce *see* Silver Pine Needle Oil

Silver Wattle Tree   *see* Mimosa

'Silvestre'   A trend-setting eau de cologne in the lavender family of fragrances for men, first issued by Victor in 1946. Its principal constituents are lavender and bergamot in the top note, pine and Douglas fir oil (oregano) in the middle note and cedarwood, vetiver and musk in the base.

Simmondsia californica   *see* Jojoba Oil

Simsim   *see* Sesame Oil

'Sir Irisch Moos'   A chypre-type fragrance for men devised by 4711 Mülhens in 1969. Its main ingredients are bergamot, lemon and galbanum, providing a fresh, green and herbaceous top note, with jasmine, patchouli and vetiver in the middle note and tonka and vanilla in the base.

Sirium myrtifolium   *see* Sandalwood

Skatole   A crystalline substance which is one of the chemical compounds of civet and is occasionally used in diluted form instead of civet as a fixative. It is also contained in some woods and is made synthetically from coal-tar.

Skimmia laurelifolia   *see* Nair Oil

Smallage   *see* Celery Seed Oil

Smelling Strip   *see* Fragrance Blotter

Smoky Note   A term used in perfumery to denote the slight smell of smoke created in a perfume by certain oils such as Birch Tar Oil. It is used in men's fragrances to provide a leathery effect. See Perfume Notes.

Smooth Lawsonia   *see* Cyprinum

Sofia   *see* Ginger Grass Oil

'Soir de Paris'   A fragrance which set a trend in the development of sweet floral perfumes. Created by Ernest Beaux and introduced by Bourjois in 1929, 'Soir de Paris' has a predominantly violet top note, with a heart of tilleul supported by suggestions of clover, lilac, rose, jasmine and other flower fragrances. The base note is chiefly composed of vetiver and styrax. The perfume is contained in a distinctive midnight blue flacon designed by Jean Helleu.

Soldier's Herb   *see* Matico

Soldier's Wound Wort   *see* Milfoil

Solidago odorata   *see* Sweet Golden Rod Oil

Solvents   *see* Volatile Solvents

Sophistication   A term used in perfumery to describe the adulteration of an essential oil by slightly increasing the amount of one of its non-odorous chemical components in order to add to its bulk.

Sorrel tree   *see* Xolisma

Souchet   *see* Cyperus

Sour Orange   *see* Bitter Orange Oil/Neroli

Sour Wood   *see* Xolisma

Southernwood   Also called Old Man and Boy's Love. A small shrub (*Artemisia abrotanum*) growing up to 4 feet high, native to southern Europe. It is closely related to Wormwood. The flowering tops provide an essential oil with a lemon-like fragrance which is occasionally used in perfumery to add subtle tones, but they are more usually dried for use in sachets and pot pourri. The scent is disagreeable to bees and moths, making the dried plants useful for laying in clothes. Dioscorides believed it would drive off snakes. Southernwood was one of the ingredients in a Roman perfume called Melinum (q.v.).

Spartium junceum   *see* Broom

Spearmint   *see* Mint

'Special No. 127'   A fragrance originally created by Floris in 1890 for the personal use of the Russian Grand Duke Orloff, to whom it was supplied in plain, unlabelled bottles, 'No. 127' being the page number in Floris' book for special formulas for individual customers. Subsequently it became a favourite perfume of Eva Peron. It provides fresh notes based on petitgrain, neroli and orange oil in the head, rose and jasmine in the heart, and patchouli in the base.

Sphaeranthus mollis   *see* Ulmaria

Spicewood   Also called Wild Allspice. An oil distilled from the wood of the Spice Bush (*Lindera benzoin* = *Benzoin aestivalis* = *Laurus benzoin*), which is cultivated in the USA. Its leaves are used as a tea substitute and its berries as a substitute for allspice. The oil has a fragrance similar to pimento and is used in bouquets containing lavender where a spicy note is desired.

Spicy Note   A phrase employed in perfumery to describe in general the distinctive fragrance of essential oils which have been obtained from spices. See Perfume Notes.

Spike, Oil of   *see* Lavender

Spikenard   An important perfume material since ancient times, spikenard derives from a perennial herb (*Nardostachys jatamansi*) native to high mountain areas (11 000–17 000 feet) in the Himalayas. It is also called Nard, True Spikenard, Spikenard of the Ancients, Indian Nard, Spike, Indian Spike, Sumbul and Jatamansi (which is its usual name in India). Spikenard Oil is steam-distilled from the roots and has a strong odour reminiscent of patchouli and valerian with a faint background of musk. It is used in modern perfumes, especially in oriental-type ones, and is an excellent fixative, but is becoming increasingly rare and therefore extremely expensive. It is much prized in India as a perfume for the hair.

Nard from India was known to Theophrastus and became an important import from the earliest days of the Roman Empire, when sea trade with India developed. To the Romans it was a highly prized ingredient

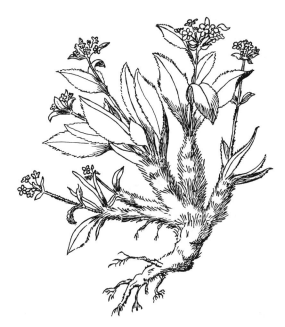

Spikenard (*Nardostachys jatamansi*).

of oils and unguents (see Roman Perfumes). The early Arab perfume makers also made considerable use of it, and its later popularity in Europe is testified by its appearance in an early work on distillation.

A closely related plant called Celtic Spikenard (*Valeriana celtica*), which grows in Alpine regions, has been widely used to provide a substitute for Spikenard. The fragrance of the essential oil, distilled from the roots, resembles camomile and patchouli.

Spiraea filipendula   *see* Dropwort

ulmaria   *see* Meadow-sweet

Splash Cologne   A toilet water containing a bare minimum (1% to 3%) of perfume concentrate. See Eau de Cologne.

Spotted Gum tree   *see* Eucalyptus

Spray   *see* Atomizer

Stacte   The Greek term for Oil of Myrrh, which was an important ingredient in the perfumes of classical times. The word means 'in drops', because, according to Theophrastus, 'it comes in drops slowly' when myrrh is bruised, but he also described another method of manufacture by which stacte was squeezed out of a mucilage made from myrrh and balanos oil dissolved in hot water.

Star Anise   Also called Aniseed Stars, Chinese Anise, Badiane and Damar. An evergreen, magnolia-like tree (*Illicium verum*) growing up to 45 feet high, native to Indonesia, China and Japan and now cultivated widely in China, Vietnam, Jamaica and elsewhere. An essential oil, called Oil of Anise or Star Aniseed Oil (and, in French, *Badiane*) is distilled from the seed capsules and used in perfumes (e.g. 'Brut') and to flavour liqueurs. The dried seeds are also used, but sparingly because of their powerful aroma, in sachets and pot pourri. In Japan the pounded bark is burned as an incense. See also Japanese Star Anise.

Statice caroliniana   *see* Marsh Rosemary

Stearoptene   An odourless, waxy substance (the word derives from the Greek *stear* meaning 'suet') contained in essential oils. In the process of refining the oil by extraction, stearoptene remains in the concrete and is removed to produce the absolute.

Stephanotis   Also called Madagascar Jasmine and Creeping Tuberose. A twining shrub (*Stephanotis floribunda*) growing to about 10 feet high and native to Madagascar. It is cultivated for its highly fragrant flowers. The fragrance is included in some quality perfumes (e.g. 'Nocturnes').

Sterculia tragacantha   *see* Tragacanth
           urens   *see* Karaya Gum

Stichados   *see* Lavender

Stickadove   *see* Lavender

Stinking Gum   *see* Asafoetida

St Johns Wort   Also called Sweet Amber and Common Tutsam. A perennial herb (*Hypericum androsaemum*) which grows wild to about 3 feet high throughout Europe and Asia. The botanical name Hypericum derives from Greek meaning 'over an apparition', from the belief that its aroma drove away ghosts. It has a strong medicinal scent and has had a variety of medicinal uses. An oil with a balsamic, terebinth-like odour is obtained from the seeds and is used occasionally in high-class perfumes (e.g. 'L'Heure Bleue').

St Laurent   *see* Yves St Laurent

St Lucia Wood   *see* Magalep

St Lucie Cherry   *see* Magalep

Stock   A plant with fragrant flowers (*Matthiola incana*) native to S. European coastal regions but now cultivated widely. It is sometimes also called Gilliflower (q.v.). It was probably the flower referred to by Theophrastus (under the name Gilliflower in translated texts) from which one of the main perfumes of the ancient Greeks was made. It also appeared in early Arab perfumes. The flowers are used in pot pourri. See also Night-scented Stock.

Stoechas   *see* Lavender

Storax   Storax, also called Styrax, of modern perfumery is obtained by expression from the inner bark of the Liquidambar tree (*Liquidambar orientalis*), being mostly produced by a crude local process in Turkey. The tree grows up to 40 feet high and is native to S.W. Asia Minor and the island of Rhodes; it first came to the notice of western perfumers in about 1650. Storax is a balsamic oleo-resin, also called Liquid Storax, Levant Storax, Oriental Storax, Flussiger Amber, Rosemalloes and Oriental Sweet Gum; it has a strong cinnamon-like odour and makes an excellent fixative. Most storax is supplied to India and China. It is used in soaps, incenses and several types of perfume, sometimes to complement, or as an alternative to, vanilla, ambergris or benzoin (e.g. 'Soir de Paris'). It is among materials now synthesized for safety or environmental reasons (see Perfume Creation).

A similar product is obtained from the bark of the American Sweet Gum tree (*Liquidambar styraciflua*), also called Red Gum or Bilsted, which is native to the USA and central America; this is known as Oil of Storax, White Peru Balsam and Honduras Balsam, and is used in perfumery, particularly in jasmine compounds, and in soaps; it was at one time exported to Spain from Mexico for this purpose. It is used in some modern quality perfumes (e.g. 'Tweed').

The storax of ancient times was a sweet oleo-resin, also known as Red Storax and Jewish Frankincense, obtained from the bark of a small tree, *Styrax officinalis*, growing up to 15 feet high and native to the eastern Mediterranean region. It is little used at the present time, although it is sometimes employed in incenses. In the Middle Ages it was used in Britain both in incenses and in pomanders. This was the 'sweet storax' of the Bible (see Bible Perfumes) and an ingredient of the royal unguent of Roman times. Herodotus stated that the Arabs burned it so that the smoke would drive away snakes when they were collecting frankincense. Pliny noted that the Arabs fumigated their houses with it. Both types of the gum were used by the early Arab perfume makers.

Strewing Herb   In ancient and medieval times fragrant plants were strewn over the floors of rooms so that, when trodden on, they would perfume the air. Sometimes herbs thought to have disinfectant properties were used in this way as a protection against disease. Rosemary, rue, tansy and lavender were among plants so used from medieval times. The custom persisted until the 18th century.

Strombus lentiginosus   *see* Sweet Hoof

Styrax   *see* Storax

Styrax benzoin   *see* Benzoin

      macrothyrsus   *see* Benzoin

      officinalis   *see* Storax

      tonkinense   *see* Benzoin

Styrene   A fragrant liquid used as a fixative in floral perfumes. It is a chemical constituent of several natural balsams, notably storax, and is prepared synthetically.

Sugandh Kokila   A fragrant oil obtained from the scented wood of a species of Cinnamon tree (*Cinnamomum cecicodaphne*), also locally called Gonari, Malagiri and Rehu, which grows in N. India and the Himalayas. It is used in Indian perfumery.

Sukk   A widely used perfume of the early Arabs which was based on pounded gallnuts, raisins and pomegranate seeds, with various fragrant materials added. Sometimes it was mixed with ramik. Sukk appears in nearly one fifth of all al-Kindi's perfume recipes and was also used in Arab medical prescriptions. (See Arab Perfumes.)

Sulphur Root   *see* Peucedan Gum

Sulphur Wort   *see* Peucedan Gum

Sumbul Root   Also called Musk Root, Violet Root, Musk and Eurangium. A root with the odour of musk obtained from a species of Ferula (*Ferula sumbul*), a plant growing up to 8 feet high in mountainous areas of Turkestan, Afghanistan and Pakistan. Although not known to European botanists until 1869, it has been used in Iran and India as a perfume and incense since ancient times. An essential oil called Sumbul Oil is distilled from it. In India the name Sumbul is, however, also applied to some other aromatic roots, including Spikenard; consequently some of the material called Sumbul Root which is used in perfumery today, and which has an odour more reminiscent of angelica, may in fact derive from another species of *Ferula*, possibly *F. suaveolens*.

Surgi   *see* Nag Kesar

Surungi   *see* Nag Kesar

Susinon (Susinum) Perfume   A perfume used by the ancient Greeks and Romans. It was derived from the flowers of the lily and is mentioned (by Theophrastus) from about 300 BC. The word derives from the ancient Egyptian word for a water lily (in modern Arabic the word susān covers all types of lilies). Pliny described a perfume of this name used in Rome in his day which was based on balanos oil and also contained calamus, honey, cinnamon, saffron and myrrh.

Swamp Cedar   *see* Arbor Vitae Oil

Swamp Laurel tree   *see* Sassafras

Swamp Tea tree   *see* Cajuput

Sweet Acacia   *see* Cassie

Sweet Assa   *see* Mastic

Sweet Bark   *see* Cascarilla

Sweet Basil   *see* Basil

Sweet Bdellium   *see* Opoponax

Sweet Birch Oil   An oil distilled from the bark of the Sweet Birch tree (*Betula lenta*) found in N. America. The oil is almost identical with Gaultheria Oil and is often sold as such . It is used by perfumers in preparing Cassie Oil and perfumes with a new-mown hay fragrance.

Sweet Cane   *see* Calamus

Sweet Chervil   *see* Sweet Cicely

Sweet Cicely   Also called Garden Myrrh, British Myrrh, Sweet-scented Myrrh and Sweet Chervil. A herb *Myrrhis odorata*, growing up to 3 feet high and native to Europe and the Caucasus. The seeds have a myrrh-like scent and are used in pot pourri.

Sweet Clover   *see* Melilot

Sweet Fern Oil   An essential oil with a cinnamon-like fragrance obtained from the Sweet Fern (*Comptonia asplenifolia*) of N. America. It is occasionally used in perfumery. See also Fern.

Sweet Flag   *see* Calamus

Sweet Gale   *see* Bog Myrtle

Sweet Golden Rod Oil   An essential oil with an anise-like scent obtained from the leaves of the Sweet Golden Rod (*Solidago odorata*), also called Fragrant-leaved Golden Rod, a plant found in eastern parts of N. America. It has medicinal uses and is occasionally used in perfumery.

Sweet Grass   A grass found in Europe, Asia and N. America (*Hierochloe odorata* = *Holcus odoratus* = *Teresia odorata*). It is used in Mexico to perfume clothes and to burn as an incense. See also Woodruff.

Sweet Gum tree   *see* Storax

Sweet Hoof   A fragrant material which comes from the operculum, or plate, over the entrance to the shell of certain marine snails (*Strombus lentiginosus, Ungues odorati* and others) found on sea coasts from India to the Red Sea. It was mentioned by Dioscorides as a medicinal drug. Early Arab perfume makers used it in the preparation of incenses. It is sometimes called Onycha (q.v.); in the Old Testament onycha was an ingredient in the holy perfume (incense) of the Jews.

Sweet Lucerne   *see* Melilot

Sweet Milfoil   *see* Maudlin

Sweet Myrrh   *see* Opoponax

Sweet Nancy   *see* Maudlin

Sweet Note   A phrase used in perfumery to describe a sweet and rather sugar-like fragrance such as vanilla. See Perfume Notes.

Sweet Orange   An essential oil, also called Oil of Portugal, with a sweet and flowery perfume, extracted from the peel of the fruit of the Sweet Orange tree (*Citrus sinensis*), which probably originated in S.E. Asia but was being widely cultivated in Italy and the eastern Mediterranean by the beginning of the 1st millennium. It is used both as a flavouring and in perfumes and appears in modern quality perfumes (e.g. 'White Satin').

The flowers of this tree are also distilled, principally in Portugal, Spain and the south of France, to produce a less fragrant form of neroli oil, found in commerce under the name 'Neroli petolae', which is sometimes used to adulterate true Neroli.

The dried peel of the fruits of Sweet Orange are used in sachets and pot pourri.

Sweet Pea Oil   An essential oil extracted by enfleurage from the flowers of the Sweet Pea (*Lathyrus odoratus*), possibly native to southern Europe and now cultivated widely with many varieties. The plant was not known in early times. Its odour suggests orange blossom and hyacinth with a hint of rose, but, despite the popularity of the plant for its fragrant flowers, there has never been a great demand for this fragrance in a perfume. As the fragrance is more easily and cheaply reproduced by synthetic means, the essential oil is therefore little used in perfumery.

Sweet Reed   *see* Calamus

Sweet Root   *see* Calamus

Sweet Rush   *see* Calamus

Sweet-scented Shrub   *see* Calycanthus

Sweet Sedge   *see* Calamus

Sweet William   A garden plant (*Dianthus barbatus*) growing up to 2 feet high and related to the clove-pink (carnation). It is native to eastern Europe but is now grown widely. The clove-scented flowers are dried for use in pot pourri.

Sweetwood Bark Tree   *see* Cascarilla

Sweet Yarrow   *see* Maudlin

'Sybaris'   A men's fragrance launched by Puig in 1988. Created by Sebastian Gomez, it features herbal top notes, with bergamot, citrus leaf, tangerine, myrtle and thyme, on a spicy, floral, fruity heart containing coriander, nutmeg, and cinnamon, with patchouli, sandalwood and musk in the base notes.

Synthetic Fragrances   Synthetic fragrances are laboratory-made imitations of natural perfumes, or fragrances devised in a laboratory which do not exist in nature. They began to be manufactured for commercial perfumery (starting with mirbane essence) from the middle of the 19th century, when the popular demand for perfumes necessitated production in bulk quantity with materials which were not limited in supply, or subject to wide variations of quality and price, or prohibitively costly. Chemists, notably among them Tiemann and Baur, isolated the significant chemical elements of essential oils which provided their odour and then reproduced them. Sometimes the odoriferous elements in an oil which was expensive to produce could be found in much greater abundance and more easily available in the essential oil of other plants; hence gerianol, which provides the nucleus of the basic fragrance (the 'odorous principal') in a rose, can be more cheaply and abundantly obtained from, for example, geranium and palma rosa and is taken from these plants for use, after chemical treatment, in making synthetic rose perfumes. Among many other substances used as synthetics in perfumery are: aldehydes, citronellol, coumarin, eugenol, farnesol, heliotropin, indole, ionene, linalöol, methyl salicylate, musk ambrette, musk ketone, nerol, pinene, skatole, styrene, terpineol and vanillin. The role of all of these will be found under their respective headings. But the total range of synthetic fragrances is vast, many being made from minerals such as coal tar (e.g. benzene and methyl salycilate) and petroleum. There are very many invented fragrances in addition to the imitations of natural scents, so that perfume makers now have some four thousand different fragrant materials to choose from when selecting the ingredients for their new compositions. Most perfumes made nowadays contain a high proportion of synthetic materials.

See also Perfume Creation.

Syringa   *see* Mock Orange Blossom/Lilac
Syringa vulgaris   *see* Lilac
Syzygium aromaticum   *see* Clove

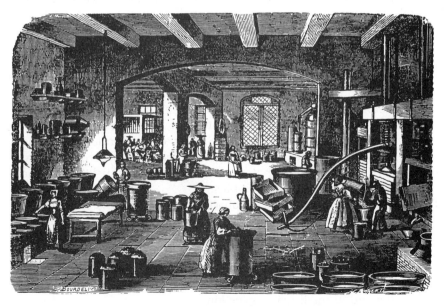

A 19th century perfume factory in Nice (*Source* Rimmel, *Book of Perfumes*, 1895).

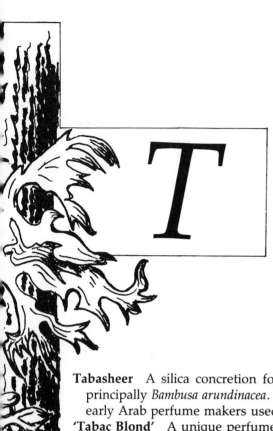

Tabasheer A silica concretion found in the hollow stems of bamboos, principally *Bambusa arundinacea*. It has for long had medicinal uses. The early Arab perfume makers used it in their recipes.

'Tabac Blond' A unique perfume produced by Caron in 1919, being the only feminine fragrance with a tobacco-scented background. The top note, principally orange blossom, and the middle note, a classic floral bouquet centred on jasmine, were unconventional, but the tobacco fragrance dominated the lower notes, with traces of cedarwood, amber, civet, benzoin, leather and moss providing an added powdery effect.

'Tabac Original' A dry, floral fragrance for men issued by Mäurer & Wirtz as an eau de cologne in 1938. Created by Firmenich, it has a fresh, citrusy top note, chiefly bergamot, lemon and neroli, with rose and orris in the middle notes and with amber, musk and tobacco fragrance included in the base notes.

Tacamahac Also called Tacka Mohacca and Elqueme. A fragrant resin principally obtained from the bark of a small tree (*Bursera gummifera* = *Elaphrium simaruba*) found in central America and the W. Indies. In the W. Indies the gum is known as West Indian Elemi. It was used by the Mayas of Mexico as an incense and was brought to Europe from the 16th century for use in incenses and sachets. Nowadays its main use is as a glue and in medicinal concoctions.

An aromatic resin called Tacamahac is also obtained from the leaf buds of the N. American Balsam Poplar (*Populus balsamifera*), a large tree introduced from S. America in the 17th century and sometimes called the Balsam of Tacamahac tree. The resin is sometimes imported into Britain under the name 'Balm of Gilead Buds' (see Balm of Gilead).

Tacka Mohacca *see* Tacamahac

Tailed Pepper *see* Cubeb

Taget Oil *see* Marigold

Tagetes minuta *see* Marigold

     patula *see* Marigold

Tagette Oil *see* Marigold

Tanacetum balsamita *see* Costmary

     vulgare *see* Tansy

Tangerine Oil Also called Mandarin Oil. An oil expressed from the fruit peel of the Tangerine Orange tree (*Citrus reticulata* var. *deliciosa*) which is cultivated widely. It provides a sharp orange fragrance used in colognes and some perfumes (e.g. 'Charles of the Ritz', 'Lace' and 'Sybaris').

Tangloo Oil An oil used in perfumery which is distilled from the flowers of the Ooka-ooka tree (*Aglaja odoratissima*), also called the Pantjal-kidang and Tangloo tree, native to Java.

Tansy A herb (*Tanacetum vulgare*), also known as Buttons, growing up to 3 feet high and common both in Europe and the USA. It has a bitter odour reminiscent of camphor. In early times it was used as a strewing herb, having the property of keeping flies away, and also as a flavouring and in medicine. The dried leaves are used in sachets and pot pourri.

Tarragon Also called Estragon, Mugwort and Little Dragon. A herb (*Artemisia dracunculus*) growing to about 2 feet high, native to the Himalayas but now cultivated widely, mainly for the leaves, which are used in cooking. The essential oil, called Tarragon Oil or Estragon Oil, which is obtained by steam-distillation of the whole plant, has a spicy, anise-like fragrance and is used not only medicinally and in flavourings but also in perfumes and colognes, particularly those of a chypre, fern or new-mown hay type. Examples of quality perfumes in which it is found are 'L'Heure Bleue' and 'Cabochard'. The dried leaves are used in sachets and pot pourri. See also Artemisia Oil.

Tea Absolute An absolute, obtained by extraction with volatile solvents and then by distillation, from the leaves of the Chinese Tea tree (*Camellia sinensis* = *Thea sinensis*). It has a warm, amber-like odour reminiscent of tobacco, and is used in leather, chypre, fougere and new-mown hay-type perfumes.

Tea Berry *see* Gaultheria

Tea tree *see* Ti-tree/Cajuput

Teisseire, Paul (1922–1986) A prominent French scientist responsible for many technical developments used in modern perfumery. He was

Director of the Roure Research Centre in Grasse from 1968 to 1982.

Terebinth Oil An essential oil, sometimes called Turpentine, obtained from the resin of the shrub-like Terebinth tree (*Pistacea terebinthus*), also called the Turpentine tree, native to the Mediterranean region but chiefly cultivated in Cyprus and Chios. Theophrastus noted that terebinth gum was one of the best resins for use in perfumery, because it set firmly and was very fragrant. In medieval times it was often an ingredient in pomanders. Oil of Terebinth is listed in Braunschweig's treatise on distillation published in 1500 AD. The plant was an important source of turpentine known as Chian Turpentine, but this should not be confused with the turpentine in general usage, which is obtained from pine trees.

Teresia odorata *see* Sweet Grass

Terpeneless Oils Essential oils separated by water or steam-distillation from which certain remaining non-odoriferous materials, chiefly resinous substances and hydrocarbon compounds called Terpenes, have been removed by a further process. The resultant oils contain only the odoriferous ingredients and are therefore much purer products and consequently highly valued by perfumers. Terpeneless oils have more 'body' than ordinary essential oils, do not decompose with age so readily, and are much more soluble in dilute alcohol.

Terpineol An alcohol with a sweet floral odour reminiscent of lilac which occurs naturally in bergamot, neroli, lime and petitgrain oils. It can also be distilled from pine oil or made chemically for use in perfumery. Discovered in 1885, it is mostly used in creating synthetic fragrances of lilac, lavender, jasmine and eucalyptus, but is also valued in making many other synthetic fragrances.

Tetraclinis articulata *see* Sandarac

Tetranthera polyantha *see* May-chang

Thanh-that tree *see* Mattipaul

Thatch Screw Pine *see* Pandanus

Thea sinensis *see* Tea Absolute

'That Man' A trend-setting chypre-type fragrance brought out by Revlon in 1961 for use in men's toiletries. The main ingredients are bergamot, petitgrain and lemon in the top note, geranium, clove-pink and cedarwood in the middle note, and moss, tonka and musk in the base.

Theophrastus An early Greek philosopher and botanist (372–287 BC). He wrote a major botanical work *An Enquiry into Plants*, produced about 295 BC, and also the first known work devoted to perfumery, a short treatise called *Concerning Odours*. These works are our most important sources on the perfumes of the ancient Greeks. See Greek Perfumes.

Thuja *see* Cedar

Thuja Leaf Oil *see* Arbor Vitae

Thuja occidentalis   *see* Cedar
Thumiaterion   *see* Turibulum
Thyme   Several species of Thyme, a plant native to the Mediterranean region and Asia Minor, are used in perfumery. Foremost is Garden Thyme (*Thymus vulgaris*), from which French perfumers manufacture most of their Oil of Thyme. The flowering tops of this are steam-distilled, 100 lb producing about $\frac{1}{2}$ to 1 lb of essential oil. In its most refined form it is called White Oil of Thyme, to distinguish it from the cruder distillate, called Red Oil of Thyme, which is sometimes sold as Oil of Origanum. White Oil of Thyme is an important component of many colognes, soaps and herb-type fragrances. Examples of modern quality fragrances which contain thyme are 'Quorum' and 'Panache'. A somewhat similar oil is also produced in Spain from *Thymus capitatus* (see Origanum Oil) and *T. zygis* var. *gracilis*. The dried leaves are used in sachets and pot pourri.

  The plant called Lemon Thyme (*T. citriodorus*) provides an essential oil which has a lemon-like fragrance and which is mostly used in soaps.

  Wild Thyme (*T. serpillum* = *T. serphyllum*), also called Creeping Thyme and Serpolet, provides an essential oil which is occasionally used in perfumery.

  A species of Thyme native to and cultivated in China (*T. quinquecostatus*) provides an oil called Thyme Linaloe Oil, which has a fragrance resembling a spicy form of rosewood; it is occasionally used in citrus-type perfumes.

  Monarda Oil, the essential oil of Bergamot, is also sometimes called Oil of Thyme.

  The name Thyme is believed to derive from a Greek word meaning 'to fumigate', as the Greeks used it as an incense in their temples. Pliny claimed that when burned it would put all venomous creatures to flight. The Greeks used a perfume based on 'tufted thyme'; this was probably Wild Thyme, which the Arabs also used in their perfume recipes.
Thymus capitatus   *see* Origanum Oil/Thyme
       mastichiana   *see* Marjoram
Ti-tree   *see* Tea tree
Tiemann, Ferdinand   A German professor of chemistry prominent in the development of synthetic perfume materials in the late 19th century. He discovered vanillin and ionone (see Synthetic Fragrances).
Tilleul   The Linden tree, or Lime tree (*Tilia europaea*), found wild in southern Europe and northern Asia, which has highly fragrant flowers. The name Tilleul is used for the tree, for an infusion made from the flowers, and in perfumery for the fragrance of the flowers, which is usually imitated synthetically in modern perfumes. Modern quality perfumes containing it include, for example, 'Soir de Paris'.

Tincture   A term applied in perfumery to the product obtained by purifying a fragrant gum or resin or other dry plant material or animal material by extraction with alcohol or some other unheated solvent. Such purification may be necessary in order to separate foreign matter, such as grit and pieces of bark, which has become embedded in the gum during the process of exudation and harvesting. After the solvent has then been removed, the resultant very pure perfume substance is known as 'clair', or 'resinodor' or 'gumodor'.

Ti-Tree Oil   Also called Melaleuca Oil. A light, nutmeg-like essential oil steam-distilled from the leaves of the Ti-(or Tea) tree (*Melaleuca alternifolia*) and Black Tea tree (*M. bracteata*) of Australia. It is closely related to Cajuput. Having good germicidal value, it is much used as a fragrance in soaps, deodorants and disinfectants.

An oil called Lemon-scented Tea Tree Oil is distilled from the leaves and twigs of *Laptospermum citratum*, found in eastern Australia, and is used similarly. It has a strong lemon-like odour.

Tobacco Notes   A phrase used in perfumery to describe fragrances resembling cured tobaccos, which are particularly popular in masculine toiletries. See Perfume Notes.

Tobacco Plant   *see* Nicotiana

Toilet Water   Also called eau de toilette. A spirit obtained by distilling fragrant materials in alcohol. Hungary Water was an early example. Toilet waters became very popular during the 19th century, in particular those known as eau de cologne, eau de portugal, florida water, honey water and lavender water. In modern perfumery, the term 'eau de toilette' signifies a preparation containing 4–8% perfume in an alcohol. See also Perfume.

Tomar Seed Oil   An oil used in Indian perfumery which is extracted from the seeds of the Wingleaf Prickly Ash tree (*Zanthoxylum alatum* = *Z. planispinum*) of N. India and China.

Tonka Bean   Also called Tonquin Bean. A bean produced by two species of a tall tree belonging to the Laburnum family:

1. the Dutch Tonka tree (*Dipteryx odorata* = *Coumarouna odorata* = *Baryosma tongo*), also called English Tonka tree, native to Brazil and Guyana and cultivated widely, especially in Brazil, Venezuela, Guyana and Martinique;
2. a closely related tree (*Dipteryx oppositifolia*) found in Brazil.

The beans of the former are also called 'Angostura Beans', and of the latter 'Para Beans'. Angostura Beans are larger and more highly valued. The beans consist of an egg-sized fruit containing seeds which are dried and then cured in rum, when they become covered with small crystals of coumarin. This is used both for flavouring and in perfumes, sometimes as a vanilla substitute. The 'new-mown hay' fragrance strengthens with age. About 10% of all modern quality perfumes contain tonka, examples being 'Je Reviens', 'Raffinée' and 'Red'. and it appears among the main ingredients of some 13% of quality fragrances for men. The dried seeds can be added to sachets and pot pourri and were once much used for laying in clothes and linen and also for scenting snuff.

Tonquin Beans *see* Tonka Beans

Tonquinol *see* Musk Baur

Top Note *see* Perfume Notes

Tragacanth Also called Gum Tragacanth, Gum Dragant, Gum Dragon, Dagaganthum and Quincy Dragagenty. A gum obtained from various species of Astragalus shrub, principally the Syrian Tragacanth (*Astragalus gummifera*) found in Asia Minor, Iran and Kurdistan. The gum, which exudes from the stem of the shrub, appears in commerce in tears, or flattened into thin, ribbon-like flakes, and is odourless. It is used as an emulsion stabilizer and for binding aromatic powders into pastes for pomander beads and incenses. See Perfume Making at Home (under Pomanders), also Appendix B recipes nos 23 and 30.

A similar gum sometimes substituted for true tragacanth is obtained from various species of Sterculia tree found in the tropics, especially the African Tragacanth tree (*Sterculia tragacantha*).

Some authorities believe that the material in the Old Testament sometimes translated from the Hebrew as 'Spices' may in fact have been tragacanth.

Treacle of Gilead *see* Balsam of Makkah

Tree Lupin A shrub (*Lupinus arboreus*) which grows up to 4 feet high, native to America but now grown widely. The flowers have a strong honey-like scent and are dried for use in pot pourri.

Tree Moss Also called Oak Moss. Two species of lichen (*Evernia furfuracea = Parmelia furfuracea* and *Usnea barbata = U. dasypoga*) are used in European perfumery under the name Tree Moss (French: *Mousse d'Arbre*) to distinguish them from Oak Moss, although in the USA the term Oak Moss covers Tree Moss as well. The Tree Moss species grow on the bark of spruce and fir trees in humid parts of central and southern Europe and N. Africa; France, Morocco and Yugoslavia are the main producers for the perfume industry. A resinoid is extracted from the lichen, and this is then further extracted to yield an absolute. The odour is powerfully tar-like. The product is used as a fixative and in many perfumes, especially of fougere and chypre type. Examples of modern quality fragrances which contain it are 'Paco Rabanne pour Homme' and 'Estée Super'. *Usnea barbarata* is also known as Bearded Usnea or Old Man's Beard; in the 16th century it was sometimes used in a toilet powder called Cyprus Powder. See also Fragrant Moss.

Trefle *see* Clover

'Trésor' A floral, semi-oriental perfume created by Sophia Grojsman of IFF for Lancôme, who launched it in 1990 (UK 1991). The same name had been used for an earlier (1952) Lancôme perfume. The top notes are principally rose, lilac and lily of the valley, introducing a heart which contains iris and heliotrope, with sandalwood, musk and amber, modified with peach and apricot, in the base. The flacon, in the form of an inverted crystal pyramid, was designed by Style Marque.

'Tsar' A spicy chypre fragrance for men introduced by Van Cleef & Arpels in 1989. Spicy top notes which include rosemary, thyme, lavender, caraway, cinnamon and juniper give way to a floral middle note of geranium, lily of the valley and jasmine, on a base containing vetivert, oak moss, patchouli and sandalwood.

Tuberose Flower Oil An essential oil, usually referred to simply as Tuberose, obtained by extraction from the flowers of the Tuberose plant (*Polianthes tuberosa* = *Hyacinthus tuberosus*), also called Night Hyacinth, native to either Indonesia or Mexico and central America, but now grown commercially for the perfume in France, Italy, Morocco, Egypt, China, Malaysia, Indonesia, India and the Comoro Islands. The flower grows from a bulb; in France a single-flower variety is cultivated for the perfume, a double-flowered one for cut flowers. The fragrance is heavy and honey-like, and has been described as like that of a well-stocked

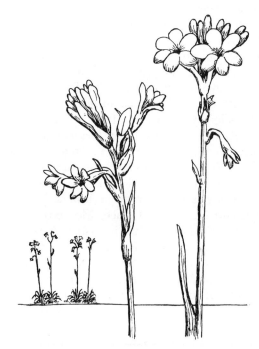

Tuberose (*Polianthes tuberosa*).

flower garden at eventide. The fragrance of the growing flowers increases after nightfall; hence in Malaysia the plant is called Mistress of the Night. Like jasmine, the flowers of tuberose are extracted by enfleurage, because they continue to produce essential oil for some 48 hours after cutting. Some 150 kilos of flowers will provide about 1 kilo of pomade, but from this the yield of absolute, extracted by volatile solvents, is so minute (about 200 g for every 1200 kilos of flowers) that it is one of the most expensive of all perfume materials, costing more than its weight in gold. Tuberose absolute is consequently now used only in very high-quality perfumes (e.g. 'Amouage' and 'Jardins de Bagatelle') where floral notes are required. But the essential oil is found as a main ingredient in some 20% of all modern quality perfumes.

Tuberose has for long been regarded as a symbol of voluptuousness and reputed to have aphrodisiac properties. It was first brought into Europe at the end of the 16th century, but for a long time was a monopoly of the Dutch, who cultivated it in hot-houses.

For Creeping Tuberose see Stephanotis.

Tulip Bottle   Also called Candlestick Bottle. A style of bottle made for eau de cologne in the late 19th century. The stopper was made like a candlestick, having a hollow on top, usually tulip or flower-shaped, into which some of the contents could be poured to give a room fragrance.

Tulip Wood Oil   *see* Rosewood Oil

'Turbulences'   A fruity–fresh floral perfume introduced by Révillon in 1981. It was created by the perfumers of Dragoco. The green, fruity accord in the top note contains touches of spearmint, cumin and bergamot, heralding a middle note dominated by rose, with woody lower notes, principally cedar and amber. The spherical glass bottle with a grey stopper is sculpted to suggest the movement of waves and was designed by Warner Schurf.

Turibulum   A portable censer of varying shape and design on which the Romans burned incense. In ancient Greece it was called a *thumiaterion* (see Perfume Containers).

Turkish Geranium Oil   *see* Ginger Grass/Palma Rose Oil

Turmeric   *see* Curcuma Oil

Tussie-Mussie   A nosegay, first popular in Elizabethan times, containing a variety of fragrant flowers or herbs selected to convey a sentiment or message through their symbolic meanings (e.g. rose for love, marjoram for happiness, daisy for faithlessness, rosemary for remembrance, rue for sorrow, etc.). Ophelia's bouquet in *Hamlet* provides a good Elizabethan example. By Victorian times almost every known plant had some such meaning. The name is also sometimes used, especially in the USA, for the miniature posy holder, usually made of silver, in which a nosegay was placed; they were designed to keep the plant stems moist. The word probably derives from Tussie, an old word for a nosegay, and Mussie, a nonce word meaning 'moss' (used for retaining moisture).

Tutsan, Common   *see* St John's Wort

'Tweed'   A classic floral aldehyde perfume first brought out by Lenthéric in 1933. Flowery and fruity top notes of bergamot, neroli, orange and violet give way to a classic floral heart which includes rose, jasmine, carnation, orris, lilac and magnolia. The base note, which is powdery, is principally musk, with nuances of vetivert, cinnamon, styrax, sandalwood, leather and civet.

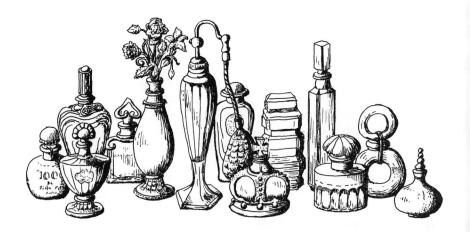

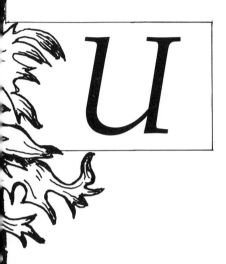

Ulmaria   *see* Meadowsweet Oil
Ulmaria filipendula   *see* Dropwort
Umari   *see* Houmiri
Ungaro, Emmanuel   *see* 'Diva'
Unguent   A semi-solid perfumed ointment or grease, often made by steeping fragrant plants or plant parts into animal fat. It contrasts with perfumed oil or water, which was more liquid. It was used in the earliest days of perfumery, when a popular way of applying perfume was to rub an unguent into the body, especially after a bath. Unguents were kept in unguent boxes made of a stone such as marble or alabaster to keep them cool, this also helping them to last. But the word unguent was also used in classical times to cover liquid perfumes (kept in a bottle) as well. See Egyptian Perfumes.
Unguent Cone   An ancient Egyptian form of pomade used by women. Perfume ingredients such as marjoram, sweet flag and myrrh were soaked in fat (see enfleurage), sometimes treated with wine, until the fat had absorbed their fragrance. The fat (probably ox tallow) was then shaped into cones. A cone would be placed on the head so that, as the heat of day melted the fat, it would trickle down over the head and body, enveloping the wearer with fragrance. See Egyptian Perfumes.
Ungues odorati   *see* Sweet Hoof
Unilever   An international conglomerate based in London which is a

major producer of detergents, household goods and toiletries and is increasing its stake in the fragrance business. Among its subsidiaries are Elizabeth Arden, Calvin Klein, Lagerfeld, Fabergé, Rimmel International, Elida Gibbs and Atkinsons.

Unona latifolia　*see* Ylang-ylang
　　　 odorata　*see* Ylang-ylang
Usnea barbata　*see* Tree Moss
　　 charypoga　*see* Tree Moss

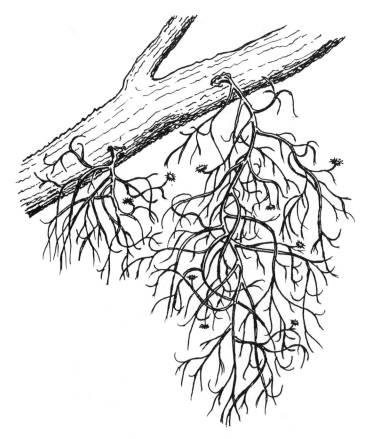

Tree Moss (*Usnea barbata*).

Uvaria odorata　*see* Ylang-ylang

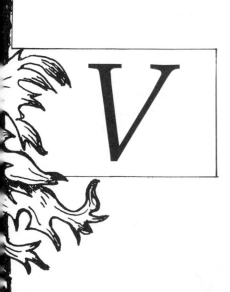

Valerian Also called All-Heal, Amantilla, Setwall, Setawale, Great Wild
Valerian and Capon's Tail. A herb (*Valeriana officinalis*) growing to about
3 feet high, native to Europe and northern Asia and cultivated in
Poland, Hungary, France, Belgium, China, Japan and the USSR. An
essential oil, Valerian Oil, is obtained from the dried roots by steam-
distillation and used in perfumery both in India and the Far East and,
to a limited extent, in the West. A variety of the plant grown in Japan
produces a variety of the oil known as Kesso Oil.

The name derives from the Latin *valere* – to be healthy – and the
plant is mainly known for its medicinal properties, for which it was
recommended by Hippocrates in the 4th/5th centuries BC. Theophrastus
mentioned a Greek perfume made from all-heal grown in Syria and
listed the plant as one of the principal ones used in perfumery at the
time, but he may have been referring in this context to galbanum. The
leaves of Valerian were used in the Middle Ages both as a spice and as
a perfume, and the roots were laid in clothes to scent them. The scent
has an extraordinary attraction to cats.

Valerian is closely related to Celtic Spikenard (see Spikenard).

A form of Valerian Oil is also obtained from *V. wallichi*, which grows
in the Himalaya region, and is used locally as a perfume.

Valeriana celtica *see* Spikenard

Van Cleef & Arpels Opening in Paris in 1906 as a jewellers, still its main business, Van Cleef & Arpels launched its first fragrance, 'First', in 1976. It has subsequently produced 'Gem' (87), together with two men's fragrances, 'Pour l'Homme' (78) and 'Tsar' (89). The company is now part of the Sanofi group.

'Vanderbilt' A quality, top-selling floral–oriental perfume named after Gloria Vanderbilt, the American high-society heiress, which was launched in the USA in 1982. The creation of Sophia Grojsman of IFF, it was introduced into Britain in 1985 by Selective Beauté International, part of Golden Limited, a subsidiary of L'Oréal. The fresh, fruity, floral top note includes jasmine, tuberose, mimosa, marigold and palma rosa combined with lemon and orange flower. The middle note is a spicy, woody blend of coriander, pimento, vetivert and oak moss, and the base contains vanilla and balsam of Tolu. The flacon, with a swan motif, was designed by Bernard Kotyuk after a design by Lalique.

'Van Gils' A men's fragrance launched in 1990 by Van Gils, the men's clothing firm established by Miel van Gils of Holland. Created by Pierre Wargnye of IFF, it contains top notes of bergamot and verbena, with middle notes which include thyme, rosemary, coriander and cardamom, and a base of amber and musk. The bottle was designed by Alain de Morgues.

Vanilla Vanilla is made from crystals which form on the surface of the fruit pods of the Vanilla Orchid Vine (*Vanilla planifolia*, also *V. pompana* and some other species). The pods are also known as Vanilloes, Vanilla Pods and Vanilla Beans. The substance was first discovered for the West in Mexico in 1520 by Cortes, who found the Aztecs using it to flavour their chocolate beverages (see Cacao). Attempts to grow it in Europe failed until it was found that pollination of the plant was achieved by an insect which lived only in tropical America. The French

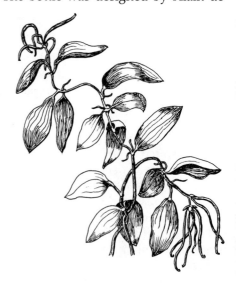

Vanilla (*Vanilla planifolia*).

learned how to pollinate the plant by hand in 1836. The crystals form during a 6-month fermentation period after the pods have been picked, and their distinctive, sweetly spicy aroma makes them an important material both in perfumery and in flavourings. In modern perfumery, vanilla was at first usually employed as a complement to extract of Tonka, but after Francois Coty used it in 'L'Aimant', it became one of the most popular of all perfume ingredients and now appears in the principal notes of 23% of all quality perfumes (e.g. 'Amouage', 'Bois des Isles', 'Jicky' and 'Habanita'). In perfumes of the highest quality Vanilla Absolute is used, but it is extremely expensive to produce. The dried pods are also used in sachets and pot pourri. Vanilla, native to Mexico and tropical America, is now cultivated in Indonesia, the W. Indies, Tahiti, the Seychelles, Réunion and Madagascar, the two latter islands producing most of the world's supply. It is often grown on Casuarina trees. See also Vanillin.

Vanilla Trilisia *see* Lacinaria

Vanillin An odorous white or yellowish-white crystalline substance found in Vanilla pods and in some other plants (including benzoin, balsam of Tolu and balsam of Peru). It is of particular value in perfumery as a fixative. However, nowadays commercial perfumers mostly use a synthetic Vanillin which has been produced from pine wood and other sources. See Tiemann.

Vaporizer *see* Atomizer

Vassoura Oil An oil with a spicy, somewhat grassy fragrance which is obtained by steam-distillation of the fresh leaves of a shrub *Baccharis dracunculifolia*, native to Brazil. It is used to give a harsh, spicy element to perfumes.

'V'E' A quality chypre perfume launched in 1990 by the fashion and costume designer Gianni Versace in association with Charles of the Ritz. Gianni Versace has also produced, in 1982, a floral perfume bearing his name. Green top notes include narcissus and hyacinth, in conjunction with bergamot and some floral notes. The heart is totally floral, principally ylang-ylang, jasmine, rose, orris and orange blossom. Woody

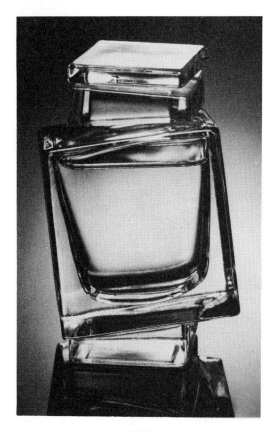

'V'E'.

and balsamic base notes include sandalwood, patchouli, frankincense, myrrh and amber. The perfume is sold in a limited-edition crystal flacon made by Baccarat to a 'tilted cube' design by Thierry Lecoule.

Velvet Dock   *see* Elecampane

'Vent Vert'   A classic Balmain perfume brought out in 1945. It was created by Germaine Sellier of Roure. Notable as the first of the 'green' perfumes (see Perfume Families), it remained the only perfume of its type for some 20 years. Its principal constituents are rose and lily of the valley, with galbanum in the top note and oak moss in the base. It was relaunched in 1991 with a revised, more floral, formula, the heart containing lily of the valley, hyacinth, rose and jasmine, with sage, sandalwood and musk in the base.

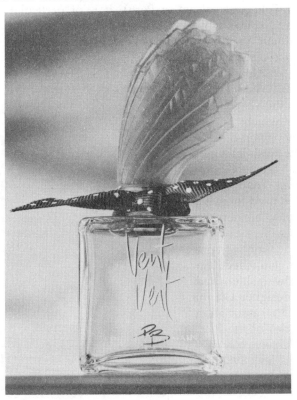

'Vent Vert'.

Verbena Oil   Sometimes called Vervain. Verbena Oil used in perfumery is distilled from the leaves of Lemon Verbena (*Lippia citriodora* = *Verbena triphylla* = *Aloysia citriodora*), known to the French as Vervaine Citronelle, a deciduous shrub growing to about 4 feet high, native to S. America, introduced into Britain at the end of the 18th century, and now cultivated in S. America, Algeria, Tunisia and the south of France. The leaves have a lemon or melissa-like fragrance which they retain for many years, and are dried for use in sachets and pot pourri. The essential oil is distilled from the leaves; it is mostly used in soaps and cosmetics, but appears occasionally in quality fragrances (e.g. 'Monsieur de Givenchy' and 'Van Gils'). See also under Lippia.

This plant should not be confused with the perennial plant known as Verbena which is found growing wild in Britain and elsewhere (*Verbena officinalis*), also called Vervain, Holy Wort and Herb Louis. This was held sacred by the Druids, had medical properties recorded by Hippocrates and was used as a protection against the plague, but it has no value in perfumery. Nor should Verbena Oil be confused with Spanish Verbena Oil, distilled from *Thymus hyemalis* for flavouring; nor with the Verbena, or Vervaine, used in Provence liqueurs, made from the dried flowers of *Dracocephalum moldavici*; nor with Indian Verbena, which is Lemon Grass.

Vervain *see* Verbena

Vesper Flower *see* Honesty Oil

'Vetiver' The brand name of a trend-setting, woody-scented men's fragrance brought out by Carven as an eau de toilette in 1957. Created by Firmenich perfumers, its principal ingredients are bergamot and lemon in the top note, vetivert in the middle note, and a number of woody and powdery elements in the base. It comes in a flask designed by Jacques Bocquet.

Vetivert Also Vetiver and Vetyver. An important essential oil distilled from the rhizomes of Khus-khus Grass, also called Vetiver Grass (*Vetiveria zizanoides = V. odorata = Andropogon muricatus*), native to tropical Asia and now cultivated for this oil in India, Malaysia, Indonesia, China, Réunion, Brazil, Angola and the W. Indies. The oil, which in India is known as *Khas*, has an earthy odour with an underlying violet and orris-like sweetness. It is very per-

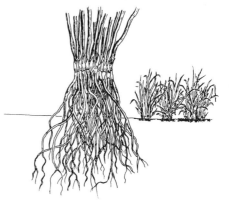

Vetivert (*Vetiveria zizanoides*).

sistent and one of the finest fixatives known. It is the basis of the Indian perfume Mousseline (q.v.) and appears as a main ingredient in some 36% of all western quality perfumes (e.g. 'Calèche', 'Chanel No. 5', 'Dioressence' and 'Parure') and 20% of all men's fragrances. The dried roots are used in sachets and pot pourri and are burned in India as an incense. An alcohol called vetiverol, extracted from the oil, is used in perfumery.

Another form of Vetivert, *Vetiveria nigritana*, is found in the Sudan and Sahara regions and used locally for perfuming clothes and fabrics.

'Vicky Tiel' A quality floral perfume introduced by the American dress designer Vicky Tiel in 1990 (UK 1991). The top notes contain bergamot and mandarin, and lead to a heart which includes narcissus, jonquil, lily of the valley and jasmine; the base, mainly sandalwood and oak moss, also has camellia and tuberose notes. An original flacon, designed by Pierre Dinand and made by Brosse, features, as part of the stopper, a classical sculptured Venus submerged in the perfume.

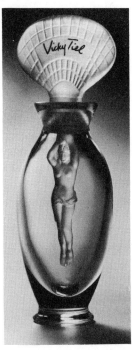

'Vicky Tiel'.

Vinaigrette A small box with a pierced inner lid containing a sponge soaked with aromatic vinegar. It was used like a smelling bottle to clear the head and counter bad smells in the air. The vinaigrette succeeded the pomander in fashionable circles in the 18th century and was popular throughout Europe until the latter part of the 19th century. Vinaigrettes, which originated in France, were usually made of silver, with a gilded interior to prevent corrosion. The vinegar base was mostly aromatized with camphor and attar of roses, or lavender, or sometimes with rosemary, sage, mint and other herbs. They were mostly flat, rectangular boxes, but other shapes were used, and were delicately worked in often elaborate designs. Birmingham 'toy-maker' silversmiths of 1800 to 1850 were particularly noted makers of vinaigrettes.

Violet Also called Sweet Violet and Sweet-scented Violet. A small, highly fragrant annual (*Viola odorata*) growing to around 5 inches high and originating in Europe, Asia and N. Africa. It is used in perfumery, medicines, love potions, sweets, hair-dressing, to make a liqueur and for cut flowers. For perfumery the essential oil is mostly obtained from plants cultivated in southern France and northern Italy, using two varieties of the plant, the Victoria violet and the Parma violet; although perfume from the latter is more highly rated, the former variety is the one mainly used, as it is more easily grown and is more disease resistant. The flowers are extracted by enfleurage, maceration or volatile solvents immediately after being picked, yielding a very small amount of extremely costly absolute. An essential oil is also obtained from the leaves and added as an absolute to a violet perfume to perfect it by providing a herbaceous, slightly earthy note. Most present day violet perfumes are made synthetically on a base of ionone or methyl-ionone, but the best have a portion of natural violet extract added to them. Modern quality fragrances using violet include, for example, 'L'Interdit', 'Nina', 'Quelques Fleurs', 'Soir de Paris' and 'Xeryus'.

The violet was well known in ancient times, the Greeks regarding it as the flower of fertility. Pliny valued its fragrance immediately after roses and lilies and observed that a garland of violets worn around the head would prevent headaches and dizziness. Both Greeks and Romans drank a wine made from violets. The early Arab perfume makers learned how to distil the oil. The violet was the floral emblem of the Bonapartes; after the Empress Marie Louise was separated from Napoleon in 1817 she established the violet industry at Parma which flourishes to this day.

Violet Root *see* Sumbul

Virgin Wax *see* Propolis

'Vivre' A classic floral aldehyde perfume first presented by Molyneux in the 1930s and relaunched in 1971 to a new formula created by perfumers of IFF. Spicy aldehyde top notes with bergamot and coriander introduce a floral heart in which rose, jasmine and orange blossom predominate, underlaid by base notes of sandalwood, vetivert and oak moss. The flacon, a strikingly modern symbolization of the human body, was designed by Serge Mansau.

Voanalakoly An aromatic shrub (*Rhinacanthus osmospermum*) found in Madagascar. The leaves are used locally to scent the hair and to make perfumed sachets.

'Vol de Nuit' A classic Guerlain oriental perfume first produced in 1933. Citrus top notes of orange, bergamot, lemon, mandarin and neroli head a body composed principally of rosewood, jasmine, palma rosa and ylang-ylang, with a strong ambery–balsamic base which includes vanilla, benzoin, balsam of Peru, sandalwood, musk, ambergris and leather fragrance.

Volatile Oil   *see* Essential Oil

Volatile Solvents   Volatile solvents first came into commercial use in perfumery at the end of the 19th century, as a means of separating the fragrant parts of an essential oil from its other parts without damaging them. To do so they must leave no residue after evaporation, must have a very low boiling point, so that fragrance components are not destroyed by the heat, and must be selective enough to extract only the substances required. Petroleum ether has been used as a volatile solvent for a long time, and more recently carbon dioxide has enabled fragrances to be extracted which were not previously obtainable (e.g. lilac). Other important volatile solvents used include hexane, benzene acetone, toluene, methanol, ethanol and butane. See Extraction.

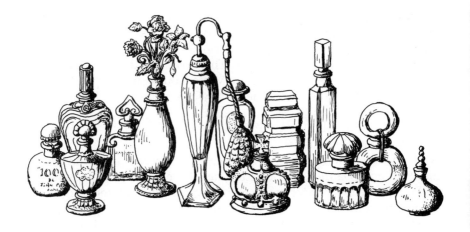

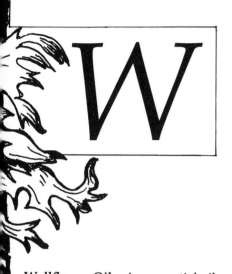

Wallflower Oil   An essential oil extracted by steam-distillation or volatile solvents from the flowers of the Wallflower (*Cheiranthus cheiri*), also called Giroflee, Giroflier, Gillyflower (q.v.), Handflower and Keiri, a perennial herb growing to about 12 inches high, native to S. Europe but now cultivated widely as a garden plant. The plant was introduced into Britain in the 17th century. The oil has a pleasing fragrance when diluted, but is disagreeable at full strength. The yield of oil, about 0.06%, is so low that in modern perfumery the fragrance is usually synthesized.

The word Cheiranthus derives from Greek meaning 'handflower', because the plant, well known to the ancient Greeks, was carried in the hand as a nosegay at festivals. Traditionally it was worn by minstrels and troubadors. Wallflower oil was used in the recipes of the early Arab perfume makers.

Walnut Oil   Walnut oil, from the nuts of the tree *Juglans regia* (English Walnut, Persian Walnut), which probably originated in Persia, was well known in classical times and was used in early Arab perfumes.

Washball   A perfumed or medicated ball of soap, sometimes containing powdered pumice or sand to provide an abrasive quality, used in Europe, particularly during the 17th and 18th centuries, for washing the face and hands and when shaving. Some were made in the home with garden herbs, others by perfumers and apothecaries. Expensive washballs were manufactured in Italy and France and sold throughout Europe. Certain essential oils were particularly suited for washballs because they remained stable when mixed with the alkaline substances of the soap, i.e. bergamot, geranium, lemon grass, palma rosa, patchouli, rosemary, sandalwood, thyme and vetivert. But early wash-ball recipes often included other expensive perfumes such as ambergris and musk. (See Appendix B, recipes nos 32 and 33.)

Wax Myrtle tree   *see* Candleberry Wax

Wax Palm   *see* Carnauba Wax

West Indian Elemi   *see* Tacamahac

White Cedar   *see* Arbor Vitae

White Cinnamon   *see* Canella

White Flower de Luce   *see* Orris

'White Linen'   A quality floral perfume introduced by Estée Lauder in 1978. The floral fragrance is principally obtained from a heart of white flowers, including jasmine, rose, honeysuckle, hyacinth, lilac and lily of the valley, with an added spicy touch from pimento. Mandarin dominates the top notes and vetivert the base. The bottle was designed by Ira Levy.

White Peru Balsam   *see* Storax

'White Satin'   A wide-selling floral perfume launched by Yardley in 1985. An unusual green top note containing grapefruit and sweet orange also includes clove, pepper and basil to provide a spicy touch. The heart is principally jasmine, geranium and ylang-ylang, and the base note mostly comes from patchouli, cedarwood and storax.

White Saunders   *see* Sandalwood

White Spruce   *see* Silver Pine Needle Oil

White Tea Tree   *see* Cajaput

Wild Allspice   *see* Spicewood

Wild Cinnamon   *see* Canella

Wild Laburnum   *see* Melilot

Wild Nard   *see* Asarabacca

Wild Rye   *see* Avens

Wild Sunflower   *see* Elecampane

Wine   Theophrastus noted that some perfume materials made wine not only smell better but also taste better. Conversely, the Greeks used wine to sweeten the odour of some perfume materials, including myrrh and various spices. The important Greek compound perfume called Kypros included among its ingredients two which were first steeped in sweet wine. The early Arab perfume makers also made use of wine in some of their perfume recipes. See also Cognac Oil.

Winter Berry   *see* Gaultheria

Winter Marjoram   *see* Origanum

Wintergreen   *see* Gaultheria

Winter's Grass   *see* Citronella

Wisteria *see* Glycine

Wisteria sinensis *see* Glycine

Wood Avens *see* Avens

Woodruff Also called Sweet Woodruff, Sweet Grass, Hay Plant, Herb Walter and Scented Hairhoof. A small member of the madder family (*Asperula odorata* = *Galium odorata*) which grows from Europe and N. Africa to Siberia. When dried it emits a 'new-mown hay' fragrance, due to a high coumarin content, and it was consequently much used in Britain at one time as a strewing herb in linen and clothes. In Old French it was known as 'Muge-de-Boys', meaning Musk of the Woods. The dried leaves are used today to provide a flavouring in some wines, liqueurs and snuffs, and in pot pourri, where the fragrance helps as a fixative.

Woody Note A phrase used in perfumery to describe fragrances reminiscent of wood. These fragrances are provided by wood oils, such as cedar, by essential oils from other plants having a wood-like aroma, such as patchouli, and by synthetics. Woody notes appear in varying degrees in most modern perfumes. See Perfume Notes.

Wormseed, American *see* Ambroisia

Wormwood Oil Also called Absinthe Oil. An oil steam-distilled from the dried leaves and flowering tops of Wormwood (*Artemisia absinthium*), also called Green Ginger, a herb growing 2 to 3 feet high, found in the Mediterranean region, Kashmir and Siberia and now also cultivated in Europe, N. Africa and the USA. A similar oil is also obtained from Roman Wormwood (*A. pontica*), which grows in S. Europe. The oil was once used in the preparation of the drink Absinthe, now no longer produced, and is still employed medicinally and in the preparation of Vermouth and some other wines. In perfumery its intense, pungent, herbaceous odour, reminiscent of cedarleaf oil, is used extensively in masculine notes and it appears in some quality perfumes (e.g. 'Ivoire').

Wormwood, Mexican *see* Ambroisia

Worth A leading Parisian fashion house formed in 1858 by Charles Worth (1826–1895), a draper born in Lincolnshire who found work in Paris. He was the first dress designer to use live models, and became court dressmaker to the Empress Eugénie of France and Empress Elizabeth of Austria. The company formed Les Parfums Worth in 1924 and produced its first perfume, 'Dans la Nuit' in that year; this perfume was initially provided as a gift to its distinguished clients. It was followed by 'Vers le Jour' in 1925, 'Sans Adieu' in 1929 and the highly successful 'Je Reviens' in 1932. Subsequent fragrances included 'Vers Toi' (34), 'Projets' (35), 'Imprudence' (38), 'Requête' (44), 'Monsieur Worth' (69), 'Miss Worth' (77) and 'Worth pour Homme' (80). The 'nose' for early Worth perfumes was Maurice Blanchet, and the flacons were by Lalique. The company ceased to be a fashion house in 1956, but continues to market perfumes, relaunching 'Dans la Nuit' in 1985.

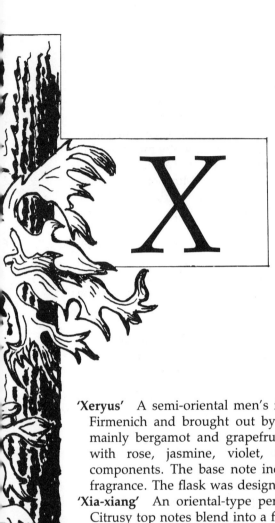

'Xeryus' A semi-oriental men's fragrance created by the fragrance firm Firmenich and brought out by Givenchy in 1986. Citrusy top notes, mainly bergamot and grapefruit, yield to a floral–spicy middle note with rose, jasmine, violet, cinnamon and coriander among its components. The base note includes musk, amber, moss and leather fragrance. The flask was designed by Pierre Dinand.

'Xia-xiang' An oriental-type perfume brought out by Revlon in 1988. Citrusy top notes blend into a floral heart containing rose, muguet and ylang-ylang, together with vanilla, tonka, camomile and fruity fragrances (plum, raspberry and peach) in the base notes. The bottle is in the form of a Chinese snuff bottle.

Ximenia A small tree (*Ximenia americana*) found in India, Sri Lanka, Malaysia, tropical Africa and tropical America. The wood has a fragrance similar to sandalwood, for which it is sometimes used in India as a substitute. The species is closely related to the Egyptian tree which produced the Balanos Oil of ancient times. The botanical name *Ximenia* comes from an early Spanish monk/botanist called Ximenes, who published works on S. American flora.

Xolisma An absolute obtained by extraction with volatile solvents from the flowers of the Xolisma bush (*Xolisma ferruginea*), also called Sourwood and Sorrel tree, a shrub growing to about 10 feet high, which resembles Sweet Myrtle and is found in parts of the southern USA. The fragrance is reminiscent of the lily.

Xylaloes *see* Aloewood

Xylobalsamum *see* Balsam of Judaea/Megaleion

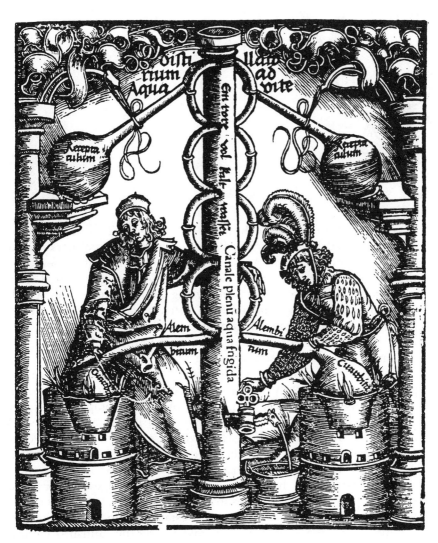

16th century distilling apparatus (*Source* Philipp Ulstadt, *Coelum Philosophorum*, 1526).

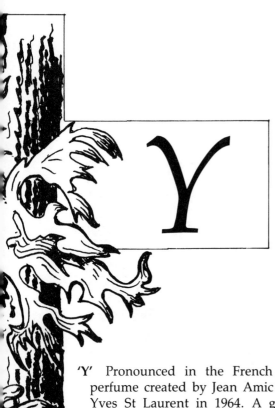

'Y' Pronounced in the French manner – 'Ee-grek'. A trend-setting perfume created by Jean Amic of Roure which was first marketed by Yves St Laurent in 1964. A green chypre fragrance, it achieved an original new effect with fruity aldehydic top notes on a floral heart dominated by jasmine, rose, ylang-ylang and tuberose. The woody lower notes are chiefly obtained from vetivert, sandalwood, patchouli and oak moss. The flacon was designed by Pierre Dinand.

Yardley One of the oldest perfume companies in the world, starting as a soap and perfume business founded in 1770 by the Cleaver family. This was taken over by William Yardley, a maker of fashionable swords, spurs and buckles, early in the 19th century in order to rescue his son-in-law William Cleaver from bankruptcy. The company remained under the control of the Yardley family until it became a joint stock company in 1890. After the Great War it expanded its production considerably, notably in products based on lavender, of which it was to become the world's largest manufacturer, with extensive lavender farms in East Anglia. Its creams were sold in Wedgewood or Royal Worcester pots and its perfumes in flacons by Baccarat. Yardley's main factory for perfumes and cosmetics was established in Basildon in 1966, at which time the company was taken over by British American Tobacco. It was subsequently acquired by the Beecham Group, and thereafter, in 1990, by the American conglomerate Wasserstein-Perella.

In 1985 the firm of Jovan, which has manufactured a wide range of fragrances for the mass market, came under the Yardley umbrella.

Famous Yardley perfumes of the past have included 'White Rose' (1910), 'Tête-à-Tête' (21) and 'Bond Street' (27). Its current fragrances include 'Lavender' (1913). 'April Violets' (23), 'Flair' (57), 'Chique' (76), 'Pure Silk' (82), 'Lace' (84), 'White Satin' (85), 'Pink Lace' (86), 'Black Velvet' (87), 'You're the Fire' (89), 'English Spring Flowers' (90), 'Chique Silver' (90), 'Nights in White Satin' (90) and 'Forever' (91). Under the Jovan label it now markets 'Pagan' and 'Musk Oil' fragrances.

Yarrow   *see* Milfoil

Yellow Bugle   *see* Ground Pine

Yellow Flag   *see* Iris, Yellow

Yellow Sanders   *see* Sandalwood

Yellow Starwort   *see* Elecampane

Yellow Sweet Clover   *see* Melilot

Yerba Mate tree   *see* Mate

Ylang-ylang   An essential oil much used in high-class perfumery. It is steam-distilled from the flowers of the Ylang-ylang Tree (*Cananga odorata = Unona odorata = Uvaria odorata*), which grows to about 60 feet high and is native to tropical S.E. Asia; also from a closely related species, locally called the Tainghe or Tho Shui Tree (*Cananga latifolia = Unona latifolia*) found principally in Malaysia. The former is cultivated

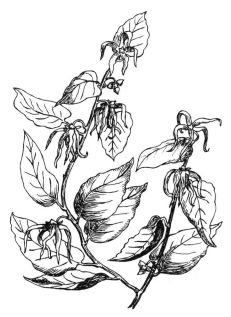

Ylang-ylang (*Cananga odorata*).

for the oil in the Philippines, Java, Madagascar, the Comoro Islands and Réunion, the best oil coming from the Philippines. The fragrance is sweet, jasmine-like and powerful and does not become apparent in the flowers until some 2–3 weeks after they have first opened, when they must be picked quickly and processed without delay; distillation and extraction of the concrete is therefore usually undertaken close to the site. One tree provides about 10 kilos of flowers a year and some 350 to 400 kilos of flowers are required to produce 1 kilo of essential oil. The oil obtained from Java, which is inferior in quality, is known as Cananga Oil and used in soaps and less expensive perfumes. Ylang-ylang was not brought into use in European perfumery until the end of the 19th century, when it was one of the ingredients of Macassar Oil. It now appears in about 40% of all quality perfumes. It is sometimes strengthened by the addition of pimento. One of its main constituents is isoeugenol.

'You're the Fire' A wide-selling spicy–floral perfume launched by Yardley in 1989. Bergamot and lavandin, with a touch of clove and nutmeg, in the top note lead to a floral heart containing jasmine, rose and orange blossom, with a woody–balsamic base note provided by patchouli, cedarwood and vanilla.

'Youth Dew' An innovative oriental perfume brought out by Estée Lauder in 1952. It was the fourth best-selling fine fragrance in 1989. It is an unusual brown in colour and the ingredients emphasize spiciness. The top notes contain orange and various spices. The heart shows a range of floral fragrances, including rose, ylang-ylang and jasmine, modified by cassie, cinnamon and a preponderating carnation. The base notes are balsamic, principally amber and balsam of Tolu. The flacon was designed by Ira Levy.

'Ysatis' A semi-oriental–floral quality perfume for wear on all occasions; it was created for Givenchy by Dominique Ropion, then with Roure, and launched in 1984. Top notes of ylang-ylang, orange blossom, mandarin and a hint of galbanum lead into a floral heart of tuberose, jasmine, rose and iris. In the base notes oak moss, patchouli, sandalwood, cloves, bay rum and frankincense are underlined by touches of castoreum, civet, ambergris and musk. The flacon was designed by Pierre Dinand.

Yu-chu-lan *see* Aglaia

Yves Rocher *see* Sanofi

Yves St Laurent A French fashion house started by the Parisian couturier Yves St Laurent in 1961 after he left Christian Dior. In 1964 the company launched its first perfume, 'Y', which has since been followed by 'Rive Gauche' (70), 'Opium' (77) and 'Paris' (83), together with three men's fragrances – 'YSL pour Homme' (71), 'Kouros' (81) and 'Jazz' (88).

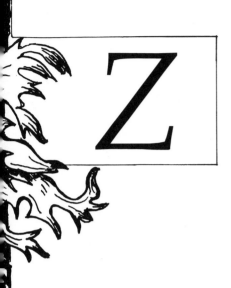

Zambac *see* Jasmine

Zdravets An essential oil with a very persistent fragrance similar to Clary Sage which is distilled from the leaves of Bigroot Geranium (*Geranium macrorhizum*). This plant, which grows to about 16 inches high, is found in central and southern Europe. It is mainly cultivated in Bulgaria, where the roots and leaves are regarded as aphrodisiacal. The oil is used occasionally in perfumery.

Zanthoxylum alatum *see* Tomar Seed Oil
     panispinum *see* Tomar Seed Oil

Zedoary Oil An essential oil distilled from the rhizomes of Zedoary (*Curcuma zeodoaria*), which has been cultivated for centuries in India and Sri Lanka for the perfume and also as a source of starch and as a condiment. The oil has a fragrance suggesting a blend of ginger and camphor, and is occasionally used in western perfumery.

Zibetha *see* Civet

Zingiber officinale *see* Ginger

'Zinnia' A quality floral perfume, launched by Floris in 1990, which has been re-created by the Floris perfumer, Douglas Cope, from a mid-18th century formula discovered in the company's archives. Top notes which include violet, galbanum and ylang-ylang lead to a heart built on a floral bouquet of rose, lily and orris, with a hint of spice from clove.

Woody base notes from sandalwood are supported by vanilla and a touch of musk.

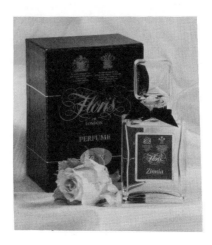

'Zinnia'.

Appendix A List of fragrances

The perfumes and fragrances in this list are mostly, though not entirely, still being marketed. Some are not sold in the UK. Those in bold type are described in more detail in the main text. Fragrances for men are indicated by 'm'. The year is mostly that of UK launching.

Name	House	Year	Family/brief description
A by Annabella	Annabella/Denis	87	Floral
m Accomplice	Coty	54	Fougere
m Acqua di Selva	Victor	47	Lavender
m Acteur	Azzaro	89	Chypre (leather, woody)
Adeline	Pola	72	Aldehyde (floral)
m Adidas	Astor/Beecham	85	Green
Adieu Sagesse	Patou	25(84)	Floral
m Admirals's Yachtman	Mas	81	Leather
Adolfo	Denney	78	Floral (sweet)
m Adolfo for Men	Denney	81	Chypre
Afghane	d'Estrées	80	Floral (sweet)
Ago	Perrin	79	Floral
m Agresste	Gal	82	Chypre
m Agua Brava	Puig	68	Lavender
m Agua Lavanda	Puig	40	Lavender
m Agua Profunda	Puig	77	Citrus
Ainsi	Atkinsons	71	Green
m Ajonc	Rocher	72	Green
Alada	Myrurgia	79	Green
m Alain Delon	Delon	80	Chypre
Alfred Sung	Riviera Concepts	86	Floral
Alliage	Lauder	72	Green
Allora	Marbert	82	Floral (fruity–fresh)
Amarige	Givenchy	91	Floral (woody)
Amazone	Hermès	75(89)	Floral (fruity–fresh)

Name	House	Year	Family/brief description
Ambush	Dana	59	Fougere
Amen Wardy	Wardy	87	Floral
Amerique	Courrèges	79	Chypre (fresh–mossy)
Amorena	Cantilène	79	Green
Amouage	Amouage	84	Floral–oriental
Amour Amour	Patou	25(84)	Floral
Amun	4711	81	Oriental
Anabella	Denis	87	Floral
Anais-Anais	Cacharel	79	Floral (fruity–fresh)
Andron	Jovan	81	Chypre (floral–musky)
m Andron for Men	Jovan	81	Chypre
Animale	S. de Lyon	87	Chypre
Anne Klein	Parlux	84	Floral
Anne Klein II	Parlux	85	Amber
An Original Perfume	Boots	81	Floral–fresh
m **Antaeus**	Chanel	81	Leather
m Antarctic	Rocher	90	Spicy–citrus
Antilope	Weil	45	Aldehyde–floral–woody
Aphrodisia	Fabergé	38	Chypre (fresh–mossy)
Apogée	Les Senteurs	89	Floral–chypre
Après l'Ondée	Guerlain	1906	Floral (green)
April Violets	Yardley	23	Floral
m Aqua Cologne Ice Blue	Williams	35	Chypre
m Aqua Velva Frost Lime	Williams	66	Citrus
Aquarius	Max Factor	69	Chypre (floral–woody)
m Aramant	Biodroga	85	Chypre
m **Aramis**	Aramis	65	Chypre
Aramis 900	Aramis	73	Floral
Aria	Missoni	88	Floral
Ariane	Avon	77	Floral
Armani	Armani	82	Floral (fresh–fruity–spicy)
m Armani pour Homme	Armani	84	Citrus

Name	House	Year	Family/brief description
m Armateur	Payot	67	Spicy
Arnold Scasi	Revlon	89	Floral
Arpège	Lanvin	27	Aldehyde (floral)
Aromatis Elixir	Clinique	72	Tobacco–leather
m Arrogance	Pikenz	82	Leather
Arrogantissima	Pikenz	88	
Audace	P. International/ Gibbs	36(88)	Oriental
m Auslese	Shiseido	78	Citrus
Aviance	Matchabelli	75	Aldehyde (floral– woody)
Azurée	Lauder	69	Chypre (floral– woody)
Azzaro	Azzaro	75	Chypre (fresh– mossy)
m **Azzaro pour Homme**	Azzaro	78	Fougere
Azzaro 9	Azzaro	85	Floral
Babe	Fabergé	76	Floral (sweet)
Babillage	Kanebo	73	Aldehyde (floral)
m Babor for Men	Babor	81	Chypre
Baboré	Babor	83	Green
Bacchus	Coty	69	
Baghari	Piguet	50	Aldehyde (floral– chypre)
Baglietto	Denis	87	
Bakir	Minteil	75	Oriental
m Balafré	Lancôme	67	Woody
Balahé	Léonard	83	Floral (fresh)
Bal à Versailles	Desprez	62	Oriental
m Balenciaga pour Homme	Balenciaga	90	Woody–spicy
Balestra	Balestra	78	Floral (fresh)
m Balestra pour Homme	Balestra	82	Chypre
m Bally Masculin	Bally	84	Fougere
Bambou	Weil	84	Floral (fruity)
Bandit	Piguet	44	Chypre (floral– mossy–leathery)
Baruffa	Atkinsons	81	Floral (fruity–fresh)
Barynia	Rubinstein	85	Floral

Name	House	Year	Family/brief description
m Basic Homme	Vichy	87	
Basile	SIRPEA	87	Green
m Basile Uomo	SIRPEA	86	Green
Bat Sheba	Muller	70	Chypre (floral)
Beautiful	Lauder	86	Floral
m Bel Ami	Hermès	86	Leather
Bellodgia	Caron	27	Floral
m Biagiotti Uomo	Biagiotti	91	Green–spicy
Bibi de Jean Bartet	COFCI	88	
Bic	Bic	88	
m Bijan for Men	Bijan	81	Woody–spicy
m Bijan Fragrance for Men	Bijan	87	Woody–spicy
Bijan Perfume for Women	Bijan	87	Floral–oriental
Bill Blass	Blass/Revlon	78	Floral
m Bill Blass for Men	Blass	70	Spicy
Bizarre	Atkinsons	79	Aldehyde (floral)
m Bjorn Borg	Borg	86	Green
m Black Belt	Coty	69	Chypre
m Black Label	Yardley	69	Fougere
m Black Suede	Avon	80	Chypre
Black Velvet	Yardley	87	Floral–chypre
Blasé	Factor	75	Floral (sweet)
Blazer	A. Klein	76	Floral (fresh)
m Blend 30	Dunhill	78	Woody
m Blenheim Bouquet	Penhaligon's	1902	Green
Bleu de Chine	Morandiere/Outline	87	Chypre
Bleu Marine	Cardin/SNDPI	86	
Bluebell	Penhaligon's	78	Green
Blue Grass	Arden	35	Floral
m Blue Stratos	Shulton	76	Fougere
Blumarine	Denis	88	
Bob Mackie	Alfin	85	
m Bogart	Bogart	78	Fougere
Bois des Îsles	Chanel	26(89)	Aldehyde (floral–woody)
m Bois de Vetiver	Bogart	82	Woody
m Bois Noir	Chanel	87	Woody

Name	House	Year	Family/brief description
Bond Street	Yardley	27	Floral–oriental
Bonne Fête	Hallden	88	
m Boss No 1	Boss	87	Chypre
m Boss Sport	Boss	89	Fougere
m Borsalino	Borsalino	84	Spicy
Boucheron	Boucheron	80	Floral–oriental
m Bowling Green	Beene	90	Green
m Braggi	Revlon	66	Chypre
m Brando	Parera	76	Fougere
m Bravas	Shiseido	69	Citrus
m Bravas Bosky	Shiseido	71	Spicy
Breathless	Avon	88	Oriental
m Brisk Spice (Wild Spice)	Avon	78	Spicy
m British Sterling	Speidel	65	Fougere
m Brummel	Williams Hispania	76	Chypre
m **Brut**	Fabergé	64	Fougere
Bulgari	Bulgari	84	Floral
m Burberrys for Men	Burberry	81	Chypre
m Burley (Bounty)	Armour	68	Floral
Byblos	Byblos	90	Floral (green, woody)
Byrsa	Palomba	87	
Byzance	Rochas	87	Oriental
Cabochard	Grès	58	Chypre (floral–mossy)
Cabotine	Grès	90	Floral
Cabriole	Arden	77	Floral (sweet)
m Cacharel pour Homme	Cacharel	81	Spicy–citrus
Cachet	Matchabelli/P. International	70	Chypre (floral–mossy)
Café	COFCI	78	
Calandre	Rabanne	69	Aldehyde (floral–woody)
Calèche	Hermès	61	Aldehyde (floral–woody)
Calendal	Molinard	29	Floral
California	Factor	90	Floral–woody

Name	House	Year	Family/brief description
Câline	Patou	64(84)	Aldehyde (floral)
m Calvin	C. Klein	81	Fougere
Calvin Klein	C. Klein	78	Green
Calyx	Prescriptives	89	Floral
m Camaro	Nerval	80	Leather
m Cambridge	Mem Comp.	81	Chypre
m Cameron	Kensington	82	Spicy
Cananga	Berger	90	Oriental
Canoe	Dana	35	Fougere
Candid	Avon	77	Floral (sweet)
Capricci	Ricci	60	Aldehyde (floral)
m Captain	Molyneux	74	Fougere
Capucci de Capucci	Capucci	87	Floral–oriental
m Capucci pour Homme	Capucci	67	Citrus–woody
m Caractère	Hechter	90	Green–spicy
Cardin	Cardin	76	Floral
m Care	Astor	79	Woody
Care No. 2	Astor	82	Chypre
Care Dynamic	Astor	88	
Carlo Corinto	Corinto	85	
Carnet du Bal	Révillon	37	Oriental
Carolina Herrera	Herrera/Puig	89	Floral
m Casablanca	Coty	83	Fougere
Casanova	Casanova	81	Chypre (floral–sweet)
Casaque	d'Albret	56	Floral (fresh)
Casmir	Chopard	91	Fruity–woody
Cassini	Cassini	90	Floral (fruity–mossy–amber)
Catherine Deneuve	Phenix	86	Chypre
m Cedarwood	Goya	58	Leather
m Cellini	Fabergé	80	Fougere
Celui	Dessès	38	Floral
Cerissa	Revlon	74	Floral (sweet)
m Cerutti Fair Play	Cerutti		
C'est Dramatique	Boots	91	Floral
C'est Irresistible	Boots	91	Oriental
C'est la Vie	Lacroix	90	Floral–amber

Name	House	Year	Family/brief description
C'est Moi	Aigner	83	Floral (fresh)
C'est Mysterieux	Boots	91	Chypre
C'est Romantique	Boots	91	Floral
C'est Sophistique	Boots	91	Floral (fruity)
Chaldee	Patou	27(84)	Floral–spicy
Chamade	Guerlain	70	Aldehyde (floral–woody)
Champagne	Monteil	83	Floral (sweet)
Chanel No. 5	Chanel	21	Aldehyde (floral)
Chanel No. 19	Chanel	71	Green
Chanel No. 22	Chanel	26(89)	Floral
Chantage	Lancaster	79	Aldehyde (floral–powdery)
Chant d'Arômes	Guerlain	62	Floral (fresh–fruity)
Chantilly	Houbigant	41	Oriental
m Chaps	Warner	79	Chypre
Charade	Factor	88	Floral (fruity)
Charisma	Avon	68	Aldehyde (floral)
Charivari	Charles of the Ritz	78	Floral
Charles of the Ritz	Charles of the Ritz	78	Floral (sweet)
Charlie	Revlon	73	Floral (fresh)
Chassrès	Pola	81	Floral
m Chaz	Revlon	75	Fougere
Chess d'Or	Chess	78	Floral
m Chevalier	d'Orsay	73	Spicy
Chiara Boni	Boni	91	Floral (fruity)
Chicane	Jacomo	73	Aldehyde (floral)
Chimère	Matchabelli	80	Chypre (floral–woody)
Chique	Yardley	76(86)	Floral–chypre
Chique Silver	Yardley	90	Chypre
Chloé	Lagerfeld	75	Floral (sweet)
Choc	Cardin	81	Chypre (fresh–mossy)
Christian Aujard	Dana	85	
m Chromatics	Aramis	74	Chypre
Chunga	Weil	78	Aldehyde (floral–powdery)
Chypre	Coty	17	Chypre (fresh–mossy)

Name	House	Year	Family/brief description
Cialenga	Balenciaga	73	Chypre (mossy–fruity)
Ciao	Houbigant	80	Chypre (mossy–fruity)
Ciara	Revson	73	Oriental
Cie	Shulton	77	Floral
Ciel	de Varens		Oriental
Cinnabar	Lauder	78	Oriental
Claiborne	Claiborne	86	Floral
Clair de Jour	Lanvin	83	Floral (fruity–fresh)
Clandestine	Laroche/L'Oréal	86	Floral
m Classic Gold	Yardley	88	Fougere
Cléa	Rocher	81	Floral (aldehyde)
Climat	Lancôme	68	Aldehyde (floral)
Clin d'Oeil	Bourjois	84	Floral (fruity)
Clinique Wrappings	Clinique	90	Floral (green)
Coca	COFCI	81	
Cocktail	Patou	30(84)	Floral (fruity)
Coco	Chanel	84	Oriental
Coeur de Ferrose	L.D. Ferro	82	
Coeurs Joie	Ricci	46	Floral
Colony	Patou	38(84)	Fruity–mossy
m Colorado Sage	Bell	78	Fougere
Colors	Benetton	87	Oriental
m Colors de Benetton Man	Benetton	88	Woody–spicy
Complice	Coty	73	Aldehyde (floral–woody)
m Contour	Gillette	80	Fougere
m Cool Sage	Avon	87	Lavender
m Cool Water	Davidoff	88	Floral–fruity–woody
m Cordovan	Avon	87	Herbal–citrus
Coriandre	Couturier	73	Chypre (fresh–mossy)
Cornubia	Penhaligon's	91	Floral
Coryssima	Coryse Salome	73	Aldehyde
Cote d'Azur	Avon	88	
m Cougar	Yardley	69	Floral
Courant	Rubinstein	72	Chypre (floral–woody)

Name	House	Year	Family/brief description
m Courrèges Homme	Courrèges	77	Chypre
Courrèges in Blue	Courrèges	83	Floral
m Cravache	Piguet	63	Leather
Creation by Ted Lapidus	Lapidus	84	Floral
Creature	Cantuel	87	
Crêpe de Chine	Millot/Desprez	25	Chypre (fresh–mossy)
Cristalle	Chanel	74	Floral (fresh)
Cuir de Russie	Chanel	24(89)	Tobacco–leather
m Cuirasse	d'Auvillers	82	Chypre
Cyane	de Varens		Citrus
m Dali pour Homme	COFCI	85	Woody–fruity–spicy
Dans la Nuit	Worth	24(85)	Floral
Darling	Elida Gibbs	81	
Davana	Berger	90	Floral
m Davidoff	Davidoff/ Lancaster	84	Leather
Daydreams	Maybelline	83	Chypre (floral–mossy)
Déchirure	ISD	89	
De Jour	Betrix	83	Oriental
Demi Jour	Houbigant	87	Floral–chypre
m Denim	Elida Gibbs	76	Chypre
m Denim Musk	Elida Gibbs	82	Musk
m Derby	Guerlain	85	Woody–spicy
m Der Mann	Jade	81	Fougere
m Derrick	Orlane	78	Spicy
m Derringer	Sans Soucis	82	Chypre
Desire	Max Factor	88	Floral–oriental
De Soir	Betrix	83	Chypre (fresh–woody)
Detchema	Révillon	53	Aldehyde (floral)
Detchema Long Time	Révillon	84	
m **Devin**	Aramis	78	Green
m De Viris	Bogart	82	Woody

Name	House	Year	Family/brief description
Diamella	Rocher	84	Chypre
Di Borghese	Borghese	78	Floral
Dilys	L. Ashley	91	Floral
m Dimensione Uomo	Ciccarelli	77	Citrus
Diorama	Dior	49	Floral
Diorella	Dior	72	Floral (fresh)
Dioressence	Dior	70	Oriental
Diorissimo	Dior	56	Floral (fresh)
Diva	Ungaro	84	Floral (amber)
Divine Folie	Patou	33(84)	Floral (spicy)
m Dollar	Coveri	84	Fougere
Donna	Gherardini/ Satinine	82	Floral
Donna R.	di Camerino	75	Aldehyde (floral– woody)
Double Jeu	M Klein	87	
m Double Mixte	Révillon	84	
Drakkar	Laroche	72	Green
m Drakkar Noir	Laroche	82	Chypre
Dune	Dior	91	Floral (green)
m Dunhill	Dunhill	34	Floral
Durer	Durer	71	Chypre (floral– balsamic)
m Eagle	Eagle	87	
m Eau Cendrée	Jacomo	74	Chypre
Eau d'Azzaro	Azzaro	87	Fruity–green
m Eau de Balenciaga Lavande	Balenciaga	73	Lavender
Eau de Caron	Caron	80	Oriental
Eau de Cologne Hermès	Hermès	79	Citrus–minty
Eau de Fleurs	Ricci	80	Floral
Eau de Fraicheur	Weil	53	Green
Eau de Givenchy	Givenchy	80	Fruity–floral
Eau de Grès	Grès	81	
Eau de Gucci	Gucci	82	Floral
m Eau de Guerlain	Guerlain	74	Herbal
m Eau de Lanvin	Lanvin	33	Spicy
Eau de Lavande	Goutal	89	Lavender

Name	House	Year	Family/brief description
m Eau de Lavanda	4711	73	Lavender
m Eau de Monsieur	Venet	71	Woody
m Eau de Monsieur Balmain	Balmain	64	Citrus
m Eau de Patou	Patou	76	Citrus
m Eau de Sport	Eckstein	84	Chypre
m Eau de Sport	Rabanne	86	Green–fresh
m Eau de Sport Lacoste	Lacoste/Patou	69	Lavender
m Eau de Sport Santos	Cartier	89	Citrus (woody)
m Eau de Vetyver	Le Galion	61	Woody
m Eau de Vetyver	Rocher	82	Woody
m Eau d'Hadrian	Goutal	80	Citrus
Eau d'Hermès	Hermès	87	Citrus-spicy
m Eau de Caporal	L'Artisan Parfumeur	85	Citrus–floral
Eau Dynamisante	Clarins	87	
Eau Fraiche	Dior	55	Citrus
Eau Fraiche	Léonard	74	Fruity–floral– woody
m Eau Fringante	d'Orsay	69	Woody
m Eau Légère	Bourjois	72	Citrus
m **Eau Sauvage**	Dior	66	Citrus
m Eau Sauvage Extrême	Dior	84	Citrus
Ébène	Balmain	84	Chypre
m Eccelente Man	Alcina	82	Chypre
Echoes	L'Arome	87	Floral
Écusson	d'Albret	56	Aldehyde (floral)
E de C du Coq	Guerlain	1894	Citrus
m **E de C Impériale**	Guerlain	1860	Citrus
m E de C Tradition	Arden	57	Citrus
m E de T Fraiche	Marbert	76	Green
m Edition	Dunhill	90	Green
Edwardian Bouquet	Floris	1901(84)	Floral
m Ego 2 Homme	Pacoma	82	Leather
Elégance	Avon	66	Aldehyde (floral)
Eleven	Atkinsons	71	Chypre (fresh–mossy)
m Elite	Floris	79	Citrus

Name	House	Year	Family/brief description
Elizabeth Taylor's Passion, *see* Passion			
Elizabethan Rose	Penhaligon's	84	Floral
Elle	Lenthéric	79	Floral (fresh)
Embrujo de Sevilla	Myrurgia	33	Aldehyde (floral–woody)
Emeraude	Coty	21	Oriental
Empreinte	Courrèges	71	Chypre (floral–woody)
Emprise	Avon	76	Floral (fresh)
English Fern	Penhaligon's	84	Fougere
English Flowers	Taylor of London	90	Floral
m **English Lavender**	Atkinsons	10	Lavender
m English Lavender	Yardley	13	Lavender
m English Leather	Mem Comp.	49	Citrus
English Rose	Yardley	89	Floral
English Spring Flowers	Yardley	90	Floral
Enigma	de Markoff	72	Oriental
Enjoli	Ritz	78	Floral (sweet)
Envol	Lapidus	81	Floral (fruity–fresh)
Epris	Max Factor	81	Chypre (floral–sweet)
m Équipage	Hermès	70	Spicy–woody
m Eroica	Kanebo	70	Floral
Escada	Escada/ Margretha Ley	90	Floral
Escape	C. Klein	91	Floral (spicy)
Espiègle	Atkinsons	73	Green
Essence Rare	Houbigant	76	Aldehyde (floral–woody)
Estée Super	Lauder	68	Floral (sweet)
Estivalia	Puig	75	Floral (fruity–fresh)
Eternity	C. Klein	89	Floral
m Eternity for Men	C. Klein	90	Fresh–green–woody
m Etienne Aigner No. 1	Aigner	75	Chypre
m Etienne Aigner No. 2	Aigner	76	Woody
Euforia	Atkinsons	85	

Name	House	Year	Family/brief description
Evolution	Guerlain	86	
Evasion	Bourjois	70	Aldehyde (floral–woody)
Exclamation	Coty	90	Floral (fruity)
m Executive	Atkinsons	72	Spicy
Exploit	Atkinsons	68	Aldehyde (floral)
Expression	Fath	77	Oriental
Facets	Avon	89	Floral
m **Fahrenheit**	Dior	88	Woody–floral–balsamic
m Fair Play	Cerruti	84	Green
Fantasque	Feraud/Avon	81	Floral
Farala	Gal	83	
Farouche	Ricci	73	Aldehyde (floral–powdery)
Fashion	Léonard	70	Aldehyde (floral)
Fashion	Lenthéric	89	Floral (woody)
Fatale	Coty	88	Floriental
F de Ferragamo	Ferragamo	71	Chypre (floral–mossy)
Femme	Rochas	42	Chypre (mossy–fruity)
Fendi	Fendi	88	Floral
m Fendi Uomo	Fendi	89	Citrus–spicy–leathery
m Fer	Feraud/Avon	82	Fougere
Ferrari Cuvée	Satinine	88	
m Ferré Uomo	Ferré	86	Woody
Ferrose	Ferro	81	Floral
Fête	Molyneux	62	Chypre (mossy–fruity)
Fête des Roses	Caron	36	Floral
Fêtiche	Pivet	86	Floral–oriental
Fidji	Laroche	66	Floral (fresh)
Filly	Capucci	83	
First	v. Cleef & Arpels	76	Floral (fresh)
Flair	Yardley	57	Chypre
Flamme	Bourjois	76	Floral (fresh)
Fleur	Lenthéric	91	Floral
Fleurs à Fleurs	Diparco	82	Floral
Fleurs de Fleurs	Ricci	80	Floral–aldehyde

Name	House	Year	Family/brief description
Fleurs de Rocaille	Caron	33	Floral
Fleurs d'Orlane	Orlane	87	Floral (spicy)
Flor de Blason	Myrurgia	26	Fougere
Flora Danica	Swank/ Worldwide	81	Floral
Florissa	Floris	78	Floral
Folies Bergère	Folies Bergère	81	Green
Forbidden	Dana	90	Floral (woody)
m For Men	Raphael	52	Citrus
Forever	Yardley	91	Floral–oriental
Forever Krystle	Charles of the Ritz	84	Chypre
Fougère Royale	Houbigant	1882	Fougere
m Fougère Royale pour Homme	Houbigant	59	Fougere
Foxfire	Avon	81	Floral (fresh)
Fracas	Piguet	48	Floral (sweet)
m Francesco Smalto	Smalto	87	Spicy–woody
Frankincense + Myrrh	Jovan	74	Oriental
Frankincense and Myrrh	Czech & Speake	83	Balsamic
Freesia	Yardley	31	Floral
m French Line	Révillon	84	Leather
French Style	Betrix	83	Aldehyde (floral–woody)
m Furyo	Bogart	88	Woody–animalic
m Futuros	Aubusson	87	
m Gallant	Avon	89	Herbaceous– woody
m Gambler	Jovan	83	Chypre
Garconne	Illuster	78	Floral (sweet)
Gardenia	Chanel	25(89)	Floral
Gardenia Passion	Goutal	89	Floral
Gauloise	Molyneux	81	Aldehyde (floral–powdery)
Gem	v. Cleef & Arpels	87	Floriental
Geminesse	Factor	74	Chypre (floral–mossy)
Genny	Hanorah	87	Floral

Name	House	Year	Family/brief description
m Gentilhomme	Weil	67	Green
m Gentleman	Givenchy	74	Woody
Germaine	Monteil	71	Floral
m Ghibli	Atkinsons	78	Chypre
Gianfranco Ferre	Ferre/de Silva	84	Floral
m Gianfranco Ferre for Man	Ferre/de Silva	84	Chypre
Gianni Versace	Versace	82	Chypre (fresh–mossy)
Gilda	Wullf	85	
m Gilvan	Kanebo	81	Floral
Ginseng	Jovan	75	Floral (sweet)
m Ginseng for Men	Jovan	75	Spicy
Giorgio Beverly Hills	Giorgio B.H.	81	Floral
m Giorgio B.H. for Men	Giorgio B.H.	84	Woody
Givenchy III	Givenchy	71	Chypre (green)
m Givenchy Gentleman	Givenchy	75	Woody
m Glacier	Jovan	82	Citrus
Glamour	Bourjois	53	Chypre (fresh–mossy)
m Globe	Rochas	90	Woody–fruity
m G-Mans	Gainsborough	71	Floral
Goce-Goce	Morris	91	Floral
Gold	Lenthéric	77	Aldehyde (floral)
m Gold	Yardley	87	Green–woody
m Gold Medal	Atkinsons	1799	Citrus
m Golf Masters	Castillac	88	Green–woody
Graffiti	Capucci	63	Green
Grain de Folie	Verfaillie	82	Oriental
Grain de Passion	Verfaillie	85	Chypre
Grain de Sable	Verfaillie	77	Floral (fresh)
Gran Palais	Raison Pure	88	Floral
m Gran Valor	Maurer & Wirtz	72	Citrus
Grapefruit	Czech & Speake	91	Citrus
Grazia	Gherardini/ Satinine	86	
m Green Water	Fath	67	Citrus
m Grès Monsieur	Grès	82	Spicy

Name	House	Year	Family/brief description
m Grès Monsieur Sport	Grès	84	Fougere
m Grès pour Homme	Grès	65	Lavender
m Grey Flannel	Beene	76	Green
Gucci No. 1	Gucci	74	Floral
Gucci No. 3	Gucci	85	Floral
m Gucci Nobile	Gucci	88	Fougere
m Gucci pour Homme	Gucci	76	Chypre (fruity–spicy)
Guirlandes	Carven	82	Floral
Habanita	Molinard	24	Floral
m Habit Rouge	Guerlain	64	Spicy–leathery
m Hai Karate	Leeming/Paquin	67	Fougere
m Hall Mark	Lenthéric	86	Fougere
Halston	Halston	75	Aldehyde (floral–woody)
m Halston 101	Halston	84	Lavender
m Halston 1–12	Halston	76	Green
m **Halston Z-14**	Halston	76	Chypre
Halston Couture	Halston	87	Chypre (green)
Halston Night	Halston	80	Floral (sweet)
m Hammam Bouquet	Penhaligon's	1872	Floral–woody
Hanae Mori	Shiseido	75	Floral (fresh)
Hanorable	Hanorah	84	Floral
Happy Diamonds	Chopard	86	Floral
m Hardy Amies	Fine Fragrances	85	Chypre
Hascish	Veejaga	83	Chypre (fresh–balsamic)
m Hascish Homme	Veejaga	84	Leather
m Hattric Extra Dry	Olivin	72	Citrus
Havoc	Quant	74	Aldehyde (floral–woody)
m Hawk	Mennen	81	Chypre
Helietta Caracciolo	Caracciolo	81	Floral (fresh)
m Heno de Pravia	Gal	55	
m Henry M Betrix City	Betrix	79	Woody

Name	House	Year	Family/brief description
m Henry M Betrix Country	Betrix	80	Green
m Henry M Betrix Party	Betrix	84	Chypre
m Herbal for Men Old Spice	Shulton	74	Green
Herbessence	Rubinstein	62	Oriental
Herbissimo	Dana	79	Lavender and others
m Hero	Fabergé	88	Green woody
Heure Exquise	Goutal	80	Floral
Heure Intime	Vigny	33	Floral
m Hidalgo	Myrurgia	71	Citrus
Hinotori	Kanebo	69	Aldehyde (floral)
Histoire d'Amour	Aubusson	84	Floral
m Ho Hang	Balenciaga	71	Spicy
m Ho Hang Club	Belenciaga	86	
m Homme	Joop	89	Oriental
Hope	Denney	57	Aldehyde (floral)
m Hud (= Clint)	Avon	76	Chypre
m Hugo Boss	Betrix/Eurocos	86	
m Hunter	Atkinsons	87	
m Hurlingham	Atkinsons	72	Citrus
m **Imperial Leather**	Cussons	76	Fougere
Impress	Kanebo	83	Floral (fruity–fresh)
Imprévu	Coty	65	Aldehyde (floral–woody)
Impromptu	Avon	89	Floral
Indra	St Pres		Floral (spicy)
Infini	Caron	70	Aldehyde (floral)
Inoui	Shiseido	76	Green
Insolent	Jourdan	86	Floral
Inspiré	4711	78	Floral (fresh)
Interlude	Denney	62	Oriental
Intimate	Revlon	55	Chypre (floral–mossy)
Intrigue	Carven	86	Floral
Intuition	Factor	88	Floral–chypre
Iola	Avon	89	Floral (woody)

Name	House	Year	Family/brief description
m Iquitos	Delon/Ultra	87	Chypre–leather
Isa	de Varens		Floral–fruity–amber
Island Gardenia	Jovan	82	Floral (sweet)
Ispahan	Rocher	82	Oriental
It	Lenthéric	78	Floral (fresh)
Italian Style	Betrix	83	Chypre (fresh–woody)
Ivoire	Balmain	79	Floral (green)
JA	Jun Ashida	83	Floral
Jacaranda	4711	71	Chypre (fresh–mossy)
m Jacomo	Jacomo	80	Spicy
m Jade East	Swank	64	Fougere
m Jaguar for Men	Frey	89	Fruity–green–spicy
J'ai Osé	Laroche	77	Oriental
Janine D	4711	76	Green
Jardanel	Desprez	73	Aldehyde (floral–woody)
Jardins de Bagatelle	Guerlain	83	Floral
Jasmin	de Varens		Floral
Jasmin de Corse	Coty	20	Floral
Jasmine	Floris	c. 1750	Floral
m Java	St Pres		Fougere
m **Jazz**	St Laurent	88	Spicy–floral
m J Casanova pour Homme	Casanova	81	Spicy
JD	Jesse Daniel	86	Floral
m Jean-Charles	Castelbajac/4711	82	Chypre
Jean Louis Scherrer	Scherrer	80	Floral (fruity–fresh)
m Jean Marie Farina	Roger & Gallet	1806	Citrus
Je Reviens	Worth	32	Aldehyde (floral)
m JHL	Aramis	82	Spicy
Jicky	Guerlain	1889	Oriental
Jil Sander	Sander	80	Green
Jil Sander No. 4	Sander	91	Floral

Name	House	Year	Family/brief description
Jitrois	Jitrois	89	Floral (fruity)
m John Weitz	Weitz	78	Fougere
Joie de Vivre	Lenthéric	85	Floral–woody
Joker	Nerval	78	Green
Jolie Madame	Balmain	53	Chypre (floral–mossy)
Jontue	Revlon	75	Floral (sweet)
Joop!	Joop/Benckiser	88	Oriental
m Jordache Man	Jordache	83	Fougere
Jordache Woman	Jordache	83	Floral (fresh)
Jour	Feraud/Avon	84	Floral
m Jovan Grass Oil	Jovan	75	Green
m Jovan Musk Oil	Jovan/Yardley	74	Floral
Joy	Patou	35	Floral
Joya	Myrurgia	50	Aldehyde (floral–woody)
Jubilee Bouquet	Penhaligon's	77	Floral–woody
Judith	Muller	75	Floral (fresh)
m Jules	Dior	80	Fougere
Jungle Gardenia	Tuvache	57	Floral (sweet)
Just Musk	Lenthéric	73	Floral (musky)
m Juvena Men	Juvena	74	Fougere
K	Krizia	87	Floral–fruity
Kalispera	Desses	62	Floral (sweet)
m Kanon	Scannon	66	Chypre
K de Krizia	Krizia	81	Floral (fresh)
Kenzo	Kenzo	88	Floral
Keora	Couturier	83	Oriental
Kew	Florini/RBG Kew	91	Floral (spicy–woody)
Khadine	Yardley	72	Floral (fresh)
Kif	Lamborghini	81	Oriental
m King David	Muller	76	Fougere
m Kipling	Weil	86	Woody–spicy
Kiry	Marbert	77	Floral (fresh)
KL	Lagerfeld	82	Oriental
m KL Homme	Lagerfeld	86	Floral (citrus)
m Knize Ten	Knize	24	Leather
m Knize Two	Knize	78	Green
Knowing	Lauder	89	Chypre

Name	House	Year	Family/brief description
Koto	Shiseido	67	Chypre (floral–leathery)
m Kouros	St Laurent	81	Fougere
m Kouros Eau de Sport	St Laurent	86	Green
m Krizia Uomo	Krizia	84	Leather
Kyoto	Kanebo	82	Aldehyde (floral–woody)
LA	Factor	80	Oriental
La Belle Vie	Sacha Distel	85	Floral
Lace	Yardley	84	Chypre
La Cor	Menard	78	Floral
m Lacoste	Lacoste/Sofipar	84	Citrus/spicy
Lady	Jovan	83	Aldehyde (floral–woody)
Lady A	Alcina	81	Floral (fresh)
Lady 80	Kanebo	80	Floral (sweet)
m Lagerfeld	Lagerfeld	78	Spicy
Laguna	Salvador Dali	91	Floral
L'Aimant	Coty	27	Aldehyde (floral)
L'Aimant Éternelle	Coty	87	Floral
L'Air du Temps	Ricci	48	Floral (spicy)
m L'Altro Uomo	di Camerino	82	Woody
La Madrague	B. Bardot	79	Floral (sweet)
m Lamborghini Convertible	Lamborghini	79	Green
m Lamborghini GT	Lamborghini	85	Fougere
Lancetti	Lancetti/Denis	76	Green
m Lancetti Uomo	Lancetti/Denis	82	Leather
m Land	Lacoste	91	Green
La Nuit	Rabanne	85	Chypre
m Lanvanda Inglesa	Gal	68	Lavender
m Lanvin for Men	Lanvin	81	Leather
La Perla	La Perla	89	Floral
m Lapidus pour Homme	Lapidus	87	Spicy–fresh
La Rose Jacqueminot	Coty	1906	Floral
m La Selva	Bouchara	87	

Name	House	Year	Family/brief description
m Lauder for Men	Lauder	85	Floral–woody
Laughter	Tuvache	75	Floral (fresh)
Laura Ashley No 1	Ashley	90	Floral
Laura Biagiotti	Biagiotti/Betrix	82	Floral (fresh)
Lauren	Lauren	78	Floral (fruity–fresh)
m Lauren by Ralf	Lauren	90	Green
m Lavande Royale	Legrain	43	Lavender
Lavender	Yardley	13	Lavender
Lavender	Floris	1730	Lavender
m Lavender	Avon	73	Lavender
Lavender-Rosemary-Thyme	Yardley	88	Traditional floral
L'Eau du Soir	Sisley	90	Floral
Le Baiser du Faune	Molinard	30	Floral
L. de Lubin	Lubin	75	Floral (fresh)
Le Dandy	d'Orsay	26	Floral
Le de Givenchy	Givenchy	57	Floral
Le Dix	Balenciaga	47	Aldehyde (floral–woody)
L'Effleurt	Coty	1909	Floral
m **L'Égoïste**	Chanel	90	Woody–spicy
Le Jardin	Factor	82	Floral (fruity-fresh)
Le Jardin d'Amour	Factor	86	Oriental–floral
L'Élisir d'Amore	Crabtree & Evelyn	89	Floral
Le Muguet du Bonheur	Caron	52	Floral (fresh)
Le Nouveau Gardenia	Coty	33	Floral
m Léonard pour Homme	Léonard	80	Leather
Les Fleurs	Houbigant	83	Floral (fresh)
Les Iscles d'Or	Molinard	30	
Le Sport	Coty	79	Floral (fruity–fresh)
Le 3e Homme de Caron	Caron	85	Citrus–spicy
Le Temps d'Aimer	Delon/Ultra	81	Chypre (mossy–fruity)

Name	House	Year	Family/brief description
Le Vertige	Coty	36	Floral
L'Heure Attendue	Patou	46(84)	Floral
L'Heure Bleue	Guerlain	12	Floral (sweet)
m L'Homme	Roger & Gallet	82	Chypre
Liberty	Yardley	82	Floral (sweet)
Lieu du Blanc	Pola	79	Floral (fresh)
m Light Musk	Avon	78	Musk
Lily of the Valley	Floris	c. 1750	Floral (single note)
Lily of the Valley	Yardley	81	Floral
m Limes	Floris	1890	Citrus
L'Insolent	Jourdan	86	
L'Interdit	Givenchy	57	Floral–aldehyde
Liu	Guerlain	29	Floral–aldehyde
Loewe	Loewe	76	Green
m Louwe para Hombre	Loewe	78	Fougere
L'Or	Coty	12	Floral
m Lordos	Shiseido	72	Fougere
m Lord de Molyneux	Molyneux	88	Chypre
m Lords	Penhaligon's	11	Citrus–woody
m Lorenzaccio	Diparco	78	Fougere
L'Orientale	Diparco/L'Oréal	81	Oriental
L'Origan	Coty	1905	Floral (sweet)
Lou-Lou	Cacharel	87	Oriental–floral
Love's Baby Soft	Love	74	Fougere
m Luciano Soprani	COPRA	87	
m Lucky	Mas	40	Fougere
m Lucky Country	Mas	77	Fougere
Lumière	Rochas	84	Floral
Lutèce	Houbigant	86	Aldehyde (floral)
Lys Bleu	d'Orleons	81	Chypre (fresh–woody)
m M	Morabito	89	Floral–oriental
m **Macassar**	Rochas	80	Leather
m Macho	Fabergé	76	Fougere
Macho Musk	Fabergé	82	Musk
Madame de Carven	Carven	79	Floral (fresh)

Name	House	Year	Family/brief description
Madame Jovan	Jovan	75	Aldehyde (floral–woody)
Madame Rochas	Rochas	60	Aldehyde (floral)
Mademoiselle Ricci	Ricci	67	Green
Maderas de Oriente	Myrurgia	18	Floral (sweet)
Madrigal	Molinard	35	Floral
Maëlle pour Enfant	Clayeux/Puig	86	Citrus–sweet
Magie Noire	Lancôme	78	Oriental
Magnolia	Rocher	83	Floral
m Magnum	Avon	89	Green–citrus
Ma Griffe	Carven	44	Chypre (fresh–mossy)
m Mahé Off Shore	Victor	82	Chypre
Mai	Shiseido	68	Floral
Maissa	Vermeil	87	Floral
Ma Liberté	Patou	87	Spicy–floral
Malmaison	Floris	early 19th c.	Spicy–floral
m Man	Jovan	77	Leather
m Man III	Sander	88	
m Man IV	Sander	91	Green
m Mandate	Shulton	77	Fougere
m Man Pure	Sander	81	Leather
m Marbert Man	Marbert	77	Fougere
Marbert Woman	Marbert	87	Floral
m Marc Cross	Cross	78	Spicy
Marilyn Monroe	East West/Colorkit	83	Floral (sweet)
Marta	Battistoni	86	
Mary Quant	Factor	81	Fruity–floral
m Masculin Acier	Bourjois	88	
m Masculin Or	Bourjois	76	
m Masculin 2	Bourjois	75	Woody
Masumi	Coty	68	Chypre (fresh–mossy)
m Matchabelli	Matchabelli	82	Leather
m Match Play	Bergerat	91	Woody
Maxi	Factor	76	Aldehyde (floral–mossy)

Name	House	Year	Family/brief description
Maxims de Paris	Cardin/SNDPIM	85	Floral
Me	Coparel	78	Floral
Megara	Le Galion	78	Floral
Mémoire	Shiseido	63	Oriental
Mémoire Chérie	Arden	57	Aldehyde (floral–powdery)
m Men	Mennen	82	Chypre
m Men's Classic	Cantilene/Payot	77	Fougere
m **Men's Club**	Rubinstein	66	Floral
m Men's Club 52	Rubinstein	72	Citrus
m Men's Cologne	Cardin	72	Spicy
m Men's Style	Juvena	82	Fougere
m Men Two	Sander	82	Woody
Mérefame	Menard	79	Aldehyde (floral)
Métal	Rabanne	79	Floral (fresh)
Métamorphose	Laporte/L'Artisan Parfumeur	79	Floral
Meteor	Coty	51	Floral
m Metropolis	Lauder	88	Woody
m MG 5	Shiseido	67	Fougere
m MG 5 Lavender	Shiseido	67	Lavender
Michelle	Balenciaga	80	Floral (sweet)
Mila Schön	Schön	81	Chypre (floral–mossy)
m Milano Cento	Milano Cento	89	Citrus–woody
Mille ('1000')	Patou	73	Floral (woody)
Millefleurs	Crabtree & Evelyn	80	Floral
m Millionaire	Menner	79	Fougere
Mimosa	Czech & Speake	82	Floral–green
m Ming	Coryse Salome	82	Fougere
Ming de Dinasty	Dinasty	83	
Mink + Pearls	Jovan	68	Chypre (floral–mossy)
Miss Balmain	Balmain	68	Chypre (floral–woody)
Miss de Rauch	de Rauch	68	Aldehyde (floral)
Miss Dior	Dior	47	Chypre (floral–woody)
Miss Factor	Factor	73	Chypre (fresh–sweet)
Missoni	Missoni	81	Chypre (fresh–mossy)

Name	House	Year	Family/brief description
m Missoni Uomo	Missoni	83	Chypre (fresh–mossy)
Miss Worth	Worth	77	Floral (sweet)
Misty Tea Rose	Jovan	83	Aldehyde (floral)
Mitsouko	Guerlain	19	Chypre (fresh–fruity–mossy)
Molinard de Molinard	Molinard	81	Citrus (fruity–fresh)
Moment Suprême	Patou	33	Floral (spicy)
Moments	Colonia/Mulhens	90	Chypre (floral)
Mon Classique	Morabito	87	Floral
m Monogram	Lauren	85	
Mon Parfum	Paloma Picasso/ L'Oréal	84	Chypre
m Monsieur Carven	Carven	78	Spicy
m Monsieur de Givenchy	Givenchy	59	Citrus–woody
m Monsieur de Grès	Grès	82	
m Monsieur de Rauch	de Rauch	73	Citrus
m Monsieur F	Ferragamo	76	Lavender
m Monsieur Houbigant	Houbigant	69	Chypre
m Monsieur Jovan	Jovan	77	Spicy
m Monsieur Lanvin	Lanvin	64	Green
m Monsieur Net	Patou	55	Citrus
m Monsieur Note Havane	Roger & Gallet	70	Spicy
m Monsieur Rochas	Rochas	69	Fougere
m Monsieur Worth	Worth	69	Fougere
Montaigne	Caron	86	
Montana	Montana	87	Chypre
m **Montana pour l'Homme**	Montana	90	Spicy–woody
Moods	Krizia	90	Floral (spicy)
Moon Drops	Revlon	70	Floral (sweet)
Moonwind	Avon	71	Aldehyde (floral–woody)
More	Shiseido	71	Aldehyde (floral)
m Moschino	Euroitalia	87	Green

Name	House	Year	Family/brief description
Moschus Love Dream	Astor	86	
Moss Rose	Floris	1850(1981)	Floral
m Motor Racing	Segura	73	Green
m Moustache	Rochas	49	Lavender
Muguet des Bois	Coty	41	Floral (fresh)
Murasaki	Shiseido	80	Green
Muse	Coty	46	Floral
m Musk Cologne	Jovan	74	Musk
m Musk English Leather	Mem Comp.	74	Musk
m Musk for Men	Avon	82	Musk
m Musk for Men	Fabergé	76	Musk
m Musk for Men	Nerval	79	Musk
m Musk for Men	Yardley	74	Musk
m Musk for Men Old Spice	Shulton	74	Musk
Musk for Women	Jovan/Yardley	76	Floriental–musk
m Musk Monsieur	Houbigant	77	Musk
Must	Cartier	81	Oriental
My Melody	4711	79	Floral (fresh)
Mystère	Rochas	78	Aldehyde (floral)
Mystique	Lenthéric	81	Aldehyde (floral)
Nahéma	Guerlain	79	Oriental (woody–floral)
Naj Oleari	Euroitalia	89	Floral
m Napoleon	Juper	47	Citrus
Narcisse Noir	Caron	12	Oriental
Neroli	Czech & Speake	84	Citrus
m New West	Aramis	90	Citrus
Night Fall	Avon	88	Floral (mossy)
Nights in White Satin	Yardley	90	Floral–oriental
Niki de Saint Phalle	PPI	84	Floral
Nina	Ricci	87	Floral (woody)
Ninja	de Coeur	81	
m Nino Cerutti	Cerutti	79	Green–floral
Nino Cerutti pour Femme	Cerutti	87	Floral

Name	House	Year	Family/brief description
Nipon	Nipon	82	Chypre (fresh–balsamic)
Nirmala	Molinard	55	Oriental
Nishiki	Shiseido	73	Aldehyde (floral–powdery)
Nitchevo	Juvena	73	Chypre (fresh–mossy)
m No. 88	Czech & Speake	81	Woody
m No. 89 for Men	Floris	58	Floral
m Nobile	Gucci	89	Citrus–tobacco
Nocturnes	Caron	81	Aldehyde (floral–powdery)
Noha-in	Perac	84	
m Noir	Roberre/Rimmel	82	Chypre
m Nomade	d'Orsay	73	Woody
Nombre Noir	Shiseido	82	Aldehyde (floral)
Nonchalance	Mäurer & Wirtz	60	Aldehyde (floral)
Norell	Revlon	69	Floral (fresh)
Norell II	Revlon	80	Chypre (green–woody)
Normandie	Patou	35	Floral
Nuance	Coty	75	Aldehyde (floral–woody)
Nueva Maja	Myrurgia	60	Chypre (fresh–balsamic)
Nuit de Longchamp	Lubin	56	Floral
Nuit de Noel	Caron	22	Oriental
Nuit d'Été	Joop	90	Floral
Number One	Betrix	77	Floral
Number Two	Betrix	78	Floral (fresh)
Number Six	Betrix	79	Oriental
Oasis	Myrurgia	80	
Obsession	C. Klein	85	Floriental
m Obsession for Men	C. Klein	88	Floriental
Occur	Avon	63	Chypre (floral–animalic)
Ô de Lancôme	Lancôme/L'Oréal	69	Fresh–citrus
Odyssey	Avon	81	Floral

Name	House	Year	Family/brief description
m Off Shore	Victor	76	Woody
Ô Intense	Lancôme/L'Oréal	86	
m Old Brown	Parera	77	Fougere
m Old Spice	Shulton	37	Spicy
m Old Spice Fresh Lime	Shulton	65	Citrus
m Oleg Cassini for Men	Jovan	79	Woody
Oleg Cassini for Women	Jovan	78	Aldehyde (floral– woody)
m Oltas	Lion	82	Green
Omar Sharif pour Femme	Prestige	90	Green–fruity
Ombre Rose	Brosseau/Patou	82	Aldehyde (floral– powdery)
m One Man Show	Bogart	80	Leather
Only	Iglesias/Myrurgia	89	Floral
m Onyx	Lenthéric	64	Floral
Open	Roger & Gallet/ Sanofi	85	Floral
Opera	Coryse Salome	32	Aldehyde (floral)
Ophelia	Avon	88	Floral
Opium	St Laurent	77	Oriental
Or	Torrente	80	Chypre (fresh– woody)
m Or Black	Morabito	82	Leather
Orfea	de Varens		Floral
Orgia	Myrurgia	73	Aldehyde (floral)
m Oriental Spice (= Eastern Spice)	Shulton	73	Chypre
m Original Musk	Mennen	82	Musk
m Or Masculin	Bourjois	72	Citrus
Ormonde	Floris	57	Fougere
Or Noir	Morabito	81	Floral
Oscar de la Renta	Sanofi	76	Floral (sweet)
m **Paco Rabanne pour Homme**	Rabanne	73	Fougere
Pagan	Jovan		Oriental
m Pagan Man	Yardley		Woody–mossy
Paillettes	Coveri	84	

Name	House	Year	Family/brief description
Panache	Lenthéric	77	Aldehyde (floral)
Panache-Evening	Lenthéric	89	Floral (green–fruity)
Pancaldi	Hanorah	88	
Panthère	Cartier	87	Floral (woody)
Paradoxe	Cardin	83	Chypre (floral–leather)
Parfum de Femme	Goutal	82	Floral
Parfum d'Elle	Montana	90	Floral
Parfum d'Hermès	Hermès	84	Floriental
Parfum Rare	Jacomo	85	Chypre
Parfum Sacré	Caron	90	Floral (amber–spicy)
Paris	Coty	21	Floral
Paris	St Laurent	83	Floral
Park Avenue	Avon	87	Citrus
Partage	Fabergé	79	Chypre (green–woody)
m Partner	Révillon	60	Spicy
Parure	Guerlain	75	Chypre (floral–fruity)
Passion	Goutal	80	Floral
Passion-El. Taylor	Chesbrough Pounds/P. International	88	Floriental
m Patou pour Homme	Patou	80	Spicy
m Patrichs	Phillipe	76	Fougere
Pavlova	Payot	76	Floral (sweet)
Pearls and Lace	Avon	85	Floral (mossy)
Pêle-Mêle	Rouff		Floral
Perry Ellis	Ellis/Stern	85	Floral
Petunia	Yardley	88	Floral
Phéromone	Miglin	78	Green
m Phileas	Ricci	84	Chypre (woody)
m Photo	Lagerfeld	90	Fresh citrus
m Pierre Cardin	Cardin	76	Citrus
m Piment	Payot	79	Spicy
Pink Lace	Yardley	88	Floral–chypre
m Pino Silvestre	Vidal	55	Lavender
m Pitralon	Lingner	70	Citrus

Name	House	Year	Family/brief description
m Pitralon Sport	Jovan	84	Fougere
Poésie	4711	83	Floral
Poison	Dior	85	Spicy–fruity–amber
m **Polo**	Warner/Lauren/ L'Oréal	78	Chypre
Pomellato	Sirpea	89	Floral
m Portos	Balenciaga	80	Chypre
m Pour Homme	Balenciaga	90	Woody–spicy
m Pour Lui	de la Renta	81	Leather
m Pour Monsieur	Chanel	61	Floral
m Pour un Homme	Caron	34	Leather
Prélude	Balenciaga	82	Oriental
Première	Castelbajac/4711	81	Floral (sweet)
Présence	Parquet	90	Floral (woody–spicy)
m **Prestige Dry Herb**	Wolff & Sohn	60	Green
m **Prestige for Men Cool Frost**	Wollf & Sohn	72	Citrus
Prêt à Porter	Perfumers Workshop	80	Floral
Princess d'Albret	d'Albret	64	Floral
Private Collection	Lauder	73	Green
Prophecy	Matchabelli	74	Aldehyde (floral)
Ptisenbon	Tartine et Choc./Givenchy	87	Floral
m Pullmann	Dana	68	Fougere
m Punjab	Capucci	79	Chypre
Pure Silk	Yardley	82	Floral–chypre
m Pyn's Colonia	Parera	69	Citrus
Quadrille	Balenciaga	55(85)	Chypre (fresh–mossy)
Quant by Quant	Quant	80	Green
Quartz	Molyneux/Sanofi	77	Floral (fruity–fresh)
Quelques Fleurs	Houbigant	12(88)	Floral
Que Sais-Je	Patou	25(84)	Floral (fruity)
m **Quorum**	Puig	82	Leather
m Racquet Club	Mem Comp.	78	Floral
Rafale	Molinard	75	Floral (fresh)

Name	House	Year	Family/brief description
m Rafale pour Homme	Molinard	80	Citrus
Raffinée	Houbigant	82	Floriental
m Raffles	Fine Fragrances	89	Floral
Raphael	Mulhens 4711	85	(Various)
m Rapport	Shulton	88	Chypre
Rare	Jacomo	88	Floral
Ravissa	Mäurer & Wirtz	79	Green
m R de Capucci	Capucci	87	Woody – fruity – spicy
Red	Giorgio Bev Hills/ Avon	89	Fleuriffe – chypre
Red	Beene	76	Chypre (fresh– mossy)
Red Door	Arden	89	Floral
Red Rose	Floris	1868	Floral
Reflections	Avon	89	Floral
Regina Schrecker	Arval	87	Floral
Regine's	Interperfume	90	Fresh – fruity
Réplique	Raphael	47	Oriental
m Reporter	Cassini	78	Fougere
Rêverie	Tuvaché	75	Chypre (floral– woody)
Révillon 4	Révillon	73	Aldehyde (floral– woody)
m Révillon pour Homme	Révillon	77	Chypre
m **Ricci Club**	Ricci	89	Fruity – woody– mossy
Risqué	Juvena	70	Aldehyde (floral)
Ritz	Charles of the Ritz	72	Floral (fresh)
Rivage	Shiseido	74	Floral
Rive Gauche	St Laurent	70	Aldehyde (floral– woody)
Robe d'un Soir	Carven	47	Aldehyde (floral– woody)
m Rockford	Atkinsons	85	Spicy
m Rodeo	Wollf & Sohn	82	Leather
Roma	Betrix/Revlon	90	Oriental (sweet– fruity)
Romeo	Romeo Gigli	91	Floral
Rose	Czech & Speake	85	Floral

Name	House	Year	Family/brief description
Rose Absolue	Goutal	82	Floral
Rose Cardin	Cardin	90	Floral
Rose de Bulgari	Bulgari	87	Floral
Rose de Noël	Caron	39	Floral
Rose de Rouge	Gemey	86	Floral
Rose Geranium	Floris	c. 1750	Floral
Roses	Yardley	81	Floral
Rosewater	Crabtree & Evelyn	87	Floral
m Rothschild	Rothschild	82	Chypre
m Rouge	Lubin	81	Leather
m **Royal Copenhagen**	Swank	70	Chypre
m Royal Copenhagen Sport	Swank	82	Chypre
m Royal Eroica	Kanebo	74	Floral
Royal Secret	Monteil	58	Oriental
m Royale Ambrée	Legrain	51	Citrus
m Royall Bay Rhum	Royall Lyme	55	Spicy
m Royall Lyme	Royall Lyme	55	Citrus
m Royall Muske	Royall Lyme	82	Musk
m Royall Spice	Royall Lyme	55	Spicy
Rubis	de Varens		Oriental
Ruffles	de la Renta	83	Floral (sweet)
m Rugger	Avon	82	Spicy
Rumba	Balenciaga	88	Floral (fruity)
m Russich Leder	Farina Gegenuber	67	Leather
Sabatini	G. Sabatini	91	Floral (green)
Safari	Lauren	90	Floral–oriental
m Sagamore	Lancôme/L'Oréal	84	Chypre
Salvador Dali	COFCI	83	Floriental
m Samarcande	Rocher	88	Woody–spicy
Samba	Perfumers Workshop	87	Floral
Samsara	Guerlain	89	Oriental
Sandalwood	Floris	1820	Oriental (woody)
m **Sandalwood**	Arden	57	Woody
m Santos	Cartier	81	Woody
Saphir	de Varens		Floral
Sarabe	Juvena	80	Oriental
Sa So	Shiseido	87	Floral (aldehyde)

Name	House	Year	Family/brief description
m SC	Beiersdorf	80	Green
Scandale	Lanvin	31	Leather
Scherrer 2	Scherrer	86	Floriental
Schön Goutte	Menard	78	Aldehyde (floral–woody)
Scoundrel	Revlon/Collins	80	Floral (fruity–fresh)
Sculptura	Jovan	81	Chypre
Secret de Venus	Weif	41	Chypre
Selection	Lancaster	77	Floral
Senchal	Charles of the Ritz	81	Chypre (floral–woody)
Sens	CMC/Vermeil	85	
Senso	Camarino	72	Chypre (floral–woody)
Senso	Ungaro	87	Floral–oriental
Septième Sens	Rykiel	79	Chypre (fruity–animalic)
Serenade	Avon	89	
m Sergio Tacchini	Tacchini/Morris	87	Green–spicy
m Sex Appeal	Jovan	76	Spicy
Sex Appeal for Women	Jovan	78	Green
Sfera	Faux	90	Floral
Shalimar	Guerlain	25	Oriental
Shalom	Muller	70	Chypre (fruity–leathery)
Shandoah	Heim	60	Floral
Sheherazade	Desprez	83	Chypre (aldehydic–sweet)
m Shendy	Roger & Gallet	70	Citrus
Shocking	Schiaparelli	35	Oriental
Shocking You	Schiaparelli	76	Green
Shuni	Goya	77	
m Sicilian Lime	Crabtree & Evelyn	77	Citrus
Signature	Hallden	88	
m Signor	Victor	74	Citrus
m Signoricci	Ricci	65	Green
m Signoricci 2	Ricci	76	Citrus
m Signor Vivara	Pucci	70	Chypre
Sikkim	Lancôme	71	Chypre (floral–animalic)
Silences	Jacomo	79	Green

Name	House	Year	Family/brief description
m Silver	Aigner	84	Chypre
Silverline	Gainsborough	72	Green
m Silver Shadow	Chantal du Monde	84	Leather
m **Silvestre**	Victor	46	Lavender
Sinan	Sinan	81(90)	Floral
m Sir Canada Ceder	4711	71	Leather
m Sir Champaca	4711	78	Fougere
m Sir Gregory	Zuma	84	
m **Sir Irisch Moos**	4711	69	Chypre
m Skin Bracer	Mennen	31	Fougere
m Skin Bracer Dry Lime	Mennen	67	Citrus
m Skin Bracer Wild Moss	Mennen	67	Fougere
m Smalto	Smalto	87	Fougere
Smitty	Coty	76	
Snob	Le Galion	37	Floral
m Snuff	Schiaparelli	77	Leather
Society	Burberry	91	Floral
Soft Musk	Avon	83	Aldehyde (floral–woody)
Soin pour Homme	Rabanne	84	
Soir de Paris	Bourjois	29	Floral (sweet)
Sonnet	Avon	72	
Sophia	Coty	80	Floral
Sortilège	Le Galion	38	Aldehyde (floral)
Sourire	Shiseido	77	Floral
Sous le Vent	Guerlain	33	Chypre
Sparta	Gal	86	
Special No. 127	Floris	1890	Floral
Spectacular	Joan Collins/ Parlux	90	Floral
Spellbound	Lauder	91	Floral–oriental
m Sport de Paco Rabanne	Rabanne	90	Fruity
m Sport Fragrance	Aigner	79	Citrus
m Sporting Club	Coryse Salome	65	Citrus
m Sport Scent for Men	Jovan	78	Fougere

Name	House	Year	Family/brief description
Sport Scent for Women	Jovan	78	Green
m Spring Water	Coryse Salome	74	Green
m Squash	Dana	84	Spicy
Stephanie	Bourjois	90	Floral
Stephanotis	Floris	pre-1800	Floral
m Stetson	Coty	81	Chypre
m Storm	Elida Gibbs	85	
Strategy	Mary Chess	35	Oriental
Style	Lenthéric	87	Chypre (floral–fruity)
Style	Avon	78	Green
Sung	Sung	89	Floral
m Sung Homme	Sung/Riviera Concepts	88	Fruity–woody
Super Fragrance	Aigner	78	Aldehyde (floral–woody)
m Super Fragrance for Men	Aigner	78	Spicy
Surreal (= Toccasa)	Avon	73	Aldehyde
Suzuro	Shiseido	76	Floral
Swann	Pacoma	84	
Sweet Honesty	Avon	73	Floral (sweet)
m **Sybaris**	Puig	88	Green–spicy
Symbiose	Stendhal	80	Floral
Tabac Blond	Caron	19	Tobacco
m **Tabac Original**	Mäurer & Wirtz	59	Floral
Tabu	Dana	31(77)	Oriental
m Tactics	Shiseido	79	Green
m Tailoring for Men	Clinique/Lauder	84	Citrus
m Tai Winds	Avon	71	Fougère
Tamango	Leonard	77	Aldehyde (floral)
Tamoré	Nerval	76	Green
m Tanamar	Parera	77	Citrus
Tapestry	Mary Chess	34	Oriental
Tasha	Avon	81	Aldehyde (floral)
Tatiana	v. Furstenberg	75	Floral
m Taxi	COFCI	86	
m Team	Femia	75	Spicy

Name	House	Year	Family/brief description
Tea Rose	Perfumers Workshop	75	Floral
Teatro alla Scala	Krizia/Florbath	86	Floral
m Tech 21	Shiseido	84	Green
m Teck	Molinard	90	Warm–woody
m Ted	Lapidus	78	Leather
m Temujin	Kanebo	78	Chypre
Tendance	Marbert	80	Aldehyde (floral–woody)
Tendresse	Atkinsons	57	Aldehyde (floral–powdery)
m Ténéré	Rabanne	88	Spicy–floral
m Terre du Sud	M. Klein	90	Spicy–amber
m **That Man**	Revlon	61	Chypre
m The Baron	Evyan	65	Floral
Theosiris	Bouchara	87	Floral
m Thor	Castillac	88	Green
Tiffany	Tiffany	87	Floral (fruity)
Tigress	Fabergé	44	Aldehyde (floral–powdery)
m Timberline	Engl. Leather Mem Comp.	68	Woody
Timeless	Avon	74	Chypre (floral–balsamic)
Tita Rossi	COFCI	87	
Toccara *see* Surreal			
Topaze	Avon	59	Aldehyde (floral)
Torrente	Torrente	77	Floral
m Toro	Marbert	80	Leather
Tosca	4711	21	Aldehyde (floral–powdery)
Touché	Jovan	80	Aldehyde (floral–powdery)
Tramp	Lenthéric	75	Floral (green)
Trance	Betrix	88	Spicy, fruity, amber
m Transart	Jouvance	88	
m Trazarra (= Nexus)	Avon	78	Spicy
Trésor	Lancôme	90	Floral–oriental

Name	House	Year	Family/brief description
Trigère	Trigère	73	Aldehyde (floral–woody)
m Trimaran	Rocher	86	
Tristano Onofri	Babor	87	Floral
m Trophée	Lancôme/L'Oréal	82	Citrus
m Trouble	Mennen/Revlon	70	Chypre
Trussardi	Trussardi	80	Chypre
Trussardi Action	Trussardi	90	Floral
m Trussardi Uomo	Trussardi	84	Leather
m **Tsar**	V. Cleef & Arpels	89	Chypre
Tubereuse	Goutal	87	Floral
Tuberose	Chess	37	Floral
m Turbo	Fabergé	80	Leather
Turbulences	Révillon	81	Floral (fruity–fresh)
m Tuscany	Aramis	84	Fougere
Tuvara	Tuvaché	65	Oriental
Tuxedo	Warner/Lauren	78	Aldehyde (floral)
Tweed	Lenthéric	33	Aldehyde (floral–powdery)
m Ulric	de Varens		Green
Ultima II	Revlon	67	Oriental
Unforgettable	Avon	66	
Unforgettable	Revlon	90	Floral–oriental
Ungaro	Ungaro	77	Floral (fruity–fresh)
Ungaro d'Ungaro	Ungaro	90	Floral
m Un Homme	Jourdan	79	Fougere
Uninhibited	Cher	88	Floral (aldehyde)
Un Jour	Jourdan	83	Floral (fruity–fresh)
Unspoken	Avon	75	Floral (sweet)
Vacances	Patou	36	Floral
m Valcan	Kanebo	76	Spicy
Valentino	Valentino/Stern	79	Floral
Vallée des Rois	Mira Takla	91	Floriental
m **Van Cleef & Arpels**	V. Cleef & Arpels	78	Leather
Vanderbilt	Vanderbilt	81	Floral (sweet)
Van Gils	Van Gils	90	Citrus–woody–spicy
m Varens for Men	de Varens		Green

Name	House	Year	Family/brief description
m Varens Rouge	de Varens		Green
m Varens Vert	de Varens		Green
m Varon Dandy	Parera	24	Woody
m V by Victor	Victor	72	Lavender
V'E	Charles of the Ritz	90	Chypre
Venise	Rocher	86	Floral–oriental
Vent Vert	Balmain	45	Green
m Verlande	Gillette	80	Chypre
Veronese	de Varens		Green
Versace	Charles of the Ritz	82	Chypre
m Versace l'Homme	Charles of the Ritz	84	Citrus–floral–spicy
m Versailles pour Homme	Desprez	80	Spicy
m Version Originale	Sinan	84	Fougere
m Vetiver	Guerlain	61	Woody
m **Vétiver pour Homme**	Carven	57	Woody
m Vetiver de Puig	Puig	78	Woody
m Vetyver	Lanvain	64	Woody
m Vetyver	Roger & Gallet	74	Woody
m Vetyver Dry	Carven	88	Woody
Via Condotti	Lancetti/Dennis	85	
Via Lanvin	Lanvin	71	Floral (sweet)
Via Passion	Diparco/L'Oréal	86	
Vicky Tiel	Tiel	90	Floral
Victorian Posy	Penhaligon's	79	Floral
Vie Privée	Rocher	89	Floral
Vincent Van Gogh	Royal Sanders	90	Floral
m Vintage	Shiseido	75	Chypre
m VIP Special Reserve	Giorgio B Hills	86	Fruity–spicy–woody
Visa	Piguet	45	Chypre
Vison	Beaulieu	86	Floral (fruity)
Vivara	Pucci	65	Green
Vivre	Molyneux	71	Aldehyde (floral)
V.O.	Sinan	84	
Voice	Lenclos	87	Floral
Volcan d'Amour	v. Furstenberg	81	Floral
Vol de Nuit	Guerlain	45	Oriental
Votre	Jourdan	78	Floral

Name	House	Year	Family/brief description
Voyou	Klein/Beaute Createurs	87	
VSP	Jovan	73	Floral
Vu	Lapidus	76	Oriental
m Wall Street	Victor/di Modrone	84	Chypre
m Weekend	Avon	78	Spicy
Weil de Weil	Weil	71	Green
m Weil pour Homme	Weil	80	Floral
m West	Fabergé	74	Fougere
m West Indian Cologne	Crabtree & Evelyn	89	Citrus
White Flowers	Astor	83	Floral (fruity–fresh)
White Lilac	Chess	32	Floral (single)
White Linen	Lauder	78	Aldehyde (floral)
White Satin	Yardley	85	Floral
White Shoulders	Evyan	45	Floral
m Wild Country	Avon	67	Fougere
Wild Hyacinth	Floris	1835	Floral
m Wild Musk	Coty	68	Musk
m Wind Drift	Mem Comp.	70	Floral
m Windjammer	Avon	68	Citrus
Wind Song	Matchabelli	53	Floral
Woman	Jovan	77	Oriental
Woman Two	Sander	83	Chypre (floral–woody)
Woman III	Sander	87	Floral
Woodhue	Fabergé	49	Oriental
m Woodhue for Men	Fabergé	38	Woody
m Worth pour Homme	Worth	80	Fougere
m **Xeryus**	Givenchy	86	Semi-oriental
Xia-Xiang	Revlon	88	Oriental
Xmas Bells	Molinard	26	Floral
Y	St Laurent	64	Green
m Yacaré	Astor	81	Woody
m Yachtman	Mas	73	Lavender

Name	House	Year	Family/brief description
m Yatagan	Caron	76	Leather
Yendi	Capucci	75	Floral (sweet)
Yesterday	Marbert	79	Aldehyde (floral)
Yolai	Cantilene	76	Floral
You're the Fire	Yardley	89	Floral
Youth Dew	Lauder	52	Oriental
Yram	Chess	38	Oriental
Ysatis	Givenchy	84	Floriental
m YSL pour Homme	St Laurent	71	Chypre
Zadig	Pucci	73	Oriental
Zagara	Zuma	43	Floral
Zany	Avon	81	Fougere
Zarolia	Barclay	81	Floral
Zen	Shiseido	64	Floral
Zibeline	Weil	28	Aldehyde (floral–woody)
Zinnia	Floris	90	Floral
m 6-0	Bjorn Borg/Romella	86	Green
Zème Sens *see* Septième Sens			
m 12	Couturier	82	Fougere
m 20–21	Fabergé	78	Chypre
273	Hayman	90	Floral (fruity)
1000 *see* Mille			
1811	Molinard	30	
1881	Cerruti	90	Chypre (citrus–woody)

Appendix B Perfume recipes and formulas

The recipes and formulas in this appendix have been selected partly to illustrate the history of perfume making and partly to provide persons wishing to try making their own fragrances with a variety of fairly simple examples (see **Perfume Making at Home**).

1. A long-lasting pot pourri

'The following mixture is said to retain its fragrance for fifty years: Gather early in the day, and when perfectly dry, a peck of Roses, pick off the petals and strew over them three-quarters of a pound of common salt. Let them remain two or three days, and if fresh flowers are added, some more salt must be sprinkled over them. Mix with the Roses half a pound of finely pounded bay salt, the same quantity of allspice, cloves and brown sugar, a quarter of a pound of gum benzoin, and two ounces of powdered orris root. Add one gill of brandy and any sort of fragrant flowers, such as Orange and Lemon flowers, Lavender and Lemon-scented Verbena, and any other sweet-scented flowers. They should be perfectly dry when added. The mixture must be occasionally stirred and kept in close-covered jars, the covers to be raised only when the perfume is desired in the room. If after a time the mixture seems to dry, moisten with brandy only, as essences soon lose their quality and injure their perfume.'

(Donald McDonald: *Fragrant Flowers and Leaves*, 1895)

2. Lavender pot pourri

To $1\frac{1}{2}$ mugsful of dried lavender flowers and leaves add 1 cupful of dried rose petals and another containing a mixture of dried and lightly crushed rosemary, bay and mint leaves, cloves and cinnamon, lemon peel and a little nutmeg. Mix into this a $\frac{1}{2}$ cupful of gum benzoin and strengthen with a few drops of lavender oil.

3. A winter pot pourri

1 quart mixed alder cones, pine cones (which may be further scented by painting their centres with pine oil), pine needles, juniper tips and

scented conifer tips; 2 oz mixed scented evergreen leaves, comprising myrtle, bay, eucalyptus and box; 1 oz fine-ground gum benzoin; 1 oz lavender; 2 teaspoon cinnamon powder; $\frac{1}{2}$ teaspoon whole cloves; $\frac{1}{2}$ vanilla pod; 2 drops each of lavender oil, pine oil and lemon oil. Add Caen anemones to decorate.

(After Penny Black: *The Book of Pot Pourri*, 1989)

4. A 'Turkish' pot pourri

1 quart mixed rose petals and buds, jasmine and orange blossom; 2 oz mixed patchouli leaves, scented geranium leaves, basil and marjoram; 1 oz lavender; peel of an orange; 1 oz cedarwood shavings; 1 oz fine-ground gum benzoin; 2 cinnamon sticks; 1 teaspoon whole cloves; $\frac{1}{2}$ teaspoon grated nutmeg; 2 drops each of lavender oil and rose oil; 1 drop each of lemon oil and patchouli oil. Add flowers to decorate.

(After Penny Black: *The Book of Pot Pourri*, 1989)

5. An 'American-Indian' pot pourri

Into 6 oz of lavender flowers mix 2 oz each of sandalwood shavings and orange leaves, 1 oz each of orris root and tonka beans, both well ground, and $\frac{1}{2}$ oz of chopped oak moss. Sprinkle with a few drops of patchouli oil.

(Adapted from Ann Tucker Fettner: *Pot Pourri*, 1983)

6. Moist pot pourri

'2 oz bay salt, $\frac{1}{2}$ oz of cloves, 6 pennyworth of musk, beat all fine together. No flowers but rose leaves and lavender. The rose leaves must be dried a little on sheets of paper before they are put into a jar. Strew in a few of the rose leaves and lavender, then a little of the mixture, and so on until the jar is filled.'

(From an English Housekeeping Book, *c.* 1840,
English Heritage (unpublished)).

7. Rose pot pourri: a Devonshire recipe

'Gather flowers in the morning when dry and lay them in the sun till the evening: Roses, Orange Flowers, Jasmine, Lavender, and, in smaller quantities, Thyme, Sage, Marjoram and Bay. Put them in an earthen wide jar or hand basin in layers. Add the following ingredients: 6 lb Bay Salt, 4 oz each of Acorus calamus root, Cassia buds and Gum Benzoin, 2 oz each of Cinnamon and Cloves, 1 oz each of Storax calamite and Otto of rose, 1 drachm Musk, $\frac{1}{2}$ oz powdered Cardamime seeds. Place the rose leaves etc. in layers in the jar. Sprinkle the Bay salt and other ingredients on each layer, press it tightly down and keep for two or three months before taking it out.'

(Lady Rosalind Northcote: *The Book of Herbs*, 1904)

8. Moist pot pourri: a piquant floral mix

1 quart crumbled petals of rose or other sweet-scented flowers or leaves; 2 oz rose geranium leaves; 1 oz lavender; 1 oz orris root powder; dried rind of $\frac{1}{2}$ lemon; 1 crushed tonquin bean; $\frac{1}{2}$ teaspoon ground allspice; $\frac{1}{2}$ teaspoon grated nutmeg; 2 drops each of lavender oil, rose geranium oil and lemon oil.

(After Penny Black: *The Book of Pot Pourri*, 1989)

9. A sleeping sachet

'A Bag to Smell Unto for Melancholy, or to Cause One to Sleep. Take drie Rose leaves (petals), keep them close in a glasse which will keep them sweet, then take powder of Mints, powder of Cloves in a grosse powder, and put the same to the Rose leaves, then put all these together in a bag, and take that to bed with you, and it will cause you to sleep, and it is good to smell unto at other times.'

(*Ram's Little Dodoen*, 1606)

10. Sweet bag for linen

'Take 1 lb each of orris roots, sweet calamus, cypress roots, dried lemon peel, dried orange peel and dried roses. Make all these into a gross powder. Take coriander seeds 4 oz, nutmegs $1\frac{1}{2}$ oz, cloves 1 oz, mix them all into a fine powder and then mix with the other. Add musk and ambergris. Then take 4 large handfuls of lavender flowers dried and rubbed, a handful each of sweet marjoram, orange leaves and walnut leaves, all dried and rubbed. Mix all together with some bits of cotton perfumed with essences and put it up into silk bags to lay with your linen.'

(from *The Compleat Housewife*, Williamsburg, 1742)

11. A lavender sachet

For a Lavender Sachet. Ground lavender flowers, 1 lb; gum benzoin in powder, $\frac{1}{2}$ lb; attar of lavender (essential oil), $\frac{1}{4}$ oz.

(G.W.S.Piesse: *The Art of Perfumery*, 1880)

12. Florida sachet

Using materials which are well dried and ground up, mix together 8 parts of orange flowers with 3 parts of coriander seeds, 6 of mint leaves, 2 each of vetiver root and calamus, and 1 each of benzoin and oak moss. Sprinkle over this a few drops of neroli oil and keep in a sealed jar, shaking occasionally, to mature before use.

(Adapted from Ann Tucker Fettner: *Pot Pourri*, 1983)

13. A sachet for scenting linen

Take 2 cupsful of dried rose petals and a $\frac{1}{2}$ cupful each of dried lavender, dried orange flowers and crushed coriander seeds, together with a teaspoonful each of orris powder, dried basil and cinnamon. Add a few cloves and a little salt and mix thoroughly.

14. An early Arab recipe for pomander beads

'Take some very green gallnuts and lay them in a frying-pan until the fat pours out. Cook them carefully until they are baked. Then let them get cold, crush them up thoroughly and sift them. Then moisten with hot water. Next, take some date syrup and put it into an earthenware cooking pot until it thickens and congeals. Then add the gallnut substance to it and pound in a mortar until it is all properly mixed. After so pounding it for one hour, sprinkle very hot water over it until the gallnut substance ceases to stick to the side of the mortar. Then take it out, put it in a large wooden bowl and knead it with your hands. Next, take a tile, spread jasmine oil over the surface and sprinkle some of the oil on your hand. Then shape the mixture into cakes, pierce them and lay them out on the tile, putting a cover over them to keep the dust off until they are dry. Then thread them on to a cord and keep them in a basket so that dust and smoke will not get into them.'

(Yaqub al-Kindi: *Book of Perfumes*, c. 850 AD)

15. Rose pomander beads

'Rose beads, or rodides, are made in this way. Of fresh roses before they become damp – 40 drachmas, spikenard – 5 drachmas, myrrh – 6 drachmas. These are beaten fine and made up into little troches, each weighing 3 oboli. These are then dried in the shade and stored in closely sealed jars. Some also add costus – 2 drachmas, and the same amount of Illyrian orris, mixing also honey, and wine from the island of Chios. They are worn about women's necks instead of necklaces to cover up the unsavoury smell of sweat.'

(Dioscorides: Materia Medica, 1st century AD)

16. A pomander recipe

'Take of lapdanum 3 drames, of the wodde of the Aloes 1 drame, of amber of grece (ambergris) 2 drames and a half, confect all these togyther with Rose water and make a ball. And this aforesayd Pomeaunder doth not onlely expell contagious ayre, but also it doth comforte the brayne.'

(Andrew Boorde: The Dyetary of Helt, 1542)

17. A recipe for pomander beads

'To make a paste for sweete Beades or Beadstones Take a pounde and a halfe of blacke earth well beaten into pouder, foure onces of Gomme dragant (Gum tragacanth), and lay it a steepe, or temper it in a mortar, with as much Rose water as wil cover the earth with the saied Gomme dragant, and stampe it well by the space of halfe an houre, with these sweete thinges folowinge. That is to say: Storax calamita, an once, powder of Cloves halfe an once, Sandalum citrinum, halfe an once; beate all into pouder very finely, and mix all together with the aforesaid paste, then take it out of the mortar, and braye it well between your hands, by the space of halfe an houre. And you may make therof Beades or Beadstones.'

(Alessio: The Secrets of Alexis of Piedmont, 1558)

18. A pomander bracelet

'Take a quarter of an ounce of Civit, a quarter and a half-quarter of an ounce of Ambergreese, not half a quarter of an ounce of ye spiritt of Roses, 7 ounces of Benjamin, almost a pound of Damask Rose buds cut. Lay gumdragon in rose water and with it make your pomander, with beads as big as nutmegs and color them with Lamp black; when you have made them up wash your hands with oyle of Jasmin to smooth them, then make them have a gloss, this quantity will make seaven Bracelets.'

(Mary Doggett: Book of Recipes, 1682)

19. Balles against the pestilence or plage, whiche also give an odour unto all things

'Take storax, one part, labdanum one parte, cloves halfe a parte, camphor at your discretion, but less than any of the other substances, of spikenard a good quantity, and of nutmegs also, of all this make paste with Rose water, in the which you shall temper gomme dragant (tragacanth) and gomme Arabic, stirring and brusyng them well. Of this paste you shall make balles to holde in your handes, and smell to.'

(Alessio: *The Secrets of Alexis of Piedmont*, 1558)

20. How to make sweet balls

'With small charge, which yet shall seem to be costly and sweet. Take one ounce of Cyprian Powder (cyperus), and Benjamin of the best mixture . . . : half an ounce of Cloves, a sufficient quantity of Illyrian Iris (orris). first, melt some Gum Tragacanth in some Rose-water: then with the former powder make it into a mass, and roll it up into little balls: bore them thorow, and fix every one on a severel tent upon the table: then take four grains of Musk, dissolve it in Rose-water, and wash the outside of the balls with it: then let them dry: afterwards wet them again, three or four times; so they will cast forth a pleasant sent about, which they will not quickly lose.'

(Giovanni Baptist della Porta: *Natural Magick*, 1658)

21. A pomander

'Heat a Mortar very hot, put in of Benjamin, Labdanum and Storax, of each one ounce; beat them to a Perfect Paste, add to them four Grains of Civet, and six of Musk; make this Paste into Beads, make Holes in them, and string them while hot.'

(Charles Carter: *The Compleat City and Country Cook*, 1732)

22. Aromatic pomander balls: a modern recipe

'Take 1 oz Benzoin, $\frac{1}{2}$ oz Olibanum, $\frac{1}{2}$ oz labdanum, $\frac{1}{2}$ oz orris powder, 3 drops oil of clary sage, 2 drops each oil of bergamot and ylang-ylang, and 5 drops essence of ambergris. Mix the resins with the orris powder and melt them by putting into a pyrex dish lined with aluminium foil and placing in a very cool oven. Add the essential oils and ambergris and work them in quickly. Divide into 2 or 3 equal portions and roll into balls, lubricating the hands with a little essential oil. When hard they can be pierced with a hot knitting needle and hung on a leather thong, or sewn into little silk or lawn bags. They will release their odour when handled.'

(After Ivan Day: *Perfumery with Herbs*, 1979)

23. Aromatic beads: a modern recipe

Make a mucilage of Gum Tragacanth by stirring $\frac{1}{2}$ pint of warm water a little at a time into 1 level tablespoon of tragacanth powder until a gelatinous mass is formed; this is poured into a bottle with the lid screwed on tightly and shaken vigourously to disperse the lumps, repeating once or twice a day for three days (if the mucilage is still lumpy, rub through a sieve). Then take 1 tablespoon each of benzoin and orris; 1 teaspoon each of cinnamon, olibanum, mace and basil; 4 powdered cloves; 2 drops each of oil of cedarwood, rhodium and verbena; and 1 drop each of essence of civet and ambergris. Reduce the dry ingredients to a powder, mix with the oil and turn all into a paste with enough mucilage of tragacanth. Form into pomanders.

(After Ivan Day: *Perfumery with Herbs*, 1979)

24. A perfume to burn

'Take Benjamin, liquid Storax, and Storax Calamita, fine, of each an Ounce; mix and dissolve them as much as you can in two Ounces of damask Rose-water; then add as much Florentine Orris in fine powder, as is sufficient to make it up into a Paste; also of Civet and Musk in fine Powder, of each a Dram; mix all these very well together, and make them up into Cakes about the Bignes of a silver Two-pence; dry them on a tin Plate, and keep them for use. These cakes are good to perfume abundance of other things, besides that they are good to burn.'

(John Nott: *The Cooks and Confectioners Dictionary*, 1723)

25. Angelica incense

'Take a root of Angelica, dry it in the oven or before the fire, then bruis it well and infuse it four or five days in white wine vinegar. To make use of it heat a brick red hot and lay the Angelica root upon the brick. The vapour that exhales therefrom is a powerful corrective of putrid air. The operation must be repeated several times.'

(*Toilet of Flora*, 1755)

26. 'Arabian incense' powder

Using coarsely ground materials, add to 5 oz of frankincense $\frac{1}{2}$ oz each of cloves, cassia and salt petre and $\frac{1}{8}$ oz of tincture of musk. Sprinkle with 1 oz of alcohol and mix thoroughly.

(Adapted from Ann Tucker Fettner: *Pot Pourri*, 1983)

27. An incense cone

Charcoal 30 parts; frankincense 2 parts; benzoin 2 parts; salt petre 1 part; sandalwood oil 3 parts; a few drops of oil of musk; mucilage of gum arabic or tragacanth. Grind the dry ingredients together until they are a fine dusty powder. Add the oils and enough mucilage to make a pliable paste. Knead for a short while on an oiled, non-porous surface and form into cones or pastilles. Cones should be about 1 inch high and $\frac{1}{4}$ inch across at the base. Dry them in a dark, well aired place. Do not enclose them in a box until thoroughly dry or they will turn mouldy.

(After Ivan Day: *Perfumery with Herbs*, 1979)

28. English incense

Parts as follows: willow charcoal 12; sandalwood powder 30; cascarilla powder 10; benzoin powder 15; saltpetre 3; cubeb powder 3; finely ground cardamom 4; myrrh 1; bergamot oil 3; rhodium oil 2; lemon oil 2; oil of musk 1; gum mucilage. Grind all the powdered ingredients together, gradually adding the oils. Mix in enough mucilage to form a firm, putty-like paste and model into small cones.

(After Ivan Day: *Perfumery with Herbs*, 1979)

29. Clove and cubeb incense

Charcoal (powdered) 30 parts; benzoin powder 2 parts; cubeb powder 2 parts; clove powder 2 parts; saltpetre 1 part; oil of bergamot 1 part; oil of clary sage 1 part; oil of mus 1 part; enough gum or mucilage to make a paste. Grind the dry ingredients together until well incorporated. Knead in the oils and make into a paste by adding a little mucilage at a time. Form into cones.

(After Ivan Day: *Perfumery with Herbs*, 1979)

30. A cassolette recipe

'Take Benjamin four ounces, Storax two ounces, Lignum Aloes half an ounce, Ambergris two drams, Musk twenty four grains, Civet one dram, twenty Cloves, Cinnamon in powder two drams; the Pills (peels) of two Limons (cut small without touching them with your hands). Mix all these together with Rose-water, and make a paste of it with your hands; and never use it without Rosewater or other Sweet Water. You may steep Gum Tragacanth in Rose-water till it become a mucilage, and with that work the other ingredients into a Paste, and form it into Cakes for use.'

(Sir Kenelm Digby: *Choice and Experimental Receipts in Physick and Chirurgery*, 1668)

31. A pastille recipe

'Incorporate the Powders of Florentine Orrice, Storax, Benjamin and other aromatics, with Orange Flower Water, put this Paste into a little

Silver or Copper Box lined with Tin. When you have a mind, set the Box
on a gentle fire or on hot ashes, and it will exhale a delightful odour.'
(J.P. Buc'hoz: The Toilet of Flora, 1771)

32. An Elizabethan recipe for a washball

'Take 3 ounces of Orris, $\frac{1}{2}$ an ounce of Cypress, 2 ounces of Calamus, 1
ounce of Rose Petals, 2 ounces of Lavender Flowers, beat all these
together in a mortar, searching them through a fine sieve, then scrape
some castile soap and dissolve it with some Rosewater, then incorporate
all your powders therewith by labouring them well in a mortar.'
(From Sir Hugh Platt, Delights for Ladies, 1602)

33. An 18th century recipe for a washball

'Take of the best white soap, half a pound, and shave it into thin slices
with a knife; then take two ounces and a half of Orris, three quarters of
an ounce of Calamus, and the same quantity of Elder Flowers; of Cloves,
and dried Rose Petals, each half an ounce; Coriander-seeds, Lavender
and Bay Leaves, of each a dram, with three drams of Storax. Reduce the
whole to fine powder, which knead into a paste with the soap; adding a
few grains of Musk or Ambergris. When you make this paste into
Washballs, soften it with a little Oil of Almonds to render the composition
more lenient. Too much cannot be said in favour of this washball, with
regard to its cleansing and cosmetic property.'
(From P.J. Buc'hoz, The Toilet of Flora, 1771)

34. Armenian paper

Make an alcoholic solution from 2 parts each of frankincense, storax and
gum benzoin, and $\frac{1}{2}$ part each of balsam of Peru and balsam of Tolu, with
5 parts of 90% alcohol. Add to this sufficient of a solution of potassium
nitrate in water to enable the paper to burn freely. Soak the absorbant
paper in this mixture, drain, allow to dry and cut into convenient strips.
(After E.J. Parry: Cyclopoedia of Perfumery, 1925)

35. A 16th century recipe for scented gloves

'Take Ambergris a drachm; the same quantity of civet; and of Orange
Flower Butter, a quarter of an ounce; mix these ingredients well together,
and rub them into the gloves with fine cotton wool, pressing the perfume
into them.'
(Quoted by Ivan Day: Perfumery with Herbs, 1979)

36. A perfumed powder for bellows

'Take iris root of Florence, $\frac{1}{2}$ a pound; roses, 4 oz; cyprus root, marjoram and cloves, 1 oz each; yellow sanders and benjamin, of each 4 oz; storax 1 oz; and beat them into a powder.'

(Philbert Guibert: *The Charitable Physician*, 1629)

37. Pomatum for the hair

'Of beef marrow, hogs lard and spermaceti each an ounce; of oil of ben $\frac{1}{2}$ a pint. Melt the whole together, add a tablespoonful of oil of bergamot and oil of roses and oil of nutmegs 10 drops.'

(From an English Housekeeping Book, *c.* 1840, English Heritage (unpublished)))

38. An early Arab recipe for a musk perfume

'Take as much as you want of Chinese birthwort and soak it for five days in fresh water in the shade in a glass vessel, changing the water once every day. Then take it out and dry it in the shade. Next, immerse it in fresh sheep's milk until it is fully covered for five days, again changing the milk once every day. Take out and dry thoroughly. Then crush it up with a pestle until it is finely powdered. Then sprinkle on to it a little clear jasmine oil, but not enough to break up the powder. To every ten parts of this add one part of musk, crush it up finely and pour it into a bottle. It is quite excellent; I've tested it and proved it myself.'

(Yaqub al-Kindi: *Book of Perfumes*, *c.* 850 AD)

39. An early Arab recipe for an ambergris perfume

'Take an ounce of cuttlefish powder, seven ounces of pure sandarac, four mithqals of pure aloewood, five dirhams of good nard, and two ounces of white bees' wax. Crush them all up separately and strain them with a sieve. Then mix them together into a powder and melt the beeswax in a clean iron pan, and sprinkle the ingredients on it little by little. Stir with a wooden stick until it has melted. Add this mixture to an equal amount of ambergris and it is ready to sell.'

(Yaqub al-Kindi: *Book of Perfumes*, *c.* 850 AD)

40. Henry VIII's perfume

'Take 6 spoonsful of rose oil, the same of rose water and a quarter of an ounce of sugar. Mix well together and add two grains of musk and one ounce of ambergris, then boil slowly for six hours and strain.'

(From a manuscript in the Ashmolean Museum, Oxford. Quoted by Roy Genders: *A History of Scent*, 1972)

41. A 16th century rose oil recipe

'Oyle of Roses and Floures, very parfit. Take the seeds of Millons (melons) well mundified and stamped, and laye them by rankes or by beddes, with the floures of Roses, by the space of 8 daies, then take a little linnen bagge wette in Rose water, or in the water of other floures, in the whiche bagge you shall put the seede and havyng well bounde it, put in a pressour, and presse out the oyle, which will be very precious, and the which you must keep alwaies close.'

(*The Secrets of Alexis of Piedmont*, 1558)

42. Sweet honey water: an 18th century recipe

'Take of good French brandy, a gallon, of the best Virgin Honey and Coriander Seeds, each a pound; Cloves, an ounce and a half; Nutmegs, an ounce; Gum Benjamin and Storax, of each an ounce; Vanilloes No. 4; the yellow rind of three large Lemons: bruise the Spices and Benjamin, cut the Vanilloes into small pieces, put all into a cucurbit (a still), and pour the Brandy on to them. After they have digested forty-eight hours, distil off the Spirit in a retort with a gentle heat.

To a gallon of this water, add of Damask Rosewater and Orange Flower water, of each a pint and a half; Musk and Ambergrise, of each five grains; first grind the musk and Ambergrise with some of the water, and afterwards put all into a large matrass (a vessel for digesting and distilling), shake them well together, and let them circulate three days and nights in a gentle heat. Then letting the water cool, filter and keep it for use in a bottle well stopped.

It is antiparalytic, smooths the skin and gives one of the most agreeable scents imaginable. Forty or sixty drops put into a pint of clear water, are sufficient to wash the hands and face.'

(Quoted by Ivan Day: *Perfumery with Herbs*, 1979)

43. A perfumed oil

Collect a mixture of lavender flowers, rose and carnation petals having a good scent, and other sweet-scented flower petals as may come to hand, together with a few pieces of oak moss, to a total weight of about 1 ounce. Crush these into a pulp and stir into a pint of jojoba oil. Keep in a sealed jar in sunlight in a warm spot such as a conservatory. After about 2 weeks strain into another jar ready for use.

44. A perfume oil made by simple enfleurage and distillation

This recipe requires two identical flat dishes, 10 inches or more in diameter and up to 1 inch deep, together with a plentiful supply of fragrant flower petals.

Purchase 1 lb of lard (preferably) or beef suet and melt it gently in a container placed in a saucepan of hot water over a low heat. Stir in 1 teaspoonful of alum and a few drops of benzoin oil. Pour this in equal amounts into the two flat dishes and allow to cool. Spread 1 inch or more thickness of freshly gathered, fragrant flower petals over the fat on one of the dishes. Invert the second dish over the first so that the rims touch each other. The cavity in-between should be completely full of flower petals. Keep in a warm position. Three or four times a week remove all the flower petals from the fat and replace with the same amount of fresh ones, turning the dishes over so that the top dish becomes the bottom one. This process should be continued for 2 or 3 weeks. Then remove the last charge of flowers, scrape the fat into a screw-top jar containing about the same quantity of vodka or spirits of wine, add 2 or 3 drops of sandalwood and stir. Keep this in a cool place for about 10 weeks, giving the jar a good shake daily. Finally, pour the liquid oil through a strainer into another screw-top jar ready for use. Alternatively, after adding the perfumed fat to the vodka, essential oil can be distilled from it. This requires a jar with a sealed lid pierced by a long (2 to 3 feet) copper tube bent to curve downwards, so that as the steam coming into it condenses the oil will drip into a small bottle underneath. This jar should be placed in hot water over a very low heat. Or, for better results, home distillation kits are now on the market (e.g. by Floralab Products of New York).

45. Rose water

To 1 pint of distilled water add 4 tablespoonsful of alcohol, 12 drops of rose oil and 2 drops of sandalwood oil, together with $\frac{1}{2}$ a cupful of rose petals. Keep in a sealed container for 2–3 weeks before use.

46. Rose water

To 2 pints of hot distilled water add a teaspoonful of rose oil, 4 drops of oil of cloves and 1 pint of alcohol. Stir and keep in a sealed jar for several days before use.

(Adapted from Ann Tucker Fettner: *Potpourri*, 1983)

47. Violet water

Into 1 pint of alcohol stir 2 oz of violet extract, 1 oz of cassia extract and $\frac{1}{2}$ oz each of rose oil and orris root tincture. Allow to stand for several days, then add 2 pints of distilled water, shake well and strain into a sealed jar ready for use.

(Adapted from Ann Tucker Fettner: *Potpourri*, 1983)

48. Geranium water

To 2 pints of alcohol add 4 oz of rose water, 5 drops of tincture of musk and 1 oz each of tincture of orris root and geranium oil. Strain into a sealed jar and keep for 2–3 weeks before use.

(Adapted from Ann Tucker Fettner: *Potpourri*, 1983)

49. Lavender water

'2 drachms each of oil of lavender, essence of bergamotte, essence of ambergris and rectified spirits of wine.'

(From an English Housekeeping Book, *c.* 1840, English Heritage (unpublished)).

50. Lavender water

To a pint of spirit of wine add a $\frac{1}{2}$ teaspoonful of lavender oil and a teaspoonful of oil of rosemary, together with 2 drops of patchouli oil. Stir slowly and thoroughly and keep in a sealed container for 2–3 weeks, shaking it every few days.

51. A lavender toilet water

To a pint of fairly weak alcohol and $\frac{1}{2}$ a cupful of distilled water add $\frac{1}{2}$ a teaspoonful of lavender oil, stirring slowly, and mix into this 4 or 5 drops of rose oil and rather fewer drops of cananga or ylang-ylang oil. Keep in a sealed container for 2–3 weeks before use.

52. Lavender water

Heat up a mugful of dried lavender in a pint of distilled water, keeping it just simmering without boiling for 5–10 minutes. Leave covered until it has cooled. Then, squeezing the liquid out of the lavender, strain it into a jar with $\frac{1}{2}$ a pint of fairly weak alcohol. Add 5 drops of lavender oil and 10 drops of labdanum oil (amber oil), stirring slowly. Keep in a sealed container for 2 weeks, shaking occasionally, before use.

53. Carmelite water

Chop up 4 oz of balm leaves and 2 oz of lemon peel and mix with pinches of ground cloves, black pepper, coriander, cinnamon, angelica, mint, nutmeg and origanum. Stir these slowly into 1 pint of alcohol and keep in a sealed jar for 2 days. Then stir in $\frac{1}{2}$ pint of orange flower water and keep in a sealed jar, shaking daily, for a further 2–3 weeks before use. Alternatively distil (see recipe no. 44).

54. Another Carmelite water

Take a cupful each of lemon balm leaves and angelica leaves and chop them up with the peel of a lemon. Add 1 teaspoonful of crushed coriander, 2 of crushed cinnamon and 4 of cloves. Stir these into 1 pint of fairly weak alcohol, add 4 drops of neroli oil, and leave in a warm sunny position (e.g. in a conservatory) for 3–4 weeks, shaking occasionally.

55. Hungary water

Into 1 pint of spirit of wine pour $\frac{1}{4}$ pint of orange flower water and $\frac{1}{4}$ teaspoonful of rosemary oil. Add 1 or 2 drops each of oil of lemon, marjoram, rose, lavender and orris. Keep in a sealed container for 2–3 weeks before use.

56. Rosemary water

'To Make Rosemarie Water. Take the Rosemarie, and the flowers in the middes of May, before sunne arise, and strippe the leaves and the flowers from the stalke, take four or five Alicompagne (Elecampane) rootes, and a handfull, or two of Sage, then beat the Rosemarie, the Sage and the rootes together, till they be verie small, and take three ounces of Cloves, three ounces of Mace, halfe a pound of Anniseedes and beat these spices everie one by it selfe. Then take all the Hearbes and the Spices, and put therein foure or five gallons of good white wine, then put in all these Hearbes and Spices, and Wine, into an earthen Pot, and put the same Pot in the ground the space of thirteen dayes, then take it up and still in a Still with a verie soft fire.'

(Thomas Dawson: *The Good Huswife's Jewell*, 1587)

57. Florida water

Mix 4 pints of alcohol with $1\frac{1}{2}$ pints of rose water. Add 1 oz each of tincture of musk and jasmine oil, $\frac{1}{2}$ oz each of oil of lemon and lavender, 4 drops of clove oil, 3 drops of neroli oil, $1\frac{1}{2}$ oz of bergamot oil and $\frac{1}{8}$ oz of cinnamon oil. Strain and keep in a sealed jar for a month before use.

(Adapted from Ann Tucker Fettner: *Potpourri*, 1983)

58. Florida water

To 1 pint of distilled water add $\frac{1}{8}$ pint of alcohol together with 4 drops of rose oil, 4 of lavender oil, 4 of lemon grass oil, 2 of clove oil and 1 of cassia oil. Keep in a sealed container for 2–3 weeks before use.

59. A floral cologne

To 1 pint of fairly weak alcohol add half a cupful of orange flower water together with a $\frac{1}{4}$ teaspoonful each of rose oil and bergamot oil and a few drops of carnation oil and ylang-ylang oil. These should be mixed together slowly, stirring well. Keep in a sealed jar for 2–3 weeks before use.

60. An oriental cologne

To 1 pint of fairly weak alcohol add 3–4 drops each of oil of jasmine, carnation, ylang-ylang, rose and lavender, together with 5 drops each of oil of clove, cinnamon and sandalwood. Stir these in slowly and thoroughly. Keep in a sealed jar for 2–3 weeks before use.

61. A country garden cologne

To 1 pint of fairly weak alcohol add 4 drops each of lavender oil, jasmine oil, rose oil and clove-pink (carnation) oil, together with 3 drops of rosemary oil and 2 drops of benzoin oil. Stir slowly and thoroughly and keep in a sealed container for 2–3 weeks before use.

The formulas which follow are all quoted from W.A. Poucher: *Perfumes, Cosmetics and Soaps*, 1991.

62. A synthetic lily of the valley fragrance

200 Extract of jasmine
100 Extract of ylang-ylang
200 Alcohol 95%
  5 Powdered cardamom
___
505

63. A 'brown windsor' soap perfume

150 Cassia oil
100 Clove oil
 80 Caraway oil
 20 Cinnamon leaf oil
100 Spike lavender oil
100 Red thyme oil
100 Rosemary oil
350 Bergamot oil
___
1000

64. A frangipanni formula

300 Jasmine extra synthetic
100 Lilac synthetic
 80 Muguet synthetic
200 Rose centifolia synthetic
200 Orange blossom synthetic
 10 Olibanum R
 30 Benzoin R
 10 Vetivert – Java
 20 Orris resin
 20 Coumarin
 30 Musk Ketone
___
1000

65. A fragrance using ginger grass oil in soaps

150 Ginger Grass oil
300 Palmarosa oil
100 Clove oil
 50 Cassia oil
200 Cedarwood oil
100 Spike lavender oil

     50 Styrax
　 50 Musk xylene
1000

66. Handkerchief perfumes

Alcohol to be added for dilution to the required strength.

(a) Bouquet des fleurs
   240 Bergamot oil
   120 Lemon oil
   120 Portugal oil
   150 Violet
   150 Tuberose
   150 Rose
 　70 Benzoin R.
1000

(b) Buckingham flowers
   200 Rose
   200 Jasmin
   200 Cassie
   200 Orange flower
     50 Concrete orris
     50 Rose otto, synthetic
     30 Neroli oil petals
     30 Lavender oil, English
 　40 Amber, synthetic
1000

(c) Japanese bouquet
   160 Cedarwood oil
   160 Patchouli oil
   160 Sandalwood oil
   160 Verbena oil, French
     80 Vetivert oil
 　280 Rose
1000

(d) Jockey club
   160 Bergamot oil
   200 Jasmin
   300 Rose

140 Tuberose
160 Mace oil, concrete
  40 Civet extract, 3%
1000

(e) *Leap-year bouquet*
300 Jasmin
  20 Patchouli oil
150 Sandalwood oil
200 Tuberose
  30 Verbena oil, French
150 Vetivert oil, Java
150 Rose
1000

(f) *Yacht club*
200 Orange blossom
100 Jasmin extra
  20 Cassie
200 Sandalwood oil
  50 Vanillin
100 Rose
330 Benzoin R.
1000

67. An eau de cologne

   5 Lemon oil
  10 Bergamot oil
   5 Portugal oil
   1 Melissa oil
  50 Rosemary herb
1000 Alcohol, 90%
 100 Water
1171
Macerate for 12 hours in a still and then distil slowly.
Collect 1000 cc, in which dissolve:
2   Neroli oil
3.5 Petitgrain oil
0.5 Thyme oil, rectified
4   Oleo-resin orris
10
Mature one month.

68. Another eau de cologne

```
   5 Bergamot oil
   6 Lemon oil
   7 Petitgrain-citronnier oil
   2 Rose–geranium oil
   1 Lavender oil
1000 Alcohol, 90%
 100 Water
1121
```

Distil 1000 cc and add:

```
   5 Petitgrain oil, terpeneless
   1 Neroli oil, bigarade
   2 Benzoin Resin
   8
```

Mature one month

69. Eau de portugal

```
  20 Sweet orange oil
   6 Bergamot oil
   3 Lemon oil
   1 Rose–geranium oil
   2 Benzoin resin
1000 Alcohol, 90%
1032
```

70. Opoponax perfume

```
 300 Bergamot oil, terpeneless
  50 Orris oil, concrete
  50 Opoponax R.
  20 Lemon oil, terpeneless
  50 Jasmin, synthetic
  80 Rose rouge, synthetic
  10 Ginger oil
  50 Myrrh R.
  40 Galbanum R.
  25 Frankincense R.
  50 Violet, synthetic
  25 Vetivert oil
  50 Cistus R.
 200 Amber, synthetic
1000
```

71. Santolina perfume

400	Lavender oil, French
100	Bergamot oil
75	Ylang-ylang oil
25	Clary sage oil
10	Oak moss absolute
40	Ambrette R.
50	Vetivert R.
50	Cassie, synthetic
150	Rose, synthetic
100	Benzoin R.
1000	

72. Fumigating pastilles

100	Siam benzoin
50	Tolu balsam
700	Charcoal
50	Saltpetre
50	Sandalwood oil
15	Patchouli oil
30	Cascarilla oil
5	Grain musk
–	Mucilage of acacia
1000	

73. A sachet base

200	Orris
150	Sandalwood
100	Cedarwood
100	Rosewood
70	Patchouli
50	Vetivert
80	Rose petals
100	Lavender
50	Ambrette seeds
30	Tonka beans
59	Siam benzoin
10	Clove
1	Grain musk
1000	

These substances are well mixed and passed through a coarse sieve twice. The base is stored until required in air-tight containers. Floral compounds can then be added to it, e.g.

600 Sachet base
350 Lavender flowers
 50 Lavender compound

74. A lavender sachet

 450 Lavender flowers
 200 Sandalwood
 100 Orris
 100 Tonka beans
 100 Patchouli leaves
  20 Lavender oil, M.B.
   2 Oak moss absolute, green
  10 Vanilla extract, 10%
   5 Petitgrain oil
  10 Bergamot oil
   3 Musk ketone
1000

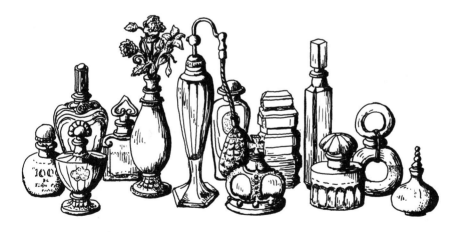

Bibliography

Arctander, Steffan (1960) *Perfume and Flavour Materials of Natural Origin*, Hoffenbergske Etablissement, Copenhagen (printed Elizabeth, NJ, USA)

Bedoukian, Paul (1967) *Perfumery and Flavouring Synthetics*, Elsevier, Amsterdam

Black, Penny (1989) *The Book of Pot Pourri*, Dorling Kindersley, London

Black, Philippa *see* Loewenfeld, Claire

Chiej, Roberto (1984) *The Macdonald Encyclopaedia of Medicinal Plants* (trans. Sylvia Mulcahy), Macdonald, London

Crone, Patricia (1987) *Meccan Trade and the Rise of Islam*, Princeton University Press

Day, Ivan (1979) *Perfumery with Herbs*, Darton, Longman & Todd and the Herb Society, London

Duff, Gail (1989) *Natural Fragrances*, Sidgwick & Jackson, London

Fettner, Ann Tucker (1983) *Pot Pourri, Incense and other Fragrant Concoctions*, Hutchinsons, London

Gaborit, Jean-Yves (1985) *Perfumes: the Essences and their Bottles*, Rizzoli, New York

Garbers, Karl (1948) *Kitab Kimiya al-'Itr wat-Tas'idat by Ya'qub bin Ishaq al-Kindi*, Deutsche Morglandische Gesellschaft Kommissionsverlag F.A. Brochhaus, Leipzig

Genders, Roy (1972) *A History of Scent*, Hamish Hamilton, London

Genders, Roy (1977) *Scented Flora of the World: an Encyclopaedia*, Robert Hale, London

Grieve, M. (1931) (ed. C.F. Leyel) *A Modern Herbal*, Cape, London reprinted Penguin, London, 1980)

Groom, Nigel (1981) *Frankincense and Myrrh: A Study of the Arabian Incense Trade*, Longman, London

Haarmann & Reimer *see* Muller, Julia

Hay, Roy (ed.) (1978) *Readers Digest Encyclopaedia of Garden Plants and Flowers*, Readers Digest, London

Hepper, F. Nigel (1990) *Pharaoh's Flowers*, HMSO, London

Hériteau, Jacqueline (1978) *Potpourris and Other Fragrant Delights*, Penguin, London

Hort, A.F. *see* Theophrastus

Huxley, Anthony and Taylor, William (1977) *Flowers of Greece and the Aegean*, Chatto & Windus, London

Huxley, Anthony *see* Polunin, Oleg

Kennett, Frances (1975) *History of Perfume*, Harrap, London

Loewenfeld, Claire and Black, Philippa (1974) *The Complete Book of Herbs and Spices*, David & Charles, Newton Abbot

Manniche, Lise (1989) *An Ancient Egyptian Herbal*, British Museum Publications, London

Matthews, Leslie G. (1973) *The Antiques of Perfume*, Bell & Sons, London

Mazuyer *see* Naves

Meyerhof, M. and Sobhy, G.P. (1932) *The Abridged Version of 'The Book of Simple Drugs' of Ahmad ibn Muhammad al-Ghafiqi, by Gregorius Abu' l-Farag (Barhebraeus)*, Faculty of Medicine, Egyptian University, Cairo

Moldenke, Harold and Alma (1952) *Plants of the Bible*, Chronica Botanica Co. Waltham, Massachusetts

Muller, Julia and others (1984) *The H & R Book of Perfume* (4 vols), English edition published by Johnson Publications, London

Naves, Y. and Mazuyer, G. (1947) *Natural Perfume Materials*, Reinhold, New York

North, Jacqueline (1986) *Perfume, Cologne and Scent Bottles*, Schiffer, Pennsylvania

Ohrbach, Barbara Milo (1986) *The Scented Room: Dried Flowers, Fragrances and Potpourri for the Home*, Sidgwick & Jackson, London

Parry, Ernest J. (1921) *The Raw Materials of Perfumery*, Pitman, London

Parry, Ernest J. (1925) *Cyclopaedia of Perfumery* (2 vols), Churchill, London

Pillivuyt, Ghislaine (1988) *Histoire du Parfum*, Denoël, Paris

Pliny *Natural History* (trans. H. Rackham, 1945), Loeb Classical Library and Harvard University Press, Cambridge, Massachusetts

Polunin, Oleg and Taylor, William (1965) *Flowers of the Mediterranean*, Chatto & Windus, London

Poucher, William A. (1991) *Perfumes, Cosmetics and Soaps*, 9th edn (3 vols), Chapman & Hall, London

Rackham, H. *see* Pliny

Rimmel, Eugene (1895) *The Book of Perfumes*, Chapman & Hall, London

Sagarin, Edward (1945) *The Science and Art of Perfumery*, Greenberg, New York

Sermadiras, Patrick (1990) *Dictionnaire des Parfums*, Sermadiras, Paris

Smith, Keith Vincent (1978) *The Illustrated Earth Garden Herbal*, Elm Tree Books, London

Sobhy, E.P. *see* Meyerhof

SPC (Soap, Perfumery and Cosmetics) (monthly), Dartford, Kent

Taylor, William *see* Huxley

Theophrastus *Enquiry into Plants* and *Concerning Odours* (trans. A.F. Hort, 1916), Loeb Classical Library and Harvard University Press, Cambridge Massachusetts

Trueman, John (1975) *The Romantic Story of Scent*, Aldus Books, London

Usher, George (1974) *A Dictionary of Plants Used by Man*, Constable, London

Warmington, E.H. (1928) *The Commerce between the Roman Empire and India*, Cambridge University Press (revised Curzon Press, London, 1974)